Textbook of
Spinal Disorders

Textbook of
Spinal
Disorders

Stephen I. Esses, MD, FRCSC, FACS

Professor of Clinical Orthopedic Surgery
Alexander and Ruth Brodsky Professorship of Spine Surgery
Director, Residency Program
Department of Orthopedic Surgery
Baylor College of Medicine
Houston, Texas

with 5 contributors

illustrated by Gino Maulucci

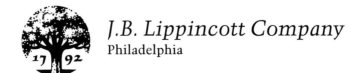

J.B. Lippincott Company
Philadelphia

Acquisitions Editor: James D. Ryan
Associate Medical Editor: Wendy Greenberger-Czarnecki
Associate Managing Editor: Elizabeth A. Durand
Indexer: Sandra King
Design Coordinator: Melissa G. Olson
Designer: William T. Donnelly
Production Manager: Caren Erlichman
Production Coordinator: David Yurkovich
Pre-press: Jay's Publishers Services, Inc.
Compositor: Tapsco, Incorporated
Printer/Binder: Quebecor/Kingsport

6   5   4   3   2   1

Library of Congress Cataloging-in-Publication Data

Textbook of spinal disorders/by Stephen I. Esses; with 5
   contributors; illustrated by Gino Maulucci.
      p. cm.
      Includes bibliographical references and index.
      ISBN 0-397-51346-1 (alk. paper)
      1. Spine—Diseases. 2. Spine—Abnormalities. I. Esses,
      Stephen
   I. (Stephen Ivor)
      [DNLM: 1. Spinal Diseases. 2. Spine—abnormalities.
         WE 725
   T3547   1995]
   RD768.T446   1995
   617.3'75—dc20
   DNLM/DLC
   for Library of Congress   94-32819
                                                                CIP

∞ *This book meets the requirements of ANSI/NISO Z39.48-1992 (Permanence of Paper).*

The authors and publisher have exerted every effort to ensure that drug selection and dosage set forth in this text are in accord with current recommendations and practice at the time of publication. However, in view of ongoing research, changes in government regulations, and the constant flow of information relating to drug therapy and drug reactions, the reader is urged to check the package insert for each drug for any change in indications and dosage and for added warnings and precautions. This is particularly important when the recommended agent is a new or infrequently employed drug.

*This book is
dedicated to my father,
Israel M. Esses,
who loved both to learn
and to teach.*

Contributors

Jesse H. Dickson, MD

Professor of Orthopedic Surgery
Department of Orthopedics
Baylor College of Medicine
Houston, Texas

Brian Doherty, PhD

Spine Engineer
Center for Spinal Disorders
Department of Orthopedic Surgery
Baylor College of Medicine
Houston, Texas

Wendell D. Erwin, MD

Clinical Professor
Department of Orthopedics
Baylor College of Medicine
Houston, Texas

Stephen I. Esses, MD, FRCSC, FACS

Professor of Clinical Orthopedic
   Surgery
Alexander and Ruth Brodsky
   Professorship of Spine Surgery
Director, Residency Program
Department of Orthopedic Surgery
Baylor College of Medicine
Houston, Texas

Michael H. Heggeness, MD, PhD

Assistant Professor, Department of
   Orthopedic Surgery
Baylor College of Medicine
Houston, Texas

Charles Reitman, PT, MD

Baylor College of Medicine
Houston, Texas

Foreword

It is with great pleasure that I have the opportunity to review *Textbook of Spinal Disorders.* Dr. Esses and his colleagues have taken on a tremendously difficult task and produced a very friendly and usable book. I believe that medical students, residents, fellows, and practitioners of spinal care in all fields will find this book useful. The book is concise, straightforward, and easy to follow and gives the reader a brief overview of each topic. Dr. Esses' colleague Gino Maulucci has provided outstanding artwork that helps to bring this difficult subject into view and in this way enhances the learning process.

Chapter 1, Anatomy, has excellent descriptions with beautiful illustrations for the uninitiated as well as the expert. As Hippocrates said, "One must understand the anatomy before one can understand the function." Dr. Esses and his colleagues have brought spinal anatomy to a very understandable level. In Chapter 2, Dr. Heggeness helps one to understand the pathology of various clinical conditions and the gross aberrancies associated with various developmental anomalies. In the chapter on Spinal Imaging, Dr. Esses describes various imaging techniques and gives us a good sense of when to order a test and which test to order. Obviously, Dr. Esses' goal is to provide some insight to cost-effective care for our patients. What to know, what to order, and when to order it is critical. One of the most enjoyable chapters is the chapter regarding Nonoperative Care of the Spine. In this chapter the reader begins to understand the differences across the medical specialties between conventional and less conventional medical therapies. In a time when unconventional therapies are using large amounts of healthcare resources, it is important to discuss these therapies and be advocates of those that are efficacious. In Chapter 7, Basic Principles of Surgery, Dr. Esses advocates avoiding fads and suggests following the well documented prospective studies. He discusses surgical approaches, indications, and, more importantly, the biology associated with fusion techniques. Again, there are excellent figures within this chapter. In Chapter 8 on Degenerative Disease, Dr. Esses takes a good look at aging versus degeneration. Clearly, we are all aging, and as clinical care personnel we must distinguish between aging and disease. Throughout the remainder of the book the excellent figures help to understand the herniated disc, spondylolisthesis, and spinal stenosis. In the chapter on Infections, Dr. Esses does an excellent job of describing very briefly the importance of the MRI in patients with infection and the value of T1- and T2-weighted images.

On a personal note, Dr. Esses begins to bridge the gap in spinal medicine. He is old enough to be regarded as an expert in his field, while young enough to be part of a new generation of clinical care providers who want to have a better understanding of various spinal diseases and their treatment. Dr. Esses advocates proven paradigms, rather than antidotes, but he is willing to investigate other suggestions with an open scientific approach.

This book serves as an outstanding educational tool for students, residents, and faculty alike. I congratulate Dr. Esses and his co-authors on an outstanding contribution to the field of spinal medicine.

James Weinstein, MD

Preface

From the time I started practicing orthopedic surgery, I have had the wonderful opportunity of teaching medical students, residents, and fellows. They have often bemoaned the lack of a single concise textbook providing the information needed to deal with spine patients. The purpose of this book is to answer that request. I have attempted to present factual information concerning the spine (cervical, thoracic, and lumbosacral) in an organized and methodical manner. Many excellent books dealing with a wide variety of spinal conditions are available. This textbook is in no way an attempt to replace them. They deal, by and large, with specific disorders affecting certain areas of the spinal column. This textbook is a general guide and is most certainly not encyclopedic. It is meant to be readable, from cover to cover, in one or two weeks.

Although written primarily for students, residents, and fellows, I hope that others will find this book of value. Chiropractors, primary care physicians, and physical therapists are encouraged to use this text as a reference. The wide variety of medical, paramedical, and non-medical personnel currently engaged in the treatment of back patients should note that this book has been written with no assumption of prior medical school education.

No matter how graphic a written description is, it rarely equals a well-executed drawing. I have the distinct pleasure of including among my friends Gino Maulucci. He is an artist of the highest caliber and has brought to this book his extraordinary knowledge and talent. Any success that this book may enjoy is a reflection of his immense contribution.

Examinations are a fact of life. It would not be fair to have residents and fellows read this book without ensuring that it contained the information essential to answering their written examinations. To this end, I have reviewed the Orthopedic In-Training Examinations from the last seven years, the Orthopedic Self-Assessment Examinations since 1984, and the Self-Assessment Specialty Examination in Spine. I have made certain that the material needed in order to correctly answer questions dealing with the spine has been covered in this textbook. Indeed, at the risk of being redundant I have taken the liberty of occasionally repeating essential information twice.

At the end of each chapter there is a list of key points and a bibliography. The list of key points is meant as a pedagogical tool. It allows quick review of important information and makes scanning of the text easier. The citations in the bibliography have been chosen because they are, in my opinion, important recent contributions to the literature. They have been selected so that the reader gets an idea of where we are and where we are headed in the various aspects of spine-related issues. Important older publications have not been included as they can easily be obtained by computer search or from other texts. Many thanks to Linné Girouard, M.L.I.S., for helping with the literature reviews and for ensuring the accuracy of the citations.

I was very fortunate to have trained at the University of Toronto when it was truly the mecca of spinal surgery. Dr. John Kostuik was one of the pioneering giants practicing in Toronto at that time. He encouraged and supported my subspecialization in spinal disorders. It was he who was instrumental in providing fellowship opportunities and subsequently an academic pathway.

In 1991 I was offered, and accepted, the position of The Ruth and Alexander Brodsky Chair of Spinal Disorders at Baylor College of Medicine in Houston, Texas. The decision to move is one that I have never regretted. Dr. Hugh Tullos, Chief of the Department of Orthopedic Surgery, has created a milieu for academic productivity. I appreciate his confidence and respect his abilities as both surgeon and administrator. It has been both an honor and a pleasure to work with my colleagues Drs. Dickson, Erwin, and Heggeness in the Center for Spinal Disorders. They practice quality medicine with care and compassion.

Dr. Jesse Dickson has encouraged me from the start of this project. He has kindly read and reread all of the rough drafts. His thoughtful suggestions have added considerably to this textbook. Dr. Dickson has been both friend and mentor. He provides unflagging support, sage advice, and constant encouragement.

Dr. Wendell Erwin and Dr. Dickson wrote most of Chapter 14 on Spinal Deformities. The excellence of their clinical acumen is reflected in their lucid presentation.

Dr. Michael Heggeness wrote Chapter 2 on Embryology and Chapter 17 on Osteoporosis. He has presented both of these very complicated topics in a readable and methodical fashion.

Chapter 5 on Biomechanics was co-authored with Brian Doherty, PhD. Unlike many engineers, he is able to explain mechanical concepts in lay terms.

Charles Reitman brings the perspective of a physical therapist to the medical community. I have thoroughly enjoyed working with him on Chapter 6, Nonoperative Care.

There are many people who have read and made suggestions for improving of this book. Many physicians have kindly contributed x-rays. I would especially like to thank George Allibone, MD, Richard Duncan, MD, Robert Huler, MD, Tatsuo Itoh, MD, Phelps Kip, MD, John Kostuik, MD, Jeffrey Kozak, MD, River Oaks Imaging and Diagnostic, and Josie Timm, MD.

J.B. Lippincott Company has done an excellent job of producing this book. I would like to thank Lisa McAllister for initiating the process and Wendy Greenberger-Czarnecki and James Ryan for seeing it to completion. Elizabeth Durand is to be congratulated on a meticulous job of editing. I have appreciated both her patience and her efforts.

Through all of the drafts, rewrites, and changes Jill Rosa has performed an outstanding job in typing and keeping the manuscript organized.

My family has always encouraged learning and education. Without their encouragement this book would never have been written.

The time spent with my wife is so very special it made relinquishing any of it to write this book extremely difficult. I thank Caroline for her constant support and infectious enthusiasm. She makes it all worthwhile.

Stephen Ivor Esses, MD
1994

Contents

1   Anatomy—1

2   Embryology and Developmental Anomalies—35
Michael H. Heggeness

3   Physical Exam—49

4   Spinal Imaging—79

5   Biomechanics of the Spine—109
Stephen I. Esses • Brian Doherty

6   Nonoperative Care of the Spine—135
Stephen I. Esses • Charles Reitman

7   Basic Principles of Surgery—147

8   Degenerative Disease of the Spine—173

9   Herniated Disc Disease—185

10   Spondylolisthesis—203

11   Spinal Stenosis—215

12   Infections of the Spine—229

13   Inflammatory Diseases of the Spine—243

14   Spinal Deformity—257
Jesse H. Dickson • Wendell D. Erwin • Stephen I. Esses

15   Spinal Trauma—287

16   Tumors of the Spine—305

17   Osteoporosis—317
Michael H. Heggeness • Stephen I. Esses

18   The Future—327

Index—331

Textbook of Spinal Disorders, by Stephen I. Esses.
J. B. Lippincott Company, Philadelphia © 1995.

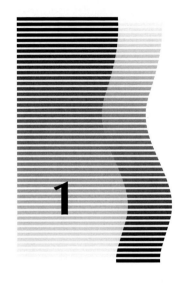

1 Anatomy

BONY ANATOMY
  Cervical Spine
  Thoracic Spine
  Lumbar Spine
  Sacrum
  Coccyx
ARTICULATIONS
  Occipitocervical
  Atlantoaxial
  Intervertebral Discs
  Uncovertebral Joints
  Facet Joints
  Ribs
LIGAMENTS
  Occipitoatlantal
  Occipito-Axial
  Atlantoaxial

MUSCLES
  Posterior
  Anterior
  Transverse
  Anterior Longitudinal
  Posterior Longitudinal
  Interspinous
  Supraspinous
  Ligamentum Flavum
  Costal
  Intertransverse
  Lumbosacral
  Iliolumbar

SPINAL CORD
  General Structure
  Cross-Sectional
    Arrangement
  Spinal Nerves
  Autonomic Nervous
    System
RELATION OF
  NEURAL
  STRUCTURES TO
  BONY STRUCTURES
  General
  Nerve Roots

NEURAL
  INNERVATION OF
  THE SPINE
  Sinuvertebral Nerve
  Posterior Primary
  Ramus
VASCULAR
  ANATOMY
  Cervical Spine
  Thoracic Spine
  Lumbosacral Spine
  Spinal Cord
  Intervertebral Disc

In discussing anatomy, certain terms must be well understood. The *sagittal* plane divides structures into a right and left side. The *coronal* or *frontal* plane divides structures into anterior and posterior sections. The *axial* or *transverse* plane lies at 90° to each of the other planes. The term *anterior* is used synonymously with *ventral* and *posterior* with *dorsal*. The term *cephalad* is used interchangeably with *superior* and *caudad* with *inferior*. These planes and terms are illustrated in Figure 1-1. *Kyphosis* is a curvature in the sagittal plane with the convexity posteriorly. *Lordosis* is a sagittal curve with the convexity anteriorly. *Scoliosis* is a curvature of the spine in the coronal plane with the convexity to the right or left.

BONY ANATOMY

The bony column of the spine is divided into five areas. From top to bottom these are the *cervical*, *thoracic*, *lumbar*, and *sacral* spine; below this lies the *coccyx* or tailbone (Fig. 1-2). Although the bones or *vertebrae* are similar throughout the spine, there are unique features that distinguish the vertebrae from one area to another. Overall, the vertebrae are ringlike structures that provide bony protection to the spinal cord and support to the trunk of the body. The segmental nature of the spine gives it flexibility.

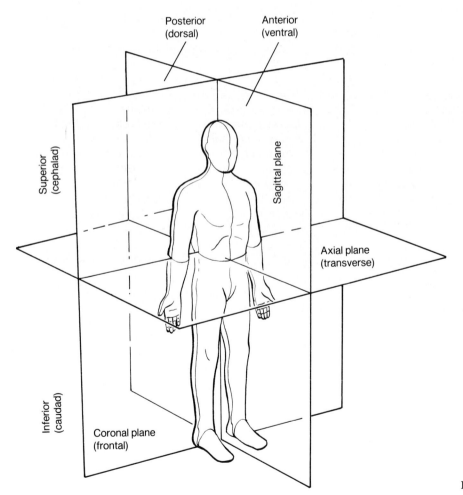

FIGURE 1–1. Anatomic planes.

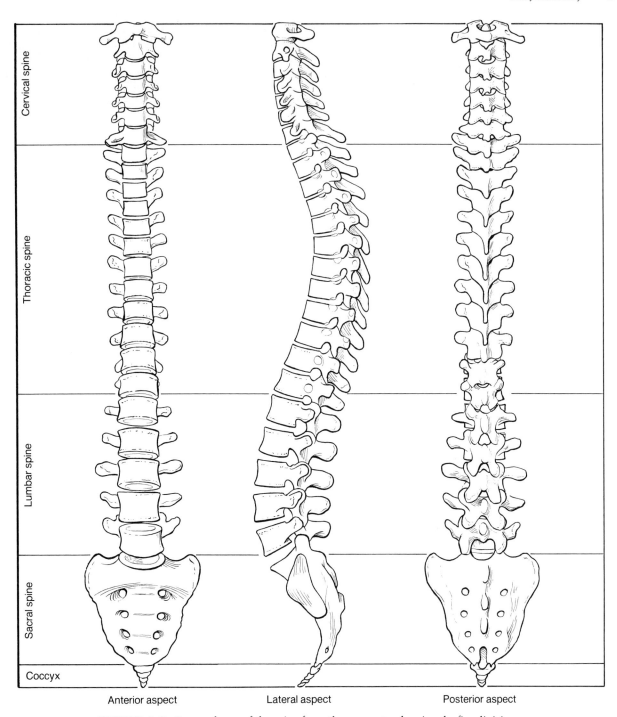

Cervical spine

Thoracic spine

Lumbar spine

Sacral spine

Coccyx

Anterior aspect   Lateral aspect   Posterior aspect

FIGURE 1–2. Bony column of the spine from three aspects, showing the five divisions.

Cervical Spine

Seven vertebrae comprise the cervical spine. They are arranged so that the neck has a *lordotic* posture (Fig. 1-3). The uppermost cervical vertebra (C1), the *atlas,* is truly a bony ring, with greater amounts of bone on the right and left sides called *lateral masses.* These lateral masses allow for articulation with the occiput above and with C2 below. These articulations are called the *superior articular facet* and the *inferior articular facet,* respectively. They are further discussed in the section on articulations. Lateral to these facets are holes or *foramina* through which the vertebral arteries pass. Each of these is called a *foramen transversarium.* Lateral to these foramina are small projections of bone called the *transverse processes.* There is a small prominence of bone both in the front and in the back of the C1 vertebral ring; these are called the *anterior* and *posterior tubercles* (Fig. 1-4).

The C2 vertebra or *axis* has a vertebral body anteriorly from which there is a projection of bone upward, called the *odontoid process* or *dens.* Occasionally it is called the *odontoid peg.*

As discussed in Chapter 2, the dens represents the body of C1 that during development becomes separated from the atlas and incorporated onto the body of the axis. On either side of the body is a lateral mass. These lateral masses differ from those at C1 in that only the superior surface is modified to become a joint. Lateral to the masses are the foramina transversarium and the transverse processes. The posterior half of C2 is different from that of C1. The bones projecting backward on the right and left sides are referred to as *laminae.* There is an inferior projection of bone from the laminae called the *inferior articular process,* which articulates with C3. The laminae meet in the midline, from where there is a projection of bone posteriorly called the *spinous process.* At C2 the spinous process is bifid (Fig. 1-5).

The third to sixth cervical vertebrae share common features. Anteriorly there is a vertebral body. When viewed from the front, there are upward projections on either side of the vertebral body called *uncinate processes.* These are further discussed in the section on articulations (uncovertebral joints). Lateral to this is a projection

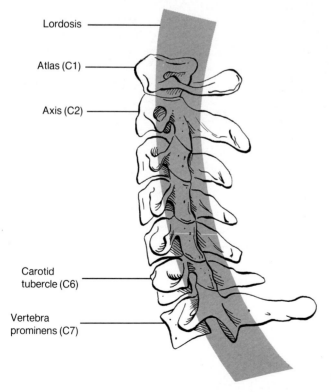

Lordosis

Atlas (C1)

Axis (C2)

Carotid tubercle (C6)

Vertebra prominens (C7)

FIGURE 1–3. Lateral aspect of the cervical spine.

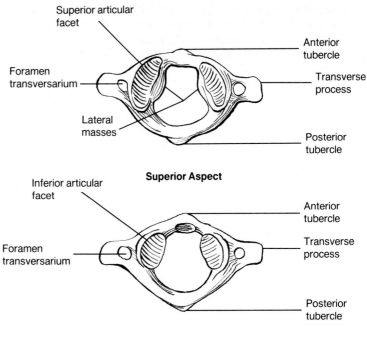

Superior Aspect

Inferior Aspect

Anterior View

FIGURE 1-4. Atlas (C1)—superior, inferior, and anterior aspects.

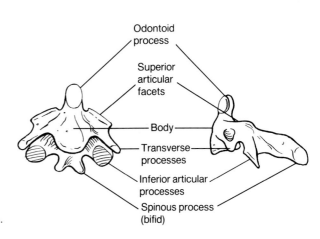

FIGURE 1-5. Axis (C2)—anterior and lateral aspects.

of bone, the foramen transversarium, through which the vertebral artery runs. The anterior bony ring of this foramen is very thin, and the posterior bone is large and truly makes up the lateral mass. The lateral masses are adapted to articulate with the vertebrae above and below. Lateral to the foramen transversarium is the transverse process. At these levels the transverse processes have both anterior and posterior tubercles. The bone in between is curved like a *sulcus* for the exiting spinal nerve. At the C6 level the anterior tubercle is large and is called the *carotid tubercle*. The spinous processes are all bifid (Fig. 1-6).

The seventh cervical vertebra, the *vertebra prominens*, is unique because it has the largest spinous process and it is not bifid. Although C7

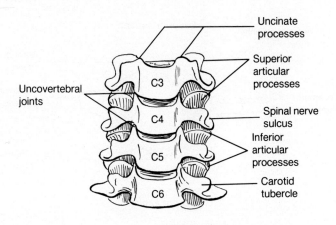

Anterior Aspect

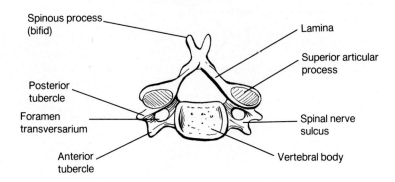

Superior Aspect

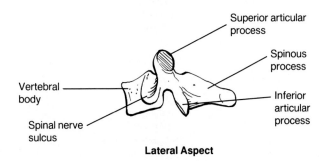

Lateral Aspect

FIGURE 1-6. Cervical vertebrae (C3–C6)— anterior, superior, and lateral aspects.

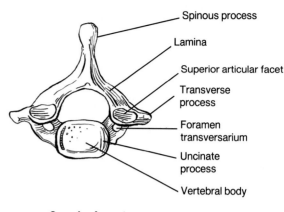

Spinous process
Lamina
Superior articular facet
Transverse process
Foramen transversarium
Uncinate process
Vertebral body

Superior Aspect

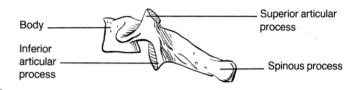

Body
Inferior articular process

Superior articular process
Spinous process

Lateral Aspect

FIGURE 1–7. Vertebra prominens (C7)—superior and lateral aspects.

has foramina transversarium, the vertebral arteries do not travel through them but rather pass anteriorly (Fig. 1-7).

Thoracic Spine

There are 12 thoracic vertebrae, which are aligned in kyphosis. There is a wide range in the thoracic kyphosis of the normal population, with a mean of 35°. The body of the thoracic vertebra is concave on all four sides. Projecting backward from the vertebral body are the *pedicles*, short tubelike structures that essentially connect the vertebral body anteriorly to the laminae and spinous process, together known as the *posterior arch*, posteriorly. Where the pedicle joins the lamina, there are projections up and down, forming the superior articular process and inferior articular process, respectively. A projection laterally forms the transverse process (Fig. 1-8).

Lumbar Spine

There are five lumbar vertebrae, aligned in lordosis, and all have similar characteristics (Fig. 1-9). The vertebral bodies are larger in the lumbar spine than in the thoracic or cervical spine. They

are concave on their lateral and anterior surfaces. The pedicles project backward, linking the bodies to the posterior arch (the laminae and spinous process). When seen in cross section, the pedicles are oval. The junction of the pedicle to the lamina is the *pars interarticularis*. The laminae are triangular in cross section. The spinous processes are larger than those in the thoracic spine and do not project downward to the same degree. The transverse processes are not as large as in the thoracic spine. At the base of each transverse process is a small prominence of bone, the *accessory* or *mammillary process*. These vary in size and position. The superior and inferior articular processes are directed such that the joint surfaces face medially and laterally, respectively. The transverse processes lie at the level of the superior aspect of the vertebral body and at the level of the facet articulating with the vertebra above (Fig. 1-10).

Sacrum

The sacrum is made up of five vertebrae that are fused together. The anterior surface is concave in both the sagittal and frontal planes. Superiorly, the sacrum is broad. The lateral surfaces

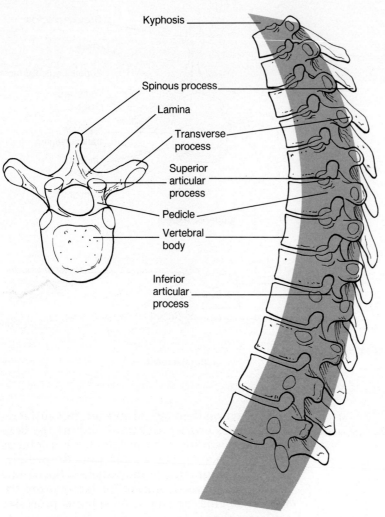

Kyphosis

Spinous process

Lamina

Transverse process

Superior articular process

Pedicle

Vertebral body

Inferior articular process

FIGURE 1–8. Thoracic vertebrae—superior aspect of vertebra and lateral aspect of thoracic column.

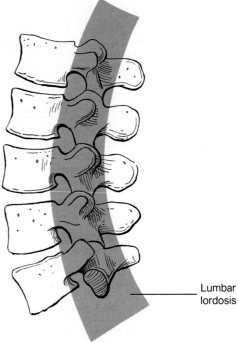

Lumbar lordosis

FIGURE 1–9. Lateral aspect of the lumbar spine.

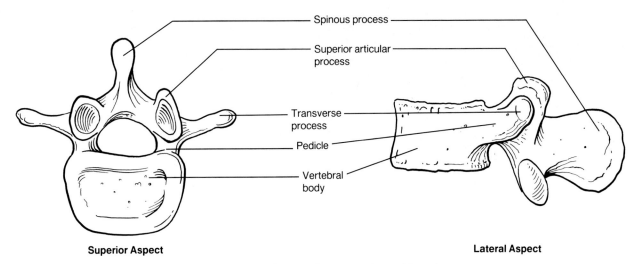

Superior Aspect

Lateral Aspect

FIGURE 1–10. Lumbar vertebra—superior and lateral aspects.

of the upper vertebrae are concave and articulate with the ilium on either side. The sacrum tapers inferiorly where it joins the coccyx.

On the anterior surface there are four pairs of foramina. Between each pair of foramina is a ridge running transversely; this is the area where the intervertebral disc was located. The upper part of the first sacral vertebra is called the *sacral promontory*. The area lateral to the pelvic foramina is called the *pars lateralis*. The pars lateralis is larger at the level of the first sacral vertebra and is referred to as the *ala* (Fig. 1-11).

The foramina are smaller on the posterior surface of the sacrum. In the midline posteriorly is the *sacral median crest*, a fusion of the spinous sacral processes. Inferiorly, some bone is absent posteriorly; this is called the *sacral hiatus*. At the cephalad end of the sacrum are two projections of bone superiorly, forming the superior articular processes. These articulate with the inferior articular processes of the fifth lumbar vertebra (Fig. 1-12).

Coccyx

The coccyx is formed from the fusion of four rudimentary vertebrae. Superiorly there are projections of bone upward and laterally, called the *coccygeal cornua* and transverse processes, respectively. Each cornu articulates with the sacrum (Fig. 1-13).

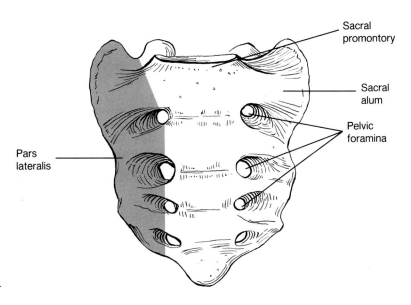

FIGURE 1–11. Sacrum—anterior aspect.

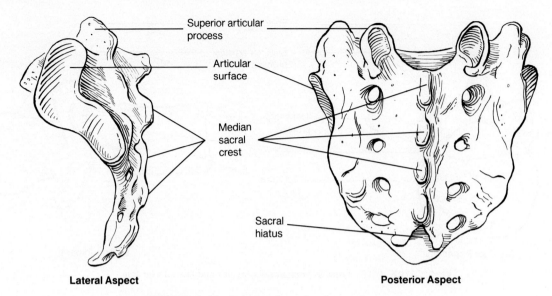

Lateral Aspect   **Posterior Aspect**

FIGURE 1–12. Sacrum—lateral and posterior aspects.

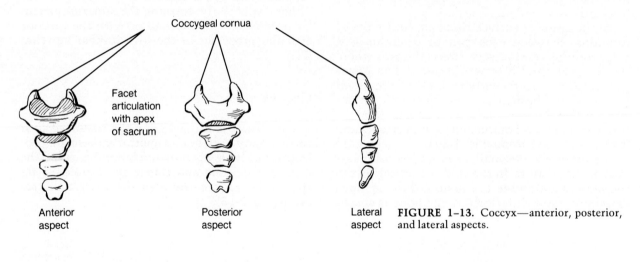

Anterior aspect   Posterior aspect   Lateral aspect

FIGURE 1–13. Coccyx—anterior, posterior, and lateral aspects.

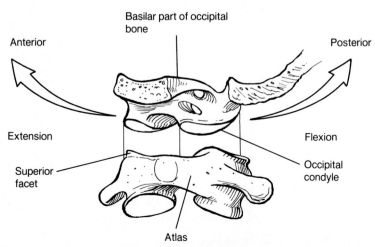

FIGURE 1–14. Occipitocervical articulations.

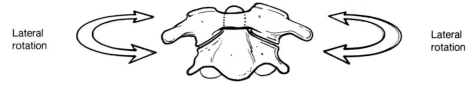

Lateral rotation

Lateral rotation

Anterior aspect of atlas and axis

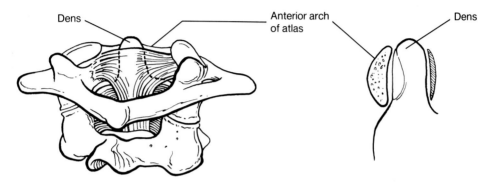

Dens

Anterior arch of atlas

Dens

FIGURE 1–15. Atlantoaxial articulations.

ARTICULATIONS

Occipitocervical

The occiput of the cranium is thickened on either side of the foramen magnum. These *condyles* match the concavities in the superior aspect of the lateral masses of the atlas. These occipitoatlantal joints allow for flexion and extension (Fig. 1-14).

Atlantoaxial

There are four articulations between C1 and C2. A small area on the posterior aspect of the anterior arch of the atlas articulates with the anterior aspect of the dens. On the posterior aspect of the dens there is a specialized surface that faces the transverse ligament. In addition to these two joints are the two facet joints, which lie laterally. They are angled slightly inferiorly in the frontal plane. Motion between the atlas and axis is lateral rotation (Fig. 1-15).

Intervertebral Discs

The intervertebral disc is a composite structure that links contiguous vertebra from C2 to the sacrum (Fig. 1-16). It is a unique joint permitting multiplanar motion. The outer part of the disc, the *annulus fibrosus*, is made up of collagen fibers arranged in layers or *lamellae*. The lamellae are thicker and more numerous anteriorly. Within each lamella, the collagen fibers are oriented obliquely about 30° to the horizontal. The orientation is reversed in contiguous layers; thus, the collagen is oriented at 120° from layer to layer. This *interstriation angle* imparts great tensile strength. The outer lamellae are thicker than those toward the center. In addition, the collagen fibers of the outer layers are anchored to the *end plate*, a 1-mm–thick layer of hyaline car-

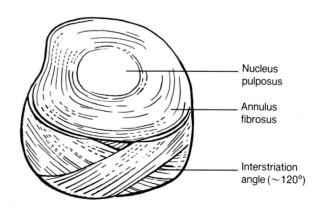

Nucleus pulposus

Annulus fibrosus

Interstriation angle (~120°)

FIGURE 1–16. Intervertebral disc.

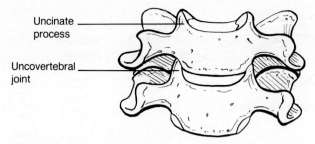

Uncinate process

Uncovertebral joint

FIGURE 1–17. Uncovertebral joints of the cervical spine.

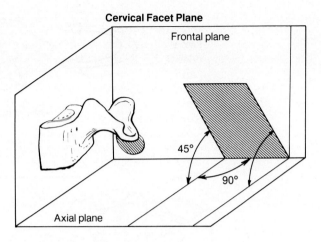

tilage attached to the inferior and superior aspects of the vertebral body. It is by this mechanism that the intervertebral disc is attached to the vertebral body. The inner lamellae of the annulus fibrosus blends with the inner *nucleus pulposus*. The nucleus is more gelatinous than the annulus and has a higher water content. The nucleus pulposus has type II collagen fibers associated with glycoproteins and proteoglycans.

Uncovertebral Joints

There are bony elevations on the lateral sides of the cervical vertebrae called uncinate processes. These articulate with the inferolateral aspect of the vertebra above to form the *uncovertebral joints*, also known as the *joints of Luschka* (Fig. 1-17).

Facet Joints

The facet or *zygoapophyseal joints* determine, to a large extent, the motion at different levels of the spine. In both the cervical and thoracic regions, the facet joint surfaces are flat. In the cervical spine, these joints are oriented at 45° to the axial plane. In the thoracic region, they are oriented 60° to the axial plane, as well as 20° to the frontal plane with the inclination medially. In the lumbar spine, the facet joint surfaces are curved, with the superior articular process concave and the inferior articular process convex. They are oriented 90° to the axial plane and 45° to the frontal plane with the inclination medially (Fig. 1-18).

Ribs

In the thoracic spine, the ribs articulate with the vertebrae at both the body and transverse

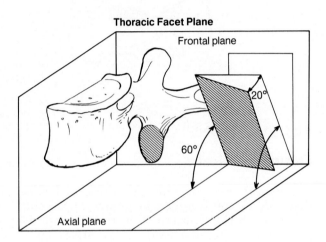

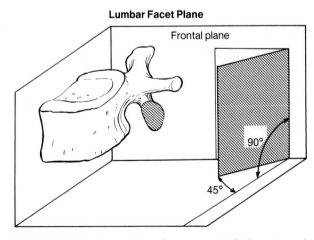

FIGURE 1–18. Facet joint planes—cervical, thoracic, and lumbar vertebrae.

processes. The second to ninth thoracic vertebrae, inclusive, have facets superiorly and inferiorly at the posterior aspect of the vertebral body. These form the *costocentral articulations*. The first, tenth, 11th, and 12th vertebral bodies have only one costal facet. In addition, at all levels there is a facet where the rib articulates with the lateral aspect of the transverse processes; these are called the *costotransverse articulations* (Fig. 1-19). The costocentral and costotransverse articulations are known collectively as the *costovertebral articulation*.

LIGAMENTS

Occipitoatlantal

The occipitoatlantal ligamentous complex consists of four components. There is an anterior and posterior *occipitoatlantal ligament*. Laterally, there are specialized thickened fibers of the occipitoatlantal joints that form the two *lateral ligaments* (Fig. 1-20).

Occipito-Axial

There are four ligaments connecting the occiput to C2. The *occipito-axial ligament* extends from the posterior surface of the body of the axis in the spinal canal to the anterior aspect of the foramen magnum. In addition to this, there are three ligaments that originate from the odontoid process. Extending laterally from the superior tip of the odontoid to the occipital condyles are the *alar ligaments*, occasionally referred to as the *check ligaments*. The *apical ligament* extends from the tip of the odontoid process to the anterior aspect of the foramen magnum (Fig. 1-21).

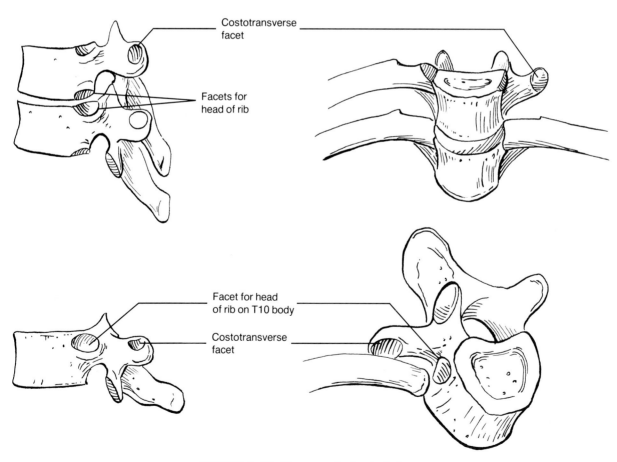

Costotransverse facet

Facets for head of rib

Facet for head of rib on T10 body

Costotransverse facet

FIGURE 1–19. Costovertebral articulations.

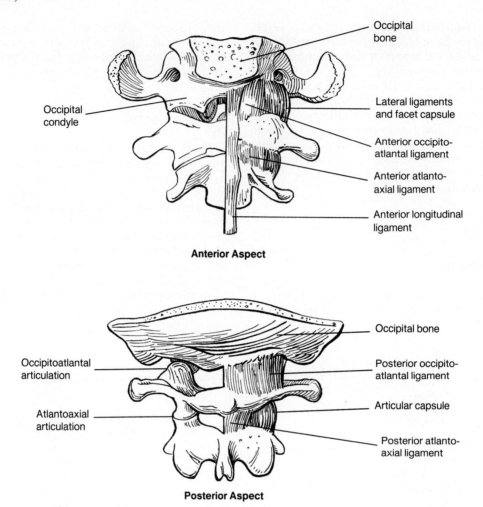

Anterior Aspect

Posterior Aspect

FIGURE 1–20. Occipitoatlantal and atlantoaxial ligaments.

Atlantoaxial

There are four major ligaments extending from the atlas to the axis: the *anterior* and *posterior atlantoaxial ligaments* and the two *lateral ligaments*. The latter are specialized thickened fibers of the atlantoaxial joint capsule (see Fig. 1-20).

Transverse

The transverse ligament stabilizes the atlantoaxial complex. The ligament extends from the anterolateral aspect of the atlas behind the dens to insert on the opposite anterolateral portion of the atlas. From its midpoint, just behind the dens, fibers extend upward to the occiput and downward to the body of the axis. These are often referred to as the *superior* and *inferior longitudinal fascicles*, respectively. The entire ligamentous complex is collectively known as the *cruciform ligament* (Fig. 1-22).

Anterior Longitudinal

The *anterior longitudinal ligament* (ALL) consists of thick, longitudinally oriented fibers extending from the axis anteriorly to the sacrum. At the levels of each vertebral body, the ALL is

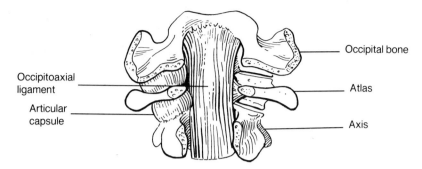

Occipitoaxial ligament

Articular capsule

Occipital bone

Atlas

Axis

Posterior Aspect—posterior part of
occipital bone and posterior arches C1
and C2 removed

Apical ligament
of dens

Alar or "check"
ligaments

C2

Posterior Aspect

FIGURE 1-21. Occipitoaxial ligaments.

broader than at the level of the intervertebral discs. At the disc level, the fibers are adherent to the annulus fibrosus. The ALL has attachments to each vertebral body superiorly and inferiorly at the levels of the end plates. Superiorly, the ALL blends intimately with the anterior atlanto-occipital ligament (Fig. 1-23).

Posterior Longitudinal

The *posterior longitudinal ligament* is weaker than the ALL. Its fibers are also longitudinally oriented but less dense. It runs from the axis caudally to the sacrum. It is the continuation of the occipitoaxial ligament. Like the ALL, it is adher-

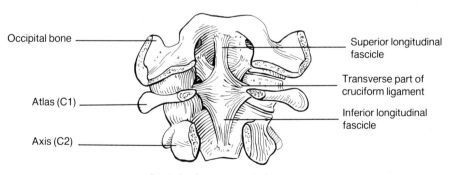

Occipital bone

Atlas (C1)

Axis (C2)

Superior longitudinal
fascicle

Transverse part of
cruciform ligament

Inferior longitudinal
fascicle

Posterior Aspect—posterior part
of occipital bone and posterior
arches of C1 and C2 removed

FIGURE 1-22. Cruciform ligament complex.

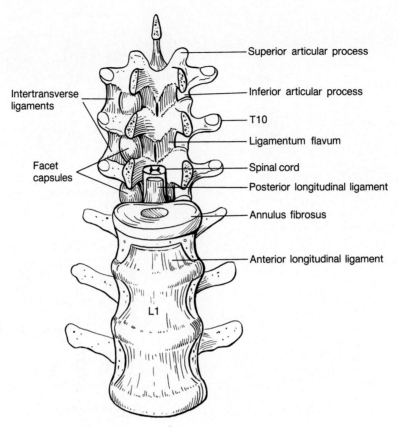

Intertransverse ligaments

Facet capsules

Superior articular process

Inferior articular process

T10

Ligamentum flavum

Spinal cord

Posterior longitudinal ligament

Annulus fibrosus

Anterior longitudinal ligament

L1

FIGURE 1–23. Anterior aspect of the spinal column.

ent to the vertebra at the superior and inferior margins and is adherent to the annular fibers of the intervertebral disc (see Fig. 1-23).

Interspinous

The *interspinous ligaments* connect each adjacent spinous process. The fibers extend from the base to the tip of each spinous process. Anteriorly, therefore, the ligament is adjacent to the ligamentum flavum and posteriorly it is adjacent to the supraspinous ligament. The interspinous ligament is well developed in the thoracic spine. In the cervical spine it becomes part of the *ligamentum nuchae*, a fibromembranous complex extending from the interspinous ligament posteriorly and cranially to insert on the occiput (Fig. 1-24).

Supraspinous

The *supraspinous ligament* is a very strong band connecting the tips of contiguous spinous processes. It extends from C7 to the sacrum. Above C7 these fibers are part of the ligamentum nuchae (see Fig. 1-24).

Ligamentum Flavum

The *ligamentum flavum*, or *yellow ligament*, consists of elastic fibers oriented longitudinally that extend from the anterior surface of the lamina above to the superior margin and posterior surface of the lamina below. There is a small space in the midline between the right and left fibers. The ligamentum flavum tends to thicken as it progresses down the spine, beginning at C2 and extending to the sacrum (see Fig. 1-23).

Costal

The *anterior costovertebral ligament complex* or *stellate ligament* connects the head of each rib to the vertebra and intervening intervertebral disc. Each costovertebral ligament complex consists of three bands or *fasciculi*. The superior fasciculus extends from the rib to the vertebral body above. The middle band connects the rib to the annulus fibrosus of the intervening disc, and the inferior fasciculus connects the head of the rib to the inferior vertebral body (Fig. 1-25).

The *costotransverse ligament complex* connects the neck of the rib to the transverse process. It also has three bands—anterior, middle, and posterior (see Fig. 1-25).

Intertransverse

The *intertransverse ligament* extends from the entire length of the transverse process inferiorly to the superior aspect of the adjacent transverse process. These ligaments are best developed in the thoracic region, where they act as attachments for muscle groups (see Figs. 1-23 and 1-25).

Lumbosacral

The *lumbosacral ligament* is a very thick band that extends from the anterior-inferior aspect of the transverse process of the last lumbar vertebra to the lateral surface of the sacrum. It becomes intimately adherent to the anterior sacroiliac ligament. The lumbosacral ligament is often referred to as the *sickle ligament* (Fig. 1-26).

Iliolumbar

The *iliolumbar ligament* extends from the transverse process of the last lumbar vertebra laterally and superiorly to the iliac crest (see Fig. 1-26).

MUSCLES

Posterior

The posterior muscle groups of the back lie under the shoulder and some upper extremity mus-

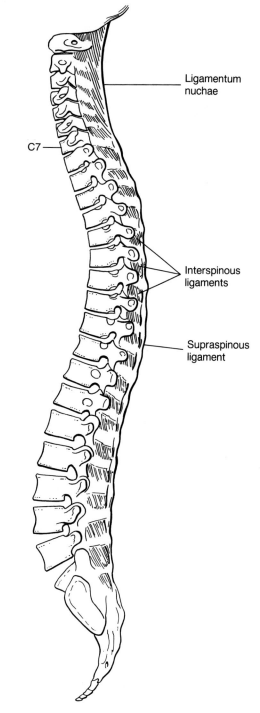

FIGURE 1–24. Nuchal, interspinous, and supraspinous ligaments.

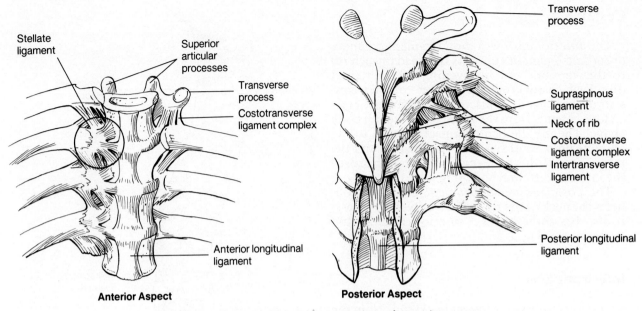

FIGURE 1–25. Costal ligaments—anterior and posterior aspects.

cle groups. The posterior back musculature can be divided into superficial, middle, and deep layers (Fig. 1-27).

The superficial posterior muscles are collectively called the *erector spinae*. There are three separate muscle groups that comprise the erector spinae—the *iliocostalis, longissimus,* and *spinalis.* The iliocostalis group, the most lateral of the erector spinae, has three segments—the *iliocostalis lumborum, iliocostalis thoracis,* and *iliocostalis cervicis.* The iliocostalis lumborum originates from the iliac crest and sacrum to extend

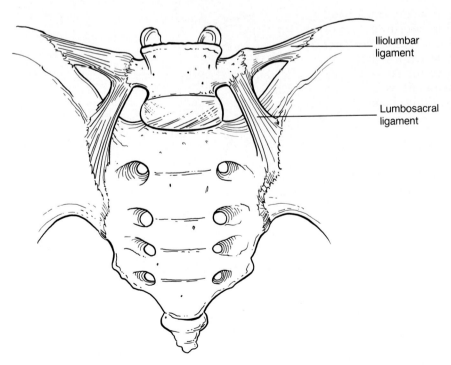

FIGURE 1–26. Lumbosacral and iliolumbar ligaments.

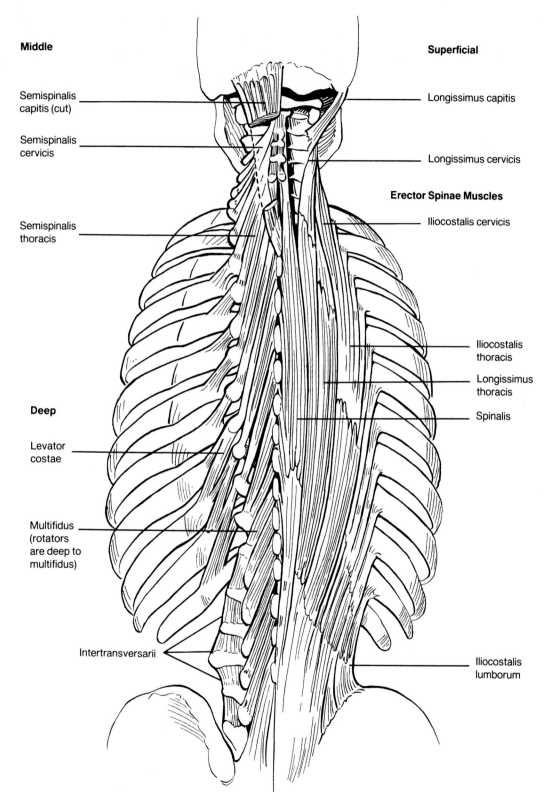

Middle

Semispinalis
capitis (cut)

Semispinalis
cervicis

Semispinalis
thoracis

Deep

Levator
costae

Multifidus
(rotators
are deep to
multifidus)

Intertransversarii

Superficial

Longissimus capitis

Longissimus cervicis

Erector Spinae Muscles

Iliocostalis cervicis

Iliocostalis
thoracis

Longissimus
thoracis

Spinalis

Iliocostalis
lumborum

FIGURE 1–27. Posterior spinal musculature.

superiorly and insert into the lower six ribs. The iliocostalis thoracis overlaps it by originating from these same ribs and inserting on the lower borders of the upper six ribs. The iliocostalis cervicis arises medial to these insertions on the upper six ribs and is directed superiorly to insert on the transverse processes of the lower cervical vertebrae.

The longissimus muscle group also has three subdivisions—the *longissimus thoracis, longissimus cervicis*, and *longissimus capitis*. Collectively, they lie medial to the iliocostalis group. They overlap, as do the iliocostalis. The longissimus capitis originates from the transverse processes of the lower cervical vertebrae to insert into the mastoid processes of the skull. The fibers of the longissimus thoracis connect adjacent transverse processes and the heads of the ribs. Similarly, the longissimus cervicis consists of fibers connecting contiguous cervical transverse processes.

The spinalis muscle, the most medial of the erector spinae muscles, arises from the lower thoracic spinous processes and is directed upward in the midline to insert on the spinous processes of the upper thoracic vertebrae.

The middle or intermediate muscle group of the back is the *semispinalis*. This muscle is subdivided into three portions—the *semispinalis thoracis, semispinalis cervicis*, and *semispinalis capitis*. The fibers are directed obliquely in the superomedial direction. This muscle has its origin on the transverse processes and inserts on the spinous processes. The semispinalis cervicis, for example, originates from the transverse processes of the thoracic vertebrae and inserts into the spinous processes of the upper cervical vertebrae. The semispinalis capitis inserts into the base of the occiput. The semispinalis thoracis inserts into the spinous processes from the sixth cervical to the fourth thoracic level.

The deepest muscle group consists of the *multifidus, intertransversarii, rotators*, and *levator costae*. The multifidus muscle has short fascicles oriented obliquely from the transverse processes upward and medially over two to four segments to insert on the spinous processes. The intertransversarii extend from transverse process to transverse process. They are best developed in the lumbar region, where they are divided into medial and lateral fascicles. In the cervical region, there are anterior and posterior bundles. The rotators are subdivided into short and long groups. The short rotators run from the transverse processes to the base of the spinous

process one level above. The long rotators are similarly oriented but extend over two vertebrae. The levator costae originate from the transverse processes. The short bundles insert inferiorly into the rib below; the long bundles insert into the second rib inferiorly.

Anterior

In the occipitocervical region are two muscle groups that lie anteriorly—the *longus capitis* and the *longus colli* (Fig. 1-28). The longus capitis originates from the anterior aspect of the foramen magnum to insert on the transverse processes of the cervical vertebrae. The longus colli has three divisions. The longitudinal bundle lies anteriorly, arising from the upper three thoracic and lower three cervical vertebrae, and inserts into the anterior bodies of the upper cervical vertebrae. The superior oblique part of the longus colli arises from the transverse processes of C3, C4, and C5 and inserts on the anterior arch of the atlas. The inferior oblique division of the longus colli arises from the upper three thoracic vertebrae anteriorly and inserts on the anterior transverse processes of C5 and C6.

There are no muscle attachments or insertions anteriorly in the upper or midthoracic spine.

In the lower thoracic and lumbar spine are two anterior muscle groups—the *psoas* and *quadratus lumborum* (Fig. 1-29). The psoas originates from the transverse processes and posterolateral aspect of the vertebral body from T12 to L5. Its fibers run inferiorly and laterally to blend with the fibers of the *iliacus* muscle and to insert on the lesser trochanter of the femur. The quadratus lumborum originates from the last rib and transverse processes of the upper four lumbar vertebrae. It inserts on the iliac crest and iliolumbar ligament.

SPINAL CORD

General Structure

The central nervous system extends distally from the brain at the superior level of the atlas as the *spinal cord*. The spinal cord descends to the level of the inferior aspect of L1. The inferior region of the spinal cord is known as the *conus medullaris*. This usually lies between T12 and L1 and is characterized by both spinal cord and spinal nerve elements. The spinal cord becomes a

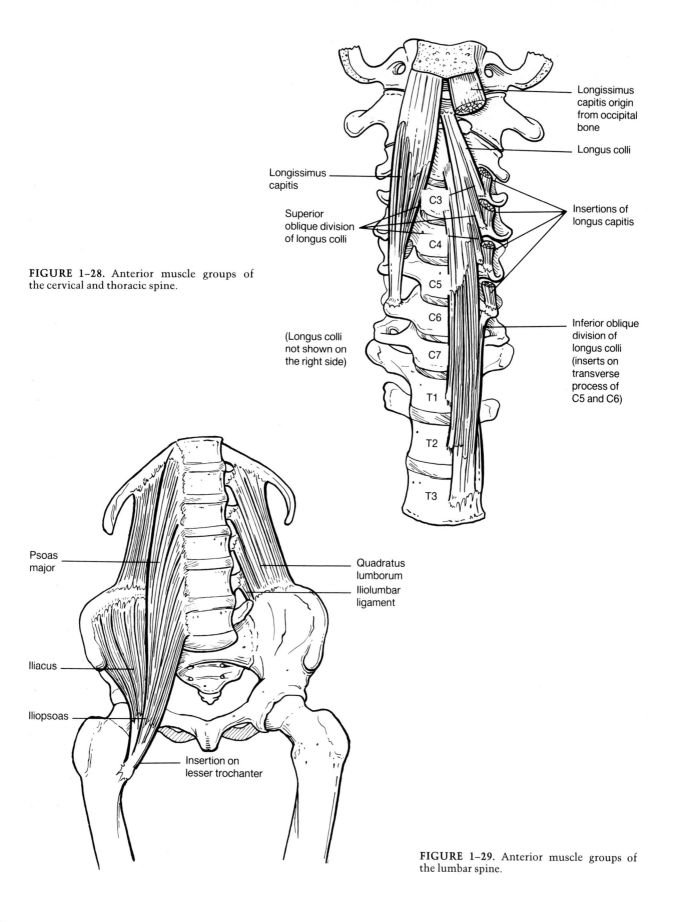

Longissimus
capitis origin
from occipital
bone

Longus colli

Longissimus
capitis

Superior
oblique division
of longus colli

Insertions of
longus capitis

C3

C4

C5

C6

Inferior oblique
division of
longus colli
(inserts on
transverse
process of
C5 and C6)

C7

(Longus colli
not shown on
the right side)

T1

T2

T3

FIGURE 1–28. Anterior muscle groups of the cervical and thoracic spine.

Psoas
major

Quadratus
lumborum
Iliolumbar
ligament

Iliacus

Iliopsoas

Insertion on
lesser trochanter

FIGURE 1–29. Anterior muscle groups of the lumbar spine.

band of tissue called the *filum terminale*, which descends and attaches at the first coccygeal segment (Fig. 1-30). Around the filum terminale are the roots of the spinal nerve, surrounded by *cerebrospinal fluid*. This arrangement of nerve roots surrounding the filum terminale is known as the *cauda equina*.

There are enlargements of the spinal cord between C3 and T2 and between T9 and T12. These areas of enlargement correspond to the large nerves supplying the upper and lower extremities, respectively, and are known as the *cervical and lumbar enlargements*.

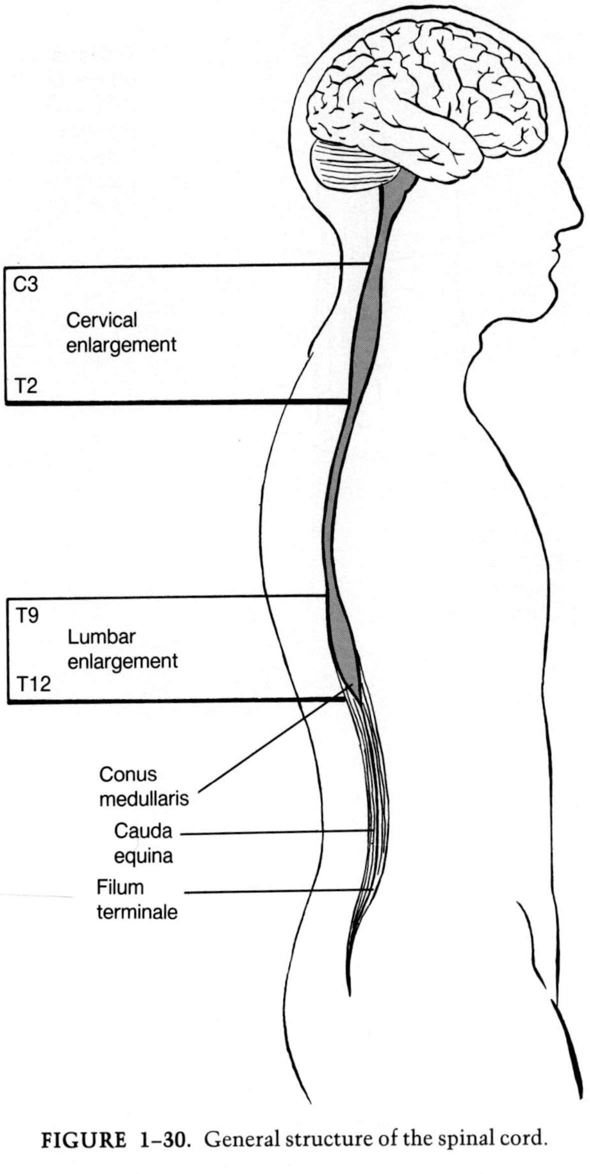

The spinal cord is surrounded by three layers of *meninges*—the *dura mater*, *arachnoid mater*, and *pia mater* (Fig. 1-31). The outermost layer, the dura mater, is a strong connective tissue structure that is continuous with the dura mater around the brain. Distally it extends to the level of the second sacral vertebra, where it ends with the filum terminale. The dura extends around each nerve root and becomes continuous with the *epineurium* of the spinal nerves. Just beneath the dura is a much thinner layer, the arachnoid mater. There is a potential space between the arachnoid and dura but it is extremely small. This interval is called the subdural space. Intimately adherent to and covering the entire surface of the spinal cord is the pia mater. Between the arachnoid and pia mater is the *subarachnoid space*, a large interval filled with cerebrospinal fluid (CSF). There are some connections or *trabeculae* connecting the arachnoid to the pia. The pia mater is vascular, and these blood vessels supply the spinal cord. There are thickenings between the nerve roots known as the *ligamentum denticulatum*. These extend laterally to adhere to the arachnoid and dura. They act as anchors, holding the spinal cord suspended within the CSF (see Fig. 1-31).

Cross-Sectional Arrangement

When viewed in cross section, the spinal cord is oval, with the anterior and posterior borders being flattened (Fig. 1-32). There are *fissures* or clefts in the midline on the anterior and posterior surfaces. These *anterior* and *posterior median fissures* extend through the greater part of the cord and incompletely divide it into right and left symmetric halves. The most central part, where these halves are united, is the *commissure*. Within the commissure and the rest of the spinal cord lies white and gray matter. The gray substance lies more centrally and is arranged in an "H" distribution, with the transverse band referred to as the *gray commissure*. The gray substance of the cord consists of nerve cells or *neurons*, nerve fibers or *axons*, blood vessels, and connective tissue. The white matter consists of nerve fibers, blood vessels, and *neuroglia*, which is supportive tissue consisting of *matrix*, *fibrils*, and small stellate cells called *neuroglial cells*.

FIGURE 1-30. General structure of the spinal cord.

(text continues on page 25)

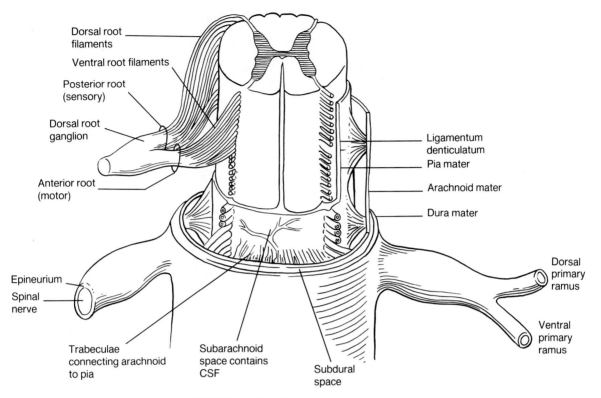

FIGURE 1-31. Meninges and spinal cord.

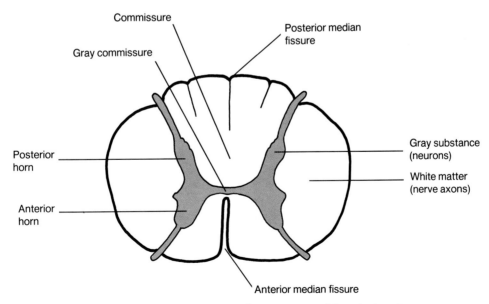

FIGURE 1-32. Cross-sectional arrangement of the spinal cord.

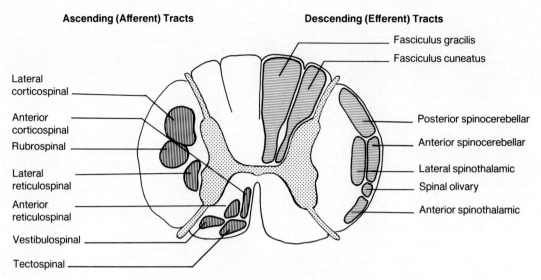

FIGURE 1–33. Ascending and descending spinal tracts.

TABLE 1–1. **Ascending Tracts**

Tract	Function	Orientation
Tracts of Goll and Burdach (Fasciculus gracilis and cuneatus)	Proprioception, vibration, discrimination	Uncrossed
Dorsal and ventral spinocerebellar tracts	Proprioception, light touch	Uncrossed
Lateral spinothalamic tract	Pain, temperature	Crossed
Spinal-olivary tract	Tendon and muscle proprioception	Crossed
Ventral spinothalamic tract	Deep tactile and pressure sensation	Crossed

TABLE 1–2. **Descending Tracts**

Tract	Function	Orientation
Lateral corticospinal tract (pyramidal)	Motor control	Crossed
Rubrospinal tract	Cerebellar reflexes	Crossed
Lateral reticulospinal tract	Inhibits locomotor control	Crossed
Reticulospinal tract	Facilitates locomotor control	Uncrossed
Vestibulospinal tract	Postural control	Uncrossed
Tectospinal tract	Eye and ear reflexes	Crossed

The nerve fibers of the white matter have a *myelin* sheath; those of the gray matter do not.

Nerve cell bodies and fibers with similar functions tend to be grouped together (Fig. 1-33). These groupings or *tracts* ascend to the brain (*afferent*), descend from the brain (*efferent*), or connect various parts of the cord to each other (see Fig. 1-33). The ascending and descending tracts may receive and transmit signals to the same side of the body (*uncrossed*) or may travel through the commissure to transmit or receive signals from the opposite side (*crossed*). This has important clinical sequelae and is discussed further in Chapters 3 and 15. Tables 1-1 and 1-2 list the major tracts and their functions.

Spinal Nerves

There are 31 pairs of spinal nerves (Fig. 1-34). There are eight cervical, 12 thoracic, five lumbar, five sacral, and one coccygeal pair from the spinal cord. Each spinal nerve has both motor and sensory fibers. Each collection of motor fibers is called a ventral or *anterior root*. The anterior root is composed of multiple filaments from the anterior horn of the gray matter of the spinal cord. Each collection of sensory fibers is called a dorsal or *posterior root*. The anterior and posterior roots perforate the dura independently. The *dorsal root ganglion* is the accumulation of the cell bodies of the sensory fibers. The ganglia are located outside but close to the spinal cord. Just beyond the spinal ganglia, the anterior and posterior roots become joined in a common dural sheath. It is at this juncture that the spinal nerve is formed (see Fig. 1-31). Nerve roots differ from peripheral nerves in that they lack a perineurium and have a very sparse epineurium.

Autonomic Nervous System

The autonomic nerve system is for the most part independent of voluntary influence (Fig. 1-35). It controls glandular and cardiac function and smooth muscle. The two components of the autonomic system are the *sympathetic* and *parasympathetic* structures. They are distinguished from the voluntary nervous system in that the bodies of the nerve cells, the ganglia, are situated outside of the central nervous system.

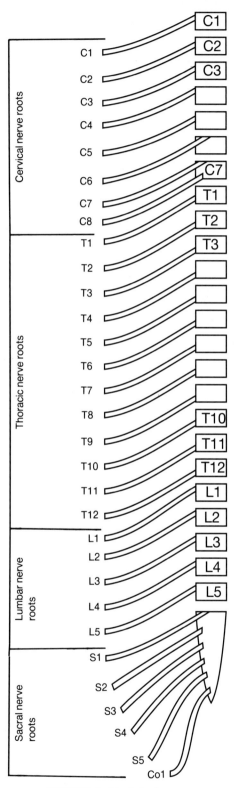

FIGURE 1–34. Spinal nerves.

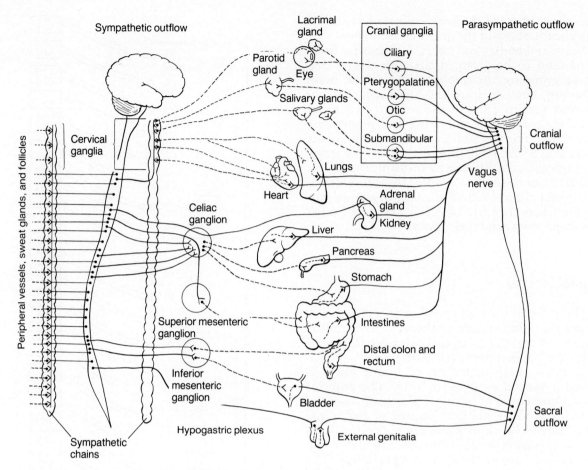

Sympathetic outflow

Lacrimal gland

Parasympathetic outflow

Parotid gland

Cranial ganglia

Eye

Ciliary

Salivary glands

Pterygopalatine

Otic

Submandibular

Cervical ganglia

Lungs

Cranial outflow

Heart

Vagus nerve

Celiac ganglion

Adrenal gland

Kidney

Liver

Pancreas

Stomach

Superior mesenteric ganglion

Intestines

Distal colon and rectum

Inferior mesenteric ganglion

Bladder

Sacral outflow

Peripheral vessels, sweat glands, and follicles

Sympathetic chains

Hypogastric plexus

External genitalia

FIGURE 1–35. Autonomic nervous system.

The sympathetic nervous system consists of a series of ganglia extending from the skull to the coccyx lying on each side of the vertebral bodies. Each sympathetic trunk ganglion gives off a *gray ramus communicans* that joins the adjacent spinal nerve just distal to the juncture of the anterior and posterior roots.

The parasympathetic nervous system has ganglia lying close to the organs they control.

RELATION OF NEURAL STRUCTURES TO BONY STRUCTURES

General

The spinal cord ends at the level of the first lumbar vertebra as the conus medullaris. In the upper spine, the cervical nerve roots arise from the spinal cord and pass laterally to exit at its corresponding level. The lumbar and sacral nerves, however, are directed distally and pass in the subarachnoid space to reach its corresponding point of exit. Thus, the dorsal and ventral roots of the lumbar and sacral nerves are long and form the cauda equina. At the level of the lower thoracic spine, the origin of the spinal nerve is two vertebral segments above its level of exit. There are eight cervical, 12 thoracic, five lumbar, and five sacral roots.

Nerve Roots

The first cervical root exits the spinal column between the occiput and the atlas. The rest of the cervical nerves, therefore, exit the spinal canal cephalad to their named and corresponding vertebra. For example, the C5 nerve root exits at the

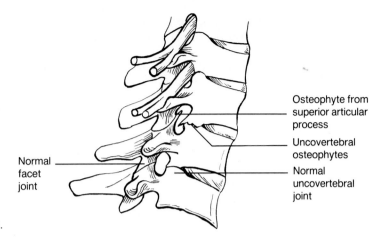

Osteophyte from superior articular process

Uncovertebral osteophytes

Normal uncovertebral joint

Normal facet joint

FIGURE 1–36. Path of the cervical nerve roots.

C4–C5 vertebral level. The difficulty in understanding the pattern of exiting nerve roots is due to the fact that there are eight cervical roots but only seven cervical vertebrae; the eighth cervical root exits cephalad to the first thoracic vertebra. All remaining nerves exit below their named vertebra.

Nerve root compression is not uncommon, and thus it is crucial to understand the path of the nerves as they exit the spinal column. The *cervical foramen*, through which the nerve roots pass, is bounded by the pars lateralis above and below, the superior articular facet posteriorly, and the posterior aspects of the vertebral bodies anteriorly with its intervening intervertebral disc (Fig. 1-36). Note the relation of the uncovertebral joint to the spinal nerve. Bony spurs or *osteophytes*, from either the uncovertebral joint

projecting posteriorly or from the facet joint projecting anteriorly, can cause compression of the nerve root. In addition, a disc protrusion can cause compression of the same nerve root. Thus, for example, the C5 nerve root can be compressed by the C4–C5 disc or the C4–C5 facet or uncovertebral joints. The cervical nerve roots tend to pass at a right angle from the cord, posterior to the vertebral artery, as they merge from the intervertebral foramina.

There are 12 thoracic nerves and the first exits between the first and second thoracic vertebrae. Thus, the 12th thoracic nerve exits at the interval between the 12th thoracic vertebra and the first lumbar vertebra. The thoracic neural foramina tend to be large and provide ample space for the nerves (Fig. 1-37). The boundaries of the thoracic neural foramina are the pedicle above and below,

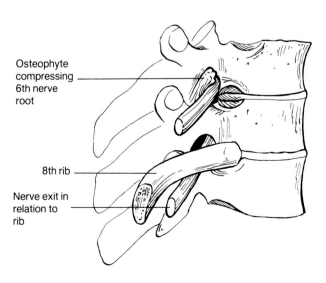

Osteophyte compressing 6th nerve root

8th rib

Nerve exit in relation to rib

FIGURE 1–37. Path of the thoracic nerve roots.

the superior articular process posteriorly, and the intervertebral disc and posterior vertebral body anteriorly.

The anatomic arrangement in the lumbar spine is unique due to the downward course of the lumbar spinal nerves (Fig. 1-38). The *lumbar neural foramina* are bounded by the pedicles above and below, the posterior vertebral body and intervertebral disc anteriorly, and the facet joint posteriorly. Because the superior articular facet wraps medially around the inferior articular facet at the level of the foramen, it is the superior articular facet that lies in closest proximity to the nerve root. The superior-inferior dimensions of the foramen are much larger than the anteroposterior. As the lumbar nerve roots descend, they exit at a right angle and are close to their corresponding pedicle; that is, the L4 nerve root exits at the L4–L5 neural foramen but tends to be closely approximated to the L4 pedicle. The L5 nerve root descends behind the L4–L5 intervertebral disc before turning laterally to exit under the L5 pedicle. Thus, a protrusion of the L4–L5 intervertebral disc can cause compression of the L5 nerve root, whereas stenosis of the L4–L5 intervertebral foramen causes L4 nerve root entrapment. The lumbar roots are large and occupy a considerable proportion of the lumbar foramina.

The sacral and coccygeal roots must travel farther from the spinal cord before exiting the spinal canal, often in excess of 20 cm. The sacral roots exit the dura at a level just above their respective foramina. The dorsal and ventral roots fuse proximal to the dorsal root ganglion. This arrangement is different than that previously discussed. The dorsal root ganglia lie within the sacral canal. Distal to this, the nerve divides into a dorsal and ventral ramus, which exits the canal through the dorsal and pelvic foramina, respectively.

NEURAL INNERVATION OF THE SPINE

In later chapters we will discuss various causes of neck and back pain. Because this is such a common problem, it is important to understand the neural innervation of various parts of the spinal column. This will allow for a more scientific understanding of symptomatic processes.

Sinuvertebral Nerve

The *sinuvertebral nerve* originates as a branch of the spinal nerve just distal to the dorsal root ganglion (Fig. 1-39). It receives a branch from the sympathetic ganglion known as the *ramus communicans*. The sinuvertebral nerve returns through the intervertebral foramen under the

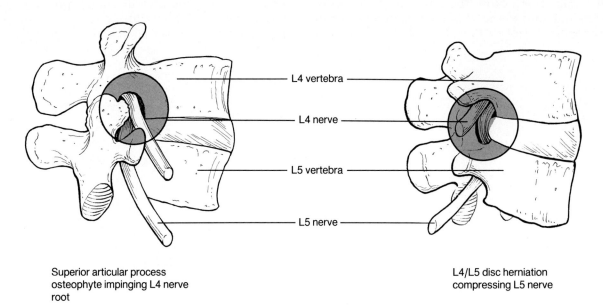

L4 vertebra

L4 nerve

L5 vertebra

L5 nerve

Superior articular process osteophyte impinging L4 nerve root

L4/L5 disc herniation compressing L5 nerve

FIGURE 1–38. Path of the lumbar nerve roots.

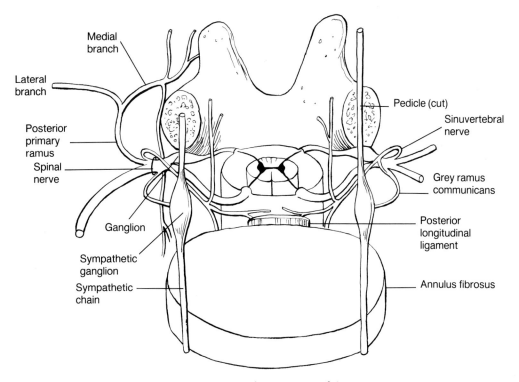

FIGURE 1–39. Neural innervation of the spine.

pedicle. As it enters the spinal canal, it divides into the ascending, descending, and transverse branches. These branches anastomose with their corresponding contralateral counterpart. In addition, the ascending and descending branches anastomose freely with branches from the sinuvertebral nerve one level above and below. These branches innervate the posterior longitudinal ligament, the annulus fibrosus, the anterior aspect of the dura, and the periosteum on the posterior aspect of the vertebral body.

Posterior Primary Ramus

After the spinal nerve leaves the canal through the intervertebral foramen, it divides into a posterior and anterior primary ramus. The *posterior primary ramus* courses directly posteriorly to divide into medial and lateral branches (see Fig. 1-39). The medial branches innervate the facet joints one level above and one level below. Medial branches also innervate the paravertebral muscles, fascia, spinous process, and laminae. In addition, there are branches to the interspinous and supraspinous ligaments. Whereas the facet

capsules and ligaments are innervated from multiple levels, the multifidus muscle has a unisegmental supply. Lateral branches of the posterior primary ramus innervate some of the paraspinal muscles and also have cutaneous distributions. The anterior ramus continues as the spinal nerve root.

VASCULAR ANATOMY

Cervical Spine

The major blood supply to the cervical spine and cord is provided by the paired *vertebral arteries* (Fig. 1-40). Branches of the right and left subclavian arteries, they ascend anterior to the foramen transversarium at C7 to course posteriorly and up through the foramina of C6 to C1. After they exit the foramina of the atlas, they travel posteriorly to enter the foramen magnum. As the vertebral arteries come together from either side, they give off a single branch anteriorly and paired branches posteriorly, which course down the spinal cord. These are the *anterior spinal* and *posterior spinal arteries*, respectively.

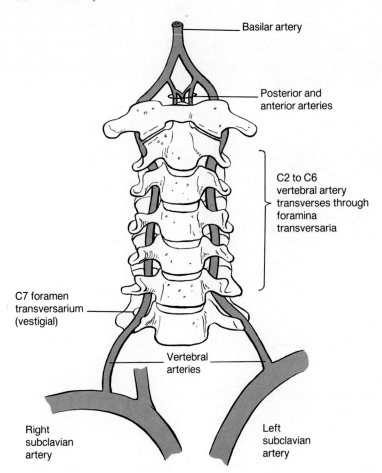

Basilar artery

Posterior and
anterior arteries

C2 to C6
vertebral artery
transverses through
foramina
transversaria

C7 foramen
transversarium
(vestigial)

Vertebral
arteries

Right
subclavian
artery

Left
subclavian
artery

FIGURE 1–40. Blood supply to the cervical spine.

The vertebral arteries, once merged, become the *basilar artery*. These spinal arteries receive anastomoses at each level of the cervical spine from branches of the vertebral artery in between the foramina transversarium.

In addition to supplying the spinal cord at the level of the cervical spine, the vertebral arteries give off lateral *spinal branches* that supply the vertebrae themselves. These branches have extensive anastomoses with branches from the arteries above and below.

Thoracic Spine

Anterior to and on the left side of the thoracic spine, between T4 and T12, lies the thoracic aorta. From the posterior aspect of this great vessel originate the *intercostal arteries* (Fig. 1-41). They are paired, with those on the right longer than those on the left because of the position of the aorta. Before coursing around the thoracic cage under the rib, each intercostal artery gives off a *posterior* and a *spinal branch*. The posterior branch passes backward to divide into an internal branch, supplying the paraspinal musculature, and an external branch, supplying the overlying skin. The spinal branch enters the spinal canal through the intervertebral foramen and supplies both the spinal cord and the vertebrae.

Lumbosacral Spine

The abdominal aorta gives off *lumbar arteries*, which are similar to the intercostals (Fig. 1-42). They run beneath the psoas muscle adherent to the vertebral bodies. Thus, the right intercostal branches run posterior to the inferior vena cava. The lumbar arteries give off posterior and abdominal branches. The *posterior branch* gives off a spinal artery, which enters the spinal canal to

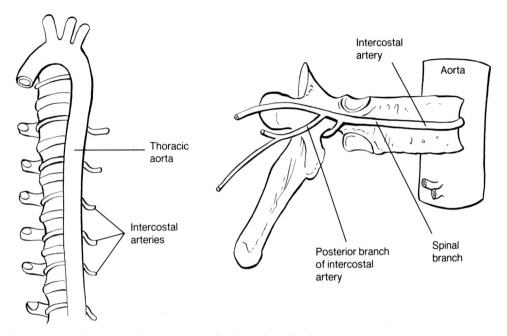

FIGURE 1–41. Blood supply to the thoracic spine.

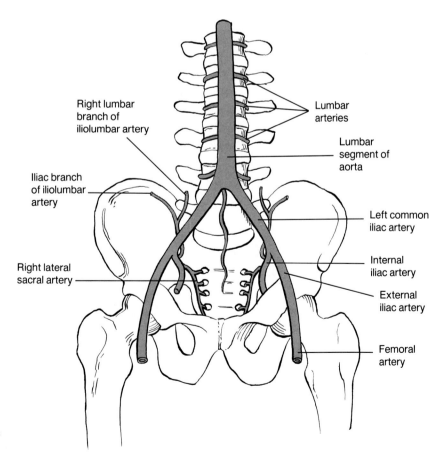

FIGURE 1–42. Blood supply to the lumbosacral spine.

supply the dura and its contents. The posterior branch continues posteriorly to give branches both to the paraspinal muscles and the skin overlying the lumbar spine.

Just before the bifurcation of the aorta is the origin of the *middle sacral artery*. It runs inferiorly over L5 and the middle of the sacrum.

The abdominal aorta usually bifurcates at the level of the fourth lumbar vertebra. The *common iliac arteries* subdivide into the *internal* and *external iliac arteries*. It is from the internal iliac artery that the *iliolumbar artery* originates. It gives rise to lumbar and iliac branches. The former supplies the last lumbar vertebra and the upper part of the sacrum. The internal iliac artery also gives rise to two *lateral sacral arteries*, which supply the rest of the sacrum and the contents of the sacral canal.

Spinal Cord

The spinal cord is supplied by three main arteries: one anterior and two posterior arteries (Fig. 1-43). The *anterior spinal artery* lies on the anterior aspect of the spinal cord in the midline from its origin to the conus medullaris. It is formed from branches of both vertebral arteries and supplies the anterior two thirds of the spinal cord. In addition, there are two *posterior spinal arteries*. They are branches of the vertebral artery inferior to the origin of the anterior spinal artery and descend on either side of the cord to the level of the conus medullaris. These arteries supply the posterior third of the spinal cord. The anterior and posterior spinal arteries anastomose with the spinal branches of the segmental vessels. These feeders are extremely variable in number and location. They are particularly important in the thoracic spine, where they usually enter the left side of the spinal canal between T9 and T11. One of these arteries may be substantially larger than the others and may provide the majority of circulation to the lower two thirds of the spinal cord. When present, this large feeder is known as the *artery of Adamkiewicz*.

There are three main pathways for venous drainage of the spine and spinal cord (Figs. 1-43 and 1-44). Segmental veins accompany the segmental arteries and drain into the *inferior vena cava*. At some levels, the segmental veins drain into the *azygous system*. In addition to this, a valveless venous network known as *Batson's plexus* permits blood flow by an alternate route when there is occlusion of the vena cava.

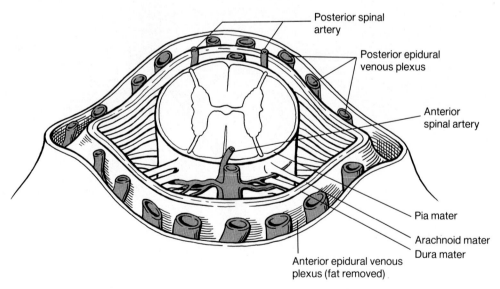

FIGURE 1–43. Arterial supply and venous drainage of the spinal cord.

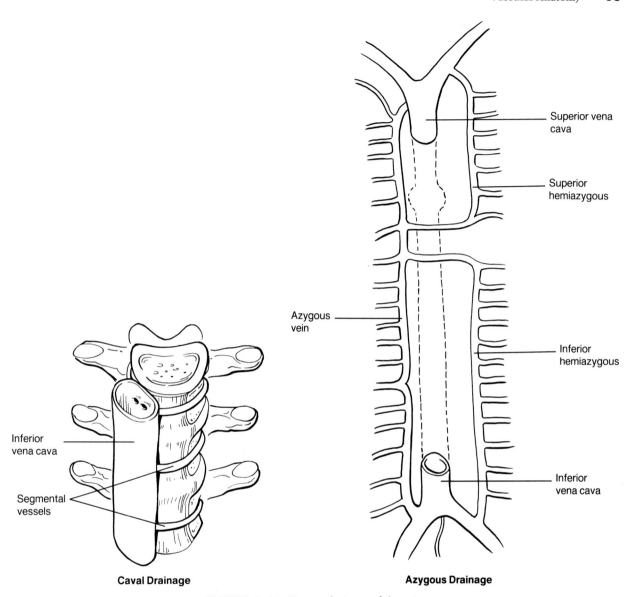

Caval Drainage   **Azygous Drainage**

FIGURE 1–44. Venous drainage of the spine.

Intervertebral Disc

Most of the adult intervertebral disc is avascular. Capillaries have been found only on histologic sections of the outer fibers of the annulus fibrosus. There are three main nutritional pathways for the intervertebral disc (Fig. 1-45). The outer annular fibers receive small arterial branches called *coronary arteries*. These perforate the outer third of the annulus fibrosus. Nutrients can diffuse inward from these vessels to the rest of the annular fibers and the periphery of the nucleus pulposus. A *nutrient artery* enters the vertebral body posteriorly in the midline. A vascular network forms within each vertebral body, terminating at the junction of the end plate and intervertebral disc. These networks are concentrated centrally and allow for diffusion of the nutrients into the nucleus pulposus. Thus, there is a centripetal, inferior, and superior nutritional pathway to each disc.

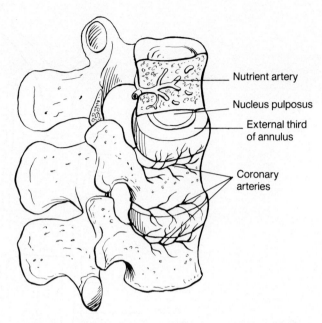

FIGURE 1-45. Nutrient supply to the intervertebral disc.

KEY POINTS

1. The 24 presacral vertebrae are divided into the cervical, thoracic, and lumbar regions, each with unique characteristics.
2. The combination of articulations, ligaments, and muscles is responsible for both the rigidity and flexibility of the spinal column.
3. The spinal cord usually ends in the upper lumbar spine as the conus medullaris, which then becomes the cauda equina. An understanding of neuroanatomy allows correlations between clinical patterns of neurologic deficit and the site of pathology.

BIBLIOGRAPHY

BOOKS

Agur A. Grant's atlas of anatomy. 9th ed. Baltimore: Williams & Wilkins, 1991.
Crock HV, Yoshizawa H. The blood supply of the vertebral column and spinal cord in man. New York: Springer-Verlag, 1977.
Giles LGF. Anatomical basis of low back pain. Baltimore: Williams & Wilkins, 1989.
Hollingshead WH. Anatomy for surgeons. The back and limbs. Vol 3. 3rd ed. New York: Harper & Row, 1982.
Schmorl G, Junghanns H. The human spine in health and disease. New York: Grune and Stratton, 1959.

JOURNALS

Bland JH, Boushey DR. New gross anatomy of the cervical spine. Arthritis Rheum 1989;32 (suppl):518.
Kikuchi S, Sato K, Konno S, Hasue M. Anatomic and radiographic study of dorsal root ganglia. Spine 1994;19:6–11.
Luk KD, Ho HC, Leong JCY. The iliolumbar ligament: A study of its anatomy, development and clinical significance. J Bone Joint Surg [Br] 1986;68:197–200.
Macintosh JE, Bogduk N. The morphology of the lumbar erector spinae. Spine 1987;12:658–668.
Macintosh JE, Bogduk N, Pearcy MJ. The effects of flexion on the geometry and actions of the lumbar erector spinae. Spine 1993;18: 884–893.
Panjabi MM, Oxland T, Takata K, Goel V, Duranceau J, Krag M. Articular facets of the human spine: Quantitative three-dimensional anatomy. Spine 1993;18:1298–1310.
Schaffler MB, Alson MD, Heller JG, Garfin SR. Morphology of the dens. A quantitative study. Spine 1992;17:738–743.
Smith GA, Aspden RM, Porter RW. Measurement of vertebral foraminal dimensions using three-dimensional computerized tomography. Spine 1993;18:629–636.
Zindrick MR, Wiltse LL, Doornik A, Widell EH, Knight GW, Patwardham AG, Thomas JC, Rothman SL, Fields BT. Analysis of morphometric characteristics of the thoracic and lumbar pedicles. Spine 1987;12:160–166.

Textbook of Spinal Disorders, by Stephen I. Esses.
J. B. Lippincott Company, Philadelphia © 1995.

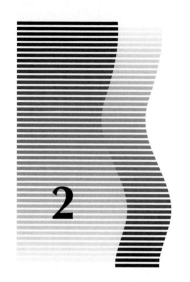

Embryology and Developmental Anomalies

Michael H. Heggeness

EMBRYOLOGY
  Pre-embryonic
  Period
  Embryonic Period
  Fetal Period
DIFFERENTIATION OF
  THE VERTEBRAE
  Mesenchymal Stage
  Chondrification
  Primary Ossification
  Secondary
  Ossification
  Development of the
  Atlas and Axis
  Development of the
  Sacrum

DEVELOPMENTAL
ANOMALIES OF
THE SPINE
  Occipitocervical
  Spine
  Thoracolumbar Spine
  Lumbosacral Junction
  Spina Bifida

EMBRYOLOGY

A detailed knowledge of the embryology of the spine is not critical to clinical practice. A basic understanding of the differentiation of the spine, however, allows the surgeon to have a better appreciation of spinal anatomy and its congenital abnormalities.

The midline structures that will differentiate into the spine are among the first to appear in an embryo. The rest of the organism will differentiate along the axis provided by these early midline structures. Thus, the development of the spine is the critical first step in the development of the organism.

Developmental biologists classify the in utero developmental process into three stages. The *pre-embryonic* period comprises the first 3 weeks after fertilization, the *embryonic* period weeks 3 to 8, and the *fetal* period week 8 to term. These stages are useful to the embryologist in marking landmarks in the development of the organism. Of course, the developmental process is a continuous process, with the organ systems undergoing differentiation with synchronized interactions with other organ systems.

The differentiation of the vertebrae also goes through defined stages that, not surprisingly, do not correspond precisely with these three stages. The differentiation of the vertebrae first involves the creation of a cellular model of the bone, the *mesenchymal* stage. The cellular model then develops into a cartilaginous model of the bone, the *chondrification* stage. The cartilage model in turn is then converted to bone in the *primary ossification* stage. The final process in the differentiation of the bone is the ossification of peripheral areas of cartilage on the periphery on the bone, the *secondary ossification* stage.

Pre-embryonic Period

After fertilization, the ovum undergoes multiple cycles of cell divisions to form a solid mass of cells, a *morula*. With time and further cell division, the morula becomes a hollow ball called a *blastocyst*, which at 7 days implants into the endometrium. On one side of the blastocyst, a cluster of cells develops and thickens, called the *embryonic disc*. The disc is initially a bilaminar structure, consisting of an upper *ectoderm* layer and a lower *endoderm* layer, which remains in contact with the yolk sac on the ventral surface (Fig. 2-1). By the third week, a distinct area of cell proliferation is evident at the caudal end of the embryonic disc. Proliferating cells from the primitive streak migrate laterally and forward between ectoderm and endoderm to form the

mesoderm layer. When the differentiation at the mesoderm is well along, an invagination of the ectoderm forms immediately cranial to the primitive streak. Cells proliferate within the invagination and migrate cranially to form a thin tube of cells, the *notochord* (Fig. 2-2). The notochord provides an axis for the differentiation of the embryo. The pre-embryonic period lasts 3 weeks.

Embryonic Period

At about 3 weeks, the midline cells of the ectoderm overlying the notochord enlarge, proliferate, and invaginate, forming the *neural folds*. Neural folds eventually unite (initially in the thoracic levels) and with complete closure form the *neural tube* (Fig. 2-3). The neural tube ultimately differentiates into the brain and spinal cord.

During differentiation of the neural tube, there is simultaneous differentiation of the mesodermal cells, which form about 43 pairs of cell aggregates, called *somites*. Somite formation is usually complete by the end of the fifth week. Cells within the somite further differentiate into the three cell types—the medial *sclerotome*, destined to become the vertebral bones; the *myotome*, destined to become muscle; and the *dermatome*, destined to become dermis and subcutaneous tissue (Fig. 2-4).

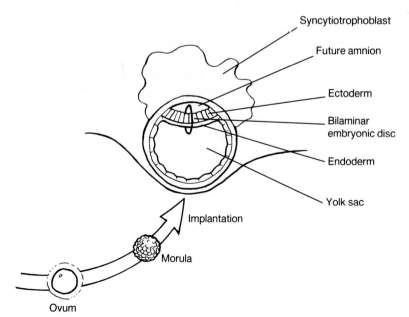

FIGURE 2–1. Early preembryonic period.

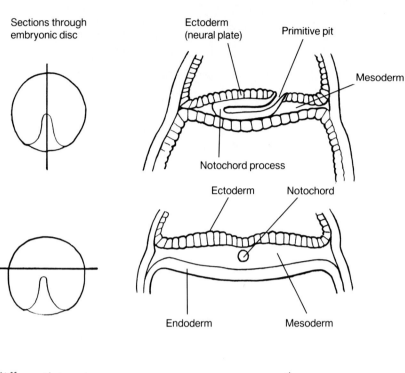

Sections through embryonic disc

Ectoderm (neural plate)

Primitive pit

Mesoderm

Notochord process

Ectoderm

Notochord

Endoderm

Mesoderm

FIGURE 2-2. Development of the notochord.

Intersegmental blood vessels differentiate at this time and penetrate between adjacent sclerotomes (somites). The primordial vertebral body forms from adjacent sclerotomes when the caudal half of one sclerotome unites with the cranial half of the subjacent sclerotome. The primitive blood vessels around the primordial vertebral bodies coalesce and persist into adulthood as the *segmental vessels*. Thus, each vertebra is composed of portions of two adjacent sclerotomes. The intervertebral disc develops from the middle portion of the sclerotomes and incorporates residual tissue from the notochord. There are vessels within the intervertebral disc at this stage of development, but by maturation the disc becomes avascular (Fig. 2-5).

As this process is occurring, the sclerotomal tissue also unites dorsally to enclose the neural tube. This is completed at about 6 weeks, at the end of the embryonic period.

Fetal Period

The fetal phase, lasting from 6 weeks to term, includes many major steps in differentiation of the spine. The differentiation of the bones in the vertebral column is usually divided into four stages: mesenchymal, chondrification, primary ossification, and secondary ossification.

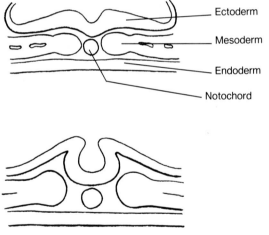

Ectoderm

Mesoderm

Endoderm

Notochord

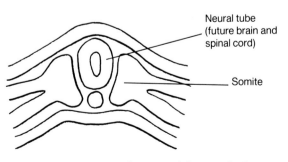

Neural tube (future brain and spinal cord)

Somite

FIGURE 2-3. Development of the neural tube.

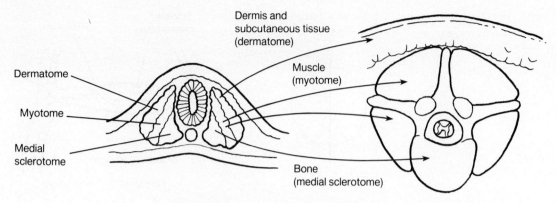

FIGURE 2–4. Development of the somite.

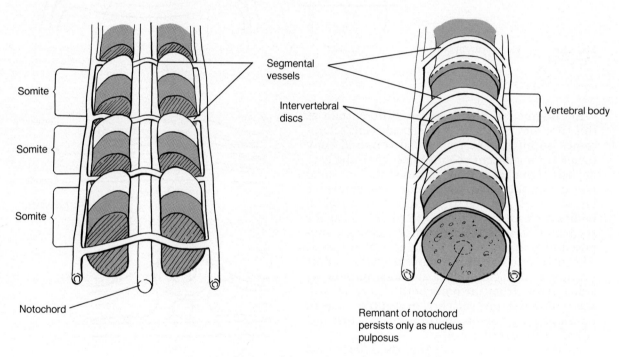

FIGURE 2–5. Development of the vertebrae and intervertebral discs.

DIFFERENTIATION OF THE VERTEBRAE

Mesenchymal Stage

The mesenchymal stage of vertebral development occurs during the embryonic period and refers to the differentiation of the cellular primordial vertebral body from the somites (Fig. 2-6). Sclerotomal cells migrate ventrally and medially to surround the notochord. Cells from the caudal and cranial halves of adjacent sclerotomes unite to form the mesenchymal vertebral body.

Chondrification

The chondrification stage begins in the fifth week. Glycosaminoglycan and cartilage matrix is synthesized, and the mesenchymal cells differentiate into a form of chondrocyte. Chondrification begins in two laterally placed fossae in the centrum, or developing vertebral body and one chondrification center in each side of the neural arch. Outgrowths from the chondrification centers in the neural arch differentiate into the cartilage anlage of the articular and transverse processes (Fig. 2-7).

Primary Ossification

Centers of primary ossification are seen within the cartilage anlage beginning at the eighth week. There is one ossification center within the centrum and one on each side of the neural arch (Fig. 2-8). The stage of primary ossification lasts well into childhood. At birth, a typical vertebra consists of a partially ossified centrum and two partially ossified arches that have not fused. An area

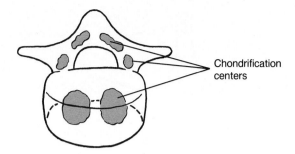

FIGURE 2–7. Stage of chondrification.

of cartilage, the *neurocentral synchondrosis*, lies between the ossified arch and the centrum. The neurocentral synchondrosis is anterior to the base of the pedicle. Thus, a good portion of the vertebral body is derived from the neural arch.

Fourth and fifth ossification centers within the cartilage anlage represent the "costal" ossification center from which the ribs are derived in the thoracic levels. In the cervical, lumbar, and sacral segments, the costal ossification center is incorporated into the vertebra as part of the lateral masses of the cervical vertebrae, the transverse processes of the lumbar vertebrae, and the ala of the sacrum.

Secondary Ossification

The formation of secondary ossification centers begins at about 8 years of age. Secondary ossification centers include the cephalad and caudad ring apophyses and separate terminal ossification centers for each transverse process and for the spinous process. The ring apophyses appear at about 8 years of age (Fig. 2-9). All other secondary ossification centers appear at about age 14. Fusion of all centers is complete at about 20 to 25 years.

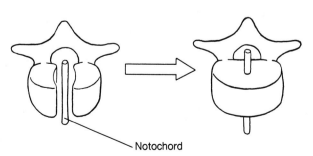

FIGURE 2–6. Mesenchymal stage.

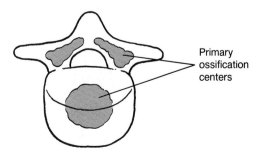

FIGURE 2–8. Stage of primary ossification.

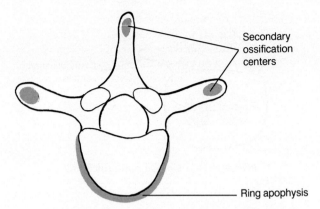

FIGURE 2–9. Stage of secondary ossification.

Development of the Atlas and Axis

Differentiation of the atlas and axis differs markedly from that of the more caudad vertebral segments. It may be grossly simplified to think of the centrum of C1 being incorporated onto the body of C2 to form the dens.

Ossification of the anterior arch of the atlas is not complete until 1 year after birth. The posterior ring of the atlas is likewise not completely ossified at birth, although it may appear so on a lateral radiograph, because the unossified segment is parallel to the x-ray beam.

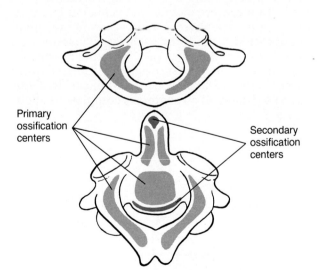

FIGURE 2–10. Ossification of the atlas and axis.

The dens anlage (representing the body of the atlas) develops from the caudal half of the fourth occipital sclerotome and the cranial half of the first cervical sclerotome. The dens ossifies from three primary centers. Two laterally placed centers appear in the sixth gestational month and join before birth. The tip of the dens is a separate ossification center that appears at about the second year and fuses with the rest of the dens at about the 12th year. The presence of a "V"-shaped notch at the tip of the dens is a normal finding in children; this may occasionally persist into adulthood as a bicornate dens called *dens bicornis*. The ossification centers of the dens fuse with the ossification centers of the centrum of the axis at about 5 years of age. This *subdental synchondrosis* is sometimes mistakenly thought to represent a fracture (Fig. 2-10).

Development of the Sacrum

Ossification of the sacrum proceeds from primary centers in the sacral centrum. No ring apophyses form caudal to the superior end plates of the first sacral segment. Each neural arch develops from two centers in the sacrum. Analogues of the costal ossification centers and of the transverse process ossification centers combine to form the sacral alae. Complete bony fusion of the sacrum does not occur until after 20 years of age.

DEVELOPMENTAL ANOMALIES OF THE SPINE

Developmental anomalies of the spine may represent completely benign incidental findings in otherwise normal people. Conversely, significant structural abnormalities in the spine may lead to profound neurologic compromise and/or devastating deformity. Structural abnormalities in the spine are also significant because of established associations with congenital abnormalities of other organ systems, especially the cardiovascular and genitourinary systems.

Many congenital spine anomalies may be classified as either failures of formation or failures of segmentation. Certain conditions (eg, sacral agenesis) are the result of the failure of a normal part of the anatomy to form and develop. Other spinal anomalies are classified as failures of segmentation if a portion of the normal anatomy develops but fails to separate normally from a neighboring structure. Examples of failure of segmentation include occipitalization of the atlas or a congenital *block vertebra*.

Occipitocervical Spine

The *Arnold-Chiari* malformation is an aberrant projection of the cerebellar tonsils into the upper cervical canal (Fig. 2-11). There are two types. Type I consists of tonsillar elongation with extension of the cerebellar tonsils into the upper cervical canal; occasionally a small portion of the inferior lobe of the cerebellum is also present in the cervical canal. This type is not associated with hydrocephalus and is often asymptomatic. Type II consists of a projection of the cerebellar tonsils and parts of the cerebellum into the cervical canal. In addition, the fourth ventricle is elongated and is also found in the upper cervical canal. In about 50% of cases, hydrocephalus is also present. With caudad migration of the brain stem

the cervical roots must course upward in the canal to exit by their proper foramina.

Arnold-Chiari malformation, when associated with brain stem compression or a spinal cord syrinx, may present indications for decompression. Associated problems of interest to the orthopedist are extremely common and include basilar impression, atlanto-occipital fusion, Klippel-Feil syndrome, and spina bifida. Syringomyelia and hydromyelia are also common.

Platybasia is a flattening of the base of the skull resulting in a more horizontal position of the plane of the clivus. This term is often wrongly used as a synonym for basilar invagination.

Basilar invagination or basilar impression is the most common congenital abnormality of the atlanto-occipital region. It may also occur as a secondary manifestation of other diseases, such as rheumatoid arthritis. Basilar invagination is an upward movement of the upper cervical spine into the foramen magnum. In this condition, the dens may assume an intracranial position, causing pressure on the brain stem. Symptomatology may manifest at any time up to the first decade of life. Usually symptoms are those of long tract involvement, as well as ataxia and lower cranial nerve dysfunction. Chamberlain's line is a line drawn from the posterior border of the hard pal-

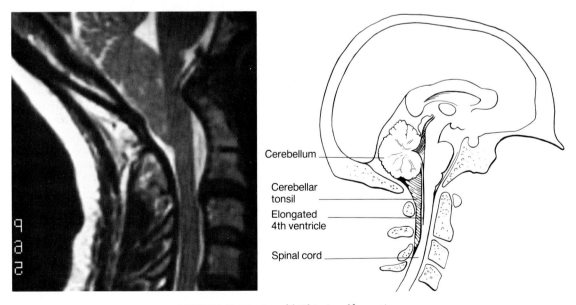

Cerebellum

Cerebellar tonsil

Elongated 4th ventricle

Spinal cord

FIGURE 2–11. Arnold-Chiari malformation.

ate to the anterior border of the posterior rim of the foramen magnum. The odontoid does not normally project more than 2 mm above this line. Plain radiographic methods are rarely definitive in the diagnosis of basilar invagination. When this diagnosis is suspected, direct imaging with magnetic resonance imaging (MRI) or computed tomographic (CT) myelography is indicated. Treatment, when significant, consists of surgical decompression and stabilization.

Occipitalization of the atlas, another common congenital abnormality of the upper cervical spine, involves fusion of one or both lateral masses to the skull, often including a fusion of the skull to the anterior arch of C1. The posterior arch is usually hypoplastic and is often tethered to the posterior rim of the foramen magnum. One report has stated that the incidence in Caucasians is in the range of 0.5% to 1%. Late development of long tract symptoms and signs in these patients is common because this lesion is frequently associated with basilar invagination.

An *arcuate foramen,* a frequent anomaly of the atlas, is ossification of the atlanto-occipital ligament as it arches over the vertebral artery. This abnormality has no clinical significance. It can assist in the assessment of C1–C2 rotation with lateral radiographs as a useful radiographic landmark.

Ossification of the *posterior arch* of the atlas is usually not complete at birth, and in about 2% of asymptomatic adults there is a lack of complete bony fusion. This abnormality is of no clinical significance unless surgery in the area is contemplated.

Torticollis, a twisting of the neck causing an abnormal position of the head, can be due to congenital deformities of the atlas. All cases of torticollis, therefore, should be investigated with x-ray. When torticollis is due to congenital vertebral anomalies, it is severe and progressive. If x-rays are normal and the deformity is rigid, it may be due to a unilateral contracture of the sternocleidomastoid muscle. This causes the head to be held tilted to the ipsilateral side and rotated to the contralateral side of the fibrotic muscle. It usually responds to stretching, range of motion, and positioning. If these measures are unsuccessful by age 24 months, surgical treatment, consisting of a resection of a portion of both heads of the sternocleidomastoid muscle, is recommended. If the torticollis is associated with a normal pas-

sive range of motion and no radiographic abnormality, the underlying cause may be ocular dysfunction.

Rarely, *agenesis of the odontoid* occurs; more frequently, a small bony remnant, termed a *hypoplastic odontoid,* remains. In these cases the transverse ligament may have no stabilizing effect on the joint, and clinically significant instability can result. In patients with severe instability, fusion may be indicated. Agenesis or hypoplasia of the odontoid is not infrequently encountered in patients with Down's syndrome, although the atlantoaxial instabilities found in 10% to 20% of Down's syndrome patients are most commonly caused by ligamentous laxity alone (Fig. 2-12).

In patients with *os odontoideum,* there is a jointlike articulation between the odontoid and the body of the axis; it appears radiologically as a wide radiolucent gap (Fig. 2-13). This gap is sometimes misinterpreted as a subdental synchondrosis, which normally lies *below* the level of the articular facets of C2. With motion between the dens and the body of C2, significant clinical instability is often present. Prevailing opinion holds that os odontoideum in most patients probably is an acquired lesion that follows nonunion of a fracture at the base of the odontoid in a young child. In patients with a relatively stable C1–C2 joint causing little compromise of the space for the cord and minimal symptomatology, nonoperative treatment is recommended. If excessive instability is demonstrated (>10 mm translation on lateral flexion-extension views) or any signs or symptoms of myelopathy are noted, surgical stabilization (a C1–C2 posterior fusion) is strongly recommended.

Klippel-Feil syndrome is an example of segmentation failure. The exact definition of the syndrome is imprecise, but most clinicians now consider any patient with a congenital fusion of the neck to have a type of Klippel-Feil syndrome (Fig. 2-14). Maurice Klippel and André Feil in 1912 described a patient with multiple congenital cervical fusions, a lower posterior hairline, and a short neck. Feil later classified these lesions into three types. Type I consists of massive fusion of many cervical and upper thoracic vertebrae. Type II patients present with fusion of one or two interspaces only. Type III patients have cervical fusions in combination with lower thoracic or lumbar fusions. This syndrome is associated with numerous other developmental ab-

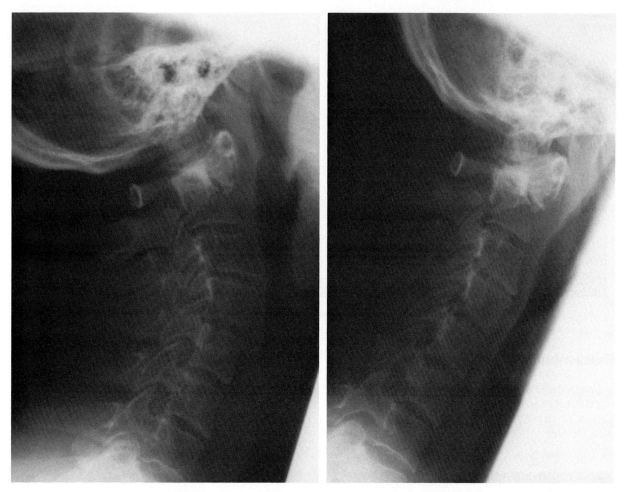

FIGURE 2–12. Atlantoaxial subluxation in Down's syndrome.

normalities, including deafness, cranial nerve palsies, cardiovascular anomalies including ventricular septal defects, Sprengel's deformity, and urogenital anomalies, which may be present in over 30% of these patients. A common physical finding in these patients is *synkinesia* (mirror motions). The most common physical finding is decreased range of motion of the neck, although in patients with multiple congenital fusions there is considerable compensatory hypermobility of the remaining open segments in many cases. The significance of this is that degenerative changes at these hypermobile levels are common.

Management of the patient with Klippel-Feil syndrome centers on a careful search for associated malformations and observation. Surgery for cosmesis is absolutely contraindicated. Rarely, degenerative change at open segments may lead to significant spondylosis or impingement on neural structures. Surgical decompression, usually with concomitant fusion, may be indicated in these rare instances.

Rarely, a patient may present with an anomalous *cervical rib* from the C7 level. This occasionally contributes to symptoms of a thoracic outlet syndrome. An anteroposterior x-ray of the cervicothoracic junction may reveal this rib. It may be identified as a cervical rib by the fact that the transverse processes of thoracic vertebrae are inclined upward; those of the cervical vertebrae are inclined downward. A rib seen emerging from in front of a downwardly inclined transverse process is probably a cervical rib.

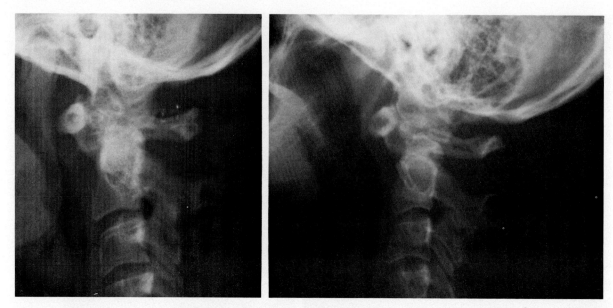

FIGURE 2–13. Two examples of os odontoideum.

Thoracolumbar Spine

Congenital scoliosis is the result of failure of segmentation, failure of formation, or a combination of these two problems during the formation of the vertebral bodies from adjacent somites. This results in anomalous vertebrae that cause deformity on the basis of asymmetric growth.

An example of a pure failure of segmentation is the congenital block vertebra. This results from the failure of a somite segment to separate

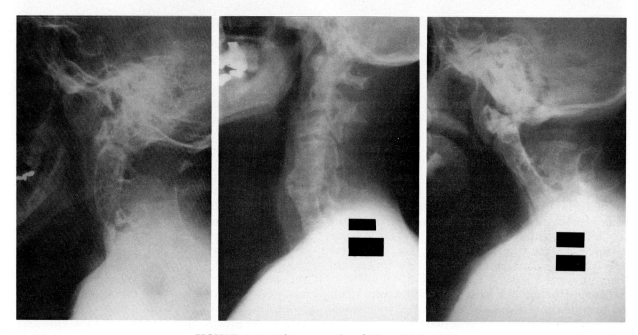

FIGURE 2–14. Three examples of Klippel-Feil syndrome.

into its cephalad and caudad halves, creating one large block vertebral body with no intervening disc. This condition rarely results in profound deformity.

A similar developmental defect that occurs on only one side of the developing vertebral segment results in the formation of a unilateral unsegmented bar. Because there are growth plates associated with each end plate, vertebral growth on the segmented half of these vertebrae proceeds, but on the unsegmented side does not. This condition often leads to asymmetric growth and severe scoliosis.

Congenital kyphosis occurs by a very similar process. Failure of segmentation across the anterior portion of adjacent vertebral segments can occur while the posterior segments of the involved vertebrae undergo segmentation. With growth of the posterior portion of the vertebra, and the tethering of the anterior unsegmented portion, progressive kyphosis results.

Failure of formation may result in the congenital absence of a complete vertebral body, although the posterior elements may be present. This situation causes congenital kyphosis.

In many cases, the right or left half of a vertebral body fails to form. The vertebral body that remains is called, appropriately, a hemivertebra. The presence of the hemivertebra and its subsequent growth causes a significant shift of the spine to the opposite side, with resulting scoliosis.

Isolated hemivertebrae, block vertebrae, and unilateral unsegmented bars are sometimes seen as isolated clinical entities. More frequently, however, multiple events of segmentation failure and formation failure coexist. This mixed type of congenital scoliosis is frequently associated with cervical Klippel-Feil findings.

Lumbosacral Junction

There are frequent segmentation abnormalities at the lumbosacral junction. Transitional vertebrae, which have accessory articulations between the transverse process of the most caudal lumbar vertebrae and either the sacrum or the ilium, have been reported in from 4% to 8% of the general population (Fig. 2-15). Frequently, a solid bony bridge is also seen linking the transverse process of the lower lumbar vertebrae to the sacrum. When this occurs, the lumbosacral disc is often seen to be smaller than normal; sometimes it is quite vestigial.

These anatomic abnormalities are generally not associated with other skeletal abnormalities, and there is no established relation with other visceral congenital defects. This condition is not thought to be a source of clinical problems but may cause confusion in the naming of the lumbar vertebrae. Different physicians may, for example, refer to such a vertebra as a "sacralized L5" or a "lumbarized S1."

Sacral agenesis, also known as caudal aplasia, is an extremely rare developmental anomaly. It is more frequent in infants of diabetic mothers. The sacral agenesis may be partial or complete. In some cases, the contralateral iliac bones actually articulate directly across the midline. The condition is associated with other conditions, including meningocele, spina bifida of neighboring portions of the spine, urinary tract abnormalities, and associated extremity developmental defects, including congenital hip anomalies and foot deformities. Affected children often are found to have an associated treatable cause for some of their neurologic dysfunctions, such as congenital spinal stenosis, a tethered spinal cord, or an intraspinal mass.

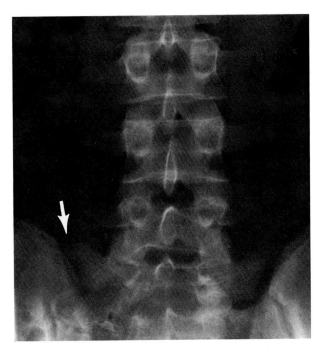

FIGURE 2-15. Segmentation abnormality at the lumbosacral junction.

Spina Bifida

Spina bifida is a term that often causes confusion, because it is used to describe a spectrum of clinical entities of varying severity. *Spina bifida occulta* is the failure of the posterior ossification centers in the lateral masses to unite. This common condition, present in about 0.5% of the population, is not normally associated with neurogenic or mechanical problems. The posterior elements of a given vertebral level may be almost completely absent, or the defect may occupy a vertical gap of less than 1 cm. The spina bifida may be present throughout the spine, may skip levels, or may be limited to a single level (Fig. 2-16). Patients with this condition may present with a hair patch on the skin overlying the spine. There is a small but significant association between this condition and problems of intradural lipoma or tethered spinal cord. In the absence of either of these complicating conditions, the principal significance of this condition is that it presents an additional hazard during surgical approaches to the spine. An anteroposterior radiograph of the spine must be closely inspected for possible posterior arch defects, or inadvertent catastrophic injury may result from routine blunt techniques for exposure of the spine.

Myelomeningocele and *spinal dysraphism* are a group of related conditions involving a dorsal defect in the neural canal. The exact cause is unknown but may involve a failure of closure of the neural tube during development or, perhaps more likely, rupture of the neural tube after normal closure and an interval of subsequent development (Fig. 2-17). There are three types of defects: meningocele, myelomeningocele, and rachischisis.

A *meningocele* is a CSF-filled sac that extends dorsally through a defect in the bony portion of the spine. It often is quite large, causing a prominent mass on the infant's back. This meningocele is invested with skin and does not contain any neural elements. Therefore, it is only very rarely associated with a neurologic deficit.

A *myelomeningocele* is a similar condition in which the sac contains neural elements. Often the neural elements are grossly abnormal and are frequently adherent to the wall of the sac. In patients with myelomeningocele, the sac is often not invested by epidermis. Severe neurologic dysfunction is common.

Rachischisis is a condition in which the neural elements of the spine are completely exposed, with no covering of overlying skin or dural material.

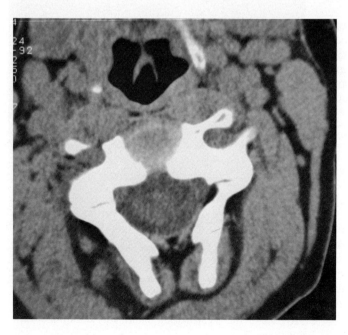

FIGURE 2-16. Spina bifida at C2.

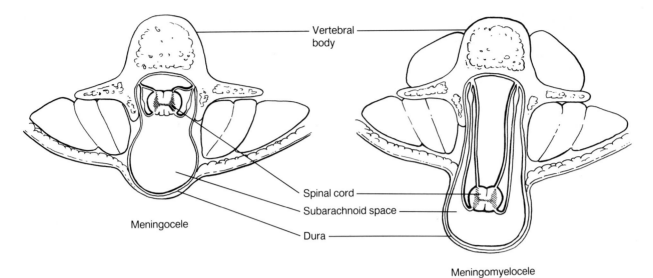

FIGURE 2–17. Meningocele and myelomeningocele.

A high percentage of infants born with myelomeningocele die in early infancy. The prognosis is much better in patients with an isolated meningocele. Such patients frequently present with other related congenital problems, including hydrocephalus. The presence of other congenital abnormalities of the spine is noted in about one fifth of patients. Tethering of the spinal cord is often noted on later growth. Surgical closure of the neural tube defect, if indicated, is frequently done very early in life.

The orthopedic management of lower extremity muscle imbalances and growth abnormalities in these patients is a complex challenge for the pediatric orthopedist. During longitudinal growth of these patients, progressive kyphosis or scoliosis is frequently encountered. Braces are ineffective, so patients often require instrumentation and fusion for progressive scoliosis. Rapidly progressive curves in such patients are often found to be associated with other neurologic conditions, such as a tethered cord, hydrocephalus, or a diastematomyelia. The suspicion for these related conditions must remain high in any patient with a spinal dysraphic condition. Progressive intractable kyphosis is often managed by a kyphectomy and fusion performed from posteriorly.

KEY POINTS

1. The vertebral bodies are derived from adjacent halves of contiguous cellular aggregates called somites.
2. Differentiation of the vertebral bodies is characterized by progression through a sequence of stages: the mesenchymal (cellular) stage, the stage of chondrification, the stage of primary ossification, and finally the stage of secondary ossification.
3. Many congenital abnormalities can be classified as failures of formation or failures of segmentation.
4. Congenital abnormalities of the spine are frequently associated with other visceral or neurologic abnormalities.

BIBLIOGRAPHY

BOOKS

Cervical Spine Research Society, Sherk H. The cervical spine. 2nd ed. Philadelphia: JB Lippincott, 1989.

Lemire RJ, Loeser JD, Leech RW, Alvord EC. Normal and abnormal development of the human nervous system. Hagerstown, MD: Harper & Row, 1976.

McLaurin RL, ed. Myelomeningocele. New York: Grune and Stratton, 1977.

Sadler TW, ed. Langman's medical embryology. 6th ed. Baltimore: Williams & Wilkins, 1990.

Winter RB. Congenital deformities of the spine. New York: Thieme, 1983.

JOURNALS

Dyste GN, Menezes AH, VanGilder JC. Symptomatic Chiari malformations. J Neurosurg 1989;71(12):159–168.

Georgopoulos G, Pizzutillo PD, Lee MS. Occipito-atlantal instability in children. J Bone Joint Surg [Am] 1987;69:429–436.

Hensinger RN. Osseous anomalies of the craniovertebral junction. Spine 1986;11:323–333.

Hensinger RN, Lang JR, MacEwen GD. Klippel-Feil syndrome: A constellation of associated anomalies. J Bone Joint Surg [Am] 1974; 56:1242–1253.

MacEwen GD, Winter RB. Evaluation of kidney anomalies in congenital scoliosis. J Bone Joint Surg [Am] 1972;54:1451–1454.

Nagib MG, Maxwell RE, Chou SN. Klippel-Feil syndrome in children: Clinical features and management. Child Neurol System 1985;1:255–263.

Tawaka T, Unthoff HK. The pathogenesis of congenital vertebral malformations. Acta Orthop Scand 1991;52:413–425.

Taylor JR. The growth of human intervertebral discs and vertebral bodies. J Anat 1975;120:49–68.

Wilkinson JA, Sedgwick EM. Occult spinal dysraphism in established congenital dislocation of the hip. J Bone Joint Surg [Br] 1988;70:744–749.

Textbook of Spinal Disorders, by Stephen I. Esses.
J. B. Lippincott Company, Philadelphia © 1995.

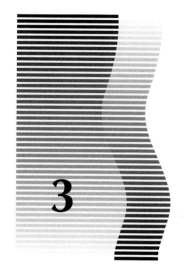

3   Physical Examination

HISTORY

ORDER OF PHYSICAL
  EXAMINATION

GENERAL
  EXAMINATION

CERVICAL SPINE
  Inspection
  Range of Motion
  Palpation
  L'Hermitte's Sign
  Compression-
    Traction Test
  Motor Examination
  Sensory Examination
  Deep Tendon
    Reflexes

THORACIC SPINE
  Inspection
  Range of Motion
  Chest Expansion
  Reflexes
  Sensory Examination

LUMBOSACRAL SPINE
  Inspection
  Range of Motion

Palpation
Motor Examination
Sensory Examination
Reflexes
Tests of Nerve Root
  Tension
Rectal Examination

SACROILIAC JOINTS
  Palpation
  Range of Motion
  Stress Test
  Fabere Test
  Gaenslen's Test

MYELOPATHY
  Spasticity
  Plantar Response
  Myelopathic Hand

TRAUMA
  Inspection
  Palpation
  Neurologic
    Evaluation

NONORGANIC
  EVALUATION

HISTORY

The patient's history is more than the sequence of events leading to medical consultation: it is the key to reaching an accurate diagnosis. The astute clinician allows the patient to recall the evolution of his or her symptoms with little interruption. Then the clinician asks specific questions to gain a perception of the patient as a person rather than simply another patient. It is important to know the patient's usual activities and how they have been altered by his or her affliction; thus, knowing the patient's work, marital status, and outside interests is crucial. If patients have difficulty articulating their complaints, the clinician may assist them by suggesting specific descriptions.

After the clinician has obtained a thorough understanding of the patient's complaints from initial presentation to the time of consultation, it is then appropriate to inquire about general health, family history, and possible related symptoms and signs. Although it may seem a cliché, the adage that the patient will tell the clinician the diagnosis if he or she listens closely is particularly true in the diagnosis of spine-related disorders. By the time the full history has been elicited, the clinician should have formulated a differential diagnosis and should have an appreciation of the patient as a person and an understanding of the extent to which the patient's problem has interfered with his or her usual activities.

It is crucial to distinguish neck pain from arm pain; similarly, it is important to distinguish between back pain and leg or radicular pain. The nature of the pain, as well as activities that precipitate symptoms, is important. These areas will be discussed along with the relevant conditions.

ORDER OF PHYSICAL EXAMINATION

As with other areas of medicine, the physical examination begins with an inspection of the affected area. This is followed by an assessment of the range of motion both actively (by the patient) and passively (by the examiner). After this, palpation, both superficial and deep, is undertaken. Special tests relevant to the area of concern and the patient's history follow.

Many patients with spinal disorders find it difficult to move from a seated to a standing position. Lying down may cause discomfort. Therefore, the examiner must develop an organized approach that minimizes the need for a patient to change position. All of the tests that can be done with the patient standing should be done together, as should the tests that require the patient to be sitting or lying down. This minimizes patient discomfort and ultimately increases patient compliance.

GENERAL EXAMINATION

The examination of the spine cannot be done in isolation. The clinician must be adept at examining not only the musculoskeletal system but also other organ systems. A general examination is done in all patients. The hip examination is mandatory in any patient presenting with lower back and buttock complaints. In patients presenting with arm pain, a cardiac examination may be appropriate. Lower paraspinal complaints may mandate a kidney examination. Evaluation of the vascular system is necessary to distinguish neurogenic from vascular claudication. All too often, missed diagnosis reflects the narrow interests of the examiner and his or her inability to consider and evaluate diagnoses outside his or her field.

CERVICAL SPINE

Inspection

Inspection of the cervical spine begins by evaluating the way the patient holds his or her head. Having the head turned to one side or tilted in a "cock-robin" fashion suggests cervical spine malalignment (Fig. 3-1). After inspecting the posture of the head, the clinician inspects the head and neck for any abnormalities. Peculiarities in the position of the ears, hairline, or webbing of the neck may be an indication of underlying congenital cervical spine deformity (Klippel-Feil syndrome, Fig. 3-2). The front and the back of the neck must be examined so as not to overlook soft tissue masses, as occur with tumors and infections.

Range of Motion

Assessment of range of motion of the cervical spine includes flexion, extension, lateral rotation to the right and left, and lateral bending to the right and left. There is an extremely wide range in these motions in the general population. With age, range of motion tends to decrease. Thus, in assessing these motions it is more important to compare the patient's excursion to one side with the other rather than the entire elicited range. Re-

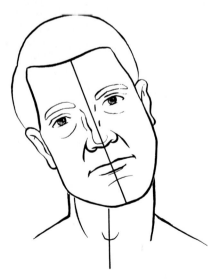

FIGURE 3–1. Cock-robin deformity.

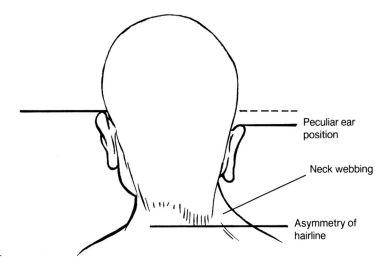

FIGURE 3–2. Klippel-Feil syndrome.

Peculiar ear position

Neck webbing

Asymmetry of hairline

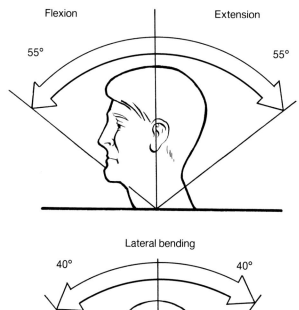

Flexion

Extension

55°

55°

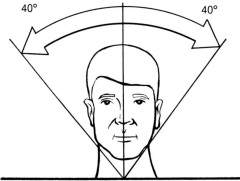

Lateral bending

40°

40°

FIGURE 3–3. Range of motion in flexion, extension, and lateral bending of the cervical spine.

duction in passive motion may indicate underlying pain, whereas reduction in both passive and active range of motion may indicate underlying malalignment. The mean forward flexion is about 55°, as is extension. Lateral bending is usually 40° to each side (Fig. 3-3). Lateral rotation in most people is 90° to each side (Fig. 3-4). The atlantoaxial joint accounts for about 47° of lateral rotation in total. Thus, a significant decrease in this direction may indicate an underlying C1–C2 abnormality. Flexion and extension occur about equally at all other levels, including the occipito-atlantal interspace. A slight increase in lateral bending occurs in the upper cervical levels compared with the lower cervical levels.

Palpation

Palpation should initially be done lightly to evaluate superficial structures and then more deeply to assess the underlying anatomy. Posteriorly, the occiput should be felt, as should each spinous process and interspinous level. The paravertebral muscles on either side should be explored for spasm, tenderness, and masses. Anteriorly, the clinician should determine whether there is spasm in the sternomastoid muscle. It is possible to gently ease one's fingers anterior to this muscle and palpate the anterior spinal column. The *carotid tubercle*, a bony prominence on the transverse process of C6, can be easily felt. Using this as a landmark for levels, the anterior

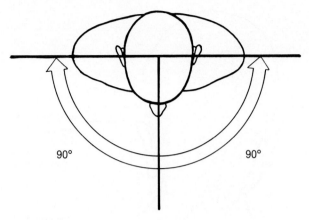

FIGURE 3–4. Range of motion in lateral rotation of the cervical spine.

cervical spine can then be evaluated for tenderness or large protruding osteophytes. By palpating the neck during motion, crepitations can be detected. The "clunk" test consists of palpating the upper cervical spine during flexion and extension. The detection of a clunk during this motion may represent underlying C1–C2 instability.

Examination of the cervical spine should be accompanied by examination of the axilla. The roots of the brachial plexus can be felt by gentle palpation of the axilla with the arm abducted 30° to 50°.

L'Hermitte's Sign

L'Hermitte's sign is pain or altered sensation radiating down the arms and legs elicited by forceful flexion of the cervical spine (Fig. 3-5). This indicates spinal cord compression, with the offending mass usually anterior to the spinal cord. Occasionally a positive L'Hermitte's sign indicates a demyelinating disease.

Compression-Traction Test

For the compression-traction test, the examiner places both hands on the patient's head (Fig. 3-6) and applies downward forceful pressure. The patient is asked whether this elicits any pain or tingling in either arm. The examiner then places one hand under the patient's chin and the other under the occiput. Gentle traction is then

exerted by lifting the head upward. The patient is asked whether this alleviates tingling or pain down either arm. This test is used to determine whether arm pain or paresthesia is a result of nerve root compression at the level of the neural foramen. Compression shortens the neck and increases the cervical lordosis. This tends to close the intervertebral foramina and increases any preexisting nerve root compression. Traction lengthens the neck, straightens the cervical lordosis, opens the posterior facet joints, and increases the intervertebral foraminal space.

Motor Examination

A thorough evaluation of the motor component of the cervical nerve roots is essential to the

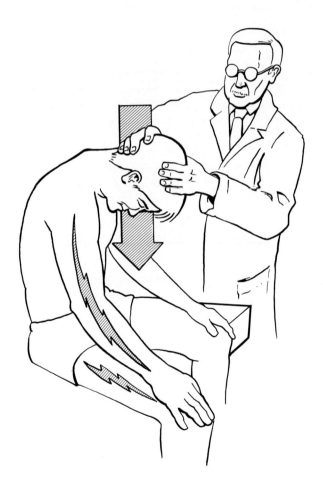

FIGURE 3–5. L'Hermitte's sign.

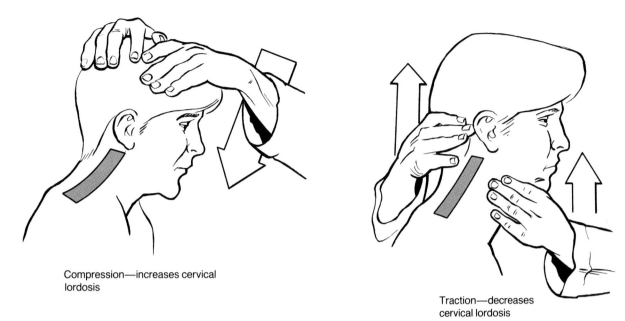

Compression—increases cervical lordosis

Traction—decreases cervical lordosis

FIGURE 3–6. Compression-traction test.

examination of the cervical spine. In many cases, weakness is not noticed by the patient but is detected on physical examination.

The standard grading scale for muscle strength is given in Table 3-1. The muscles of the shoulder girdle and upper extremity have dual and occasionally triple innervation. Therefore, to localize a specific nerve root lesion, it is necessary to test the motor strength of muscles with overlapping nerve root innervation. The major muscles and their nerve root innervation are listed in Table 3-2. Testing these muscles enables the clinician to ascertain the level or levels of nerve root involvement. No muscles are innervated by the first two cervical nerves, which are primarily sensory.

The nerve root innervation given in Table 3-2 applies to the normal situation, but many patients have a pre- or post-fixed plexus, which shifts the innervation one level proximally or distally, respectively.

Sensory Examination

The sensory distribution of the cervical nerves is shown in Figure 3-7. Examination of sensation should always include an evaluation of pain and light touch perception. If an area of altered sensibility is suspected, this area should be tested first. The usual stimulus for pain is a sharp pin. Light touch can be evaluated using a brush or a piece of gauze. It is not sufficient to simply evaluate the perception of these senses; rather, the patient should be asked to compare what he or she feels in one dermatome compared with the same dermatome on the other side. Pain and light touch sensation may be graded as normal, reduced, or increased. If there is an area of decreased pain

TABLE 3–1. **Muscle Strength Grading**

Description	Grade
No contraction	0
Flicker	1
Active movement with gravity eliminated	2
Active movement against gravity	3
Active movement against gravity and resistance	4
Normal response	5

TABLE 3–2. **Major Muscles and Their Nerve Root Innervation**

Muscle	Nerve Root Innervation*
Trapezius	C3, C4
Rhomboids	C4, <u>C5</u>
Deltoid	<u>C5</u>, C6
Biceps	C5, C6
Brachioradialis	C5, C6
Extensor carpi radialis longus and brevis	<u>C6</u>, C7
Flexor carpi radialis	<u>C6</u>, <u>C7</u>, C8
Triceps	<u>C7</u>, C8
Extensor carpi ulnaris	<u>C7</u>, C8
Extensor digitorum	<u>C7</u>, C8
Flexor digitorum profundus	<u>C8</u>, T1
Flexor pollicis longus	<u>C8</u>, T1
Intrinsics	C8, <u>T1</u>
Abductor pollicis brevis	C8, <u>T1</u>

* Major innervation is underlined.

sensation, then temperature sensibility should also be examined.

Deep Tendon Reflexes

The deep tendon reflexes are important because they represent the simplest spinal pathway. The stretch receptors of the particular muscle tendon being stimulated provide the primary sensory afferent input. There is a single synapse in the anterior gray matter of the spinal cord and an efferent motor neuron. Figure 3-8 shows this pathway for the biceps reflex. The biceps tendon is stretched at the level of the elbow and results in contraction of the muscle belly.

Table 3-3 presents the standard grading system for deep tendon reflexes. Because the normal briskness of these reflexes varies widely from person to person, it is essential to compare the deep tendon reflexes of both sides. Although many textbooks describe the deep tendon reflexes as testing a single nerve root, they obviously do not, because the stimulated muscles usually have dual innervation. Thus, a C6 nerve root deficit may result in a depression of both the

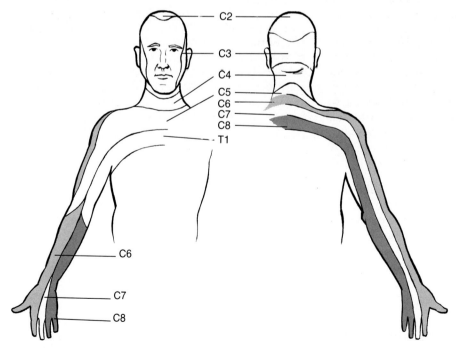

FIGURE 3–7. Sensory distribution of cervical nerves.

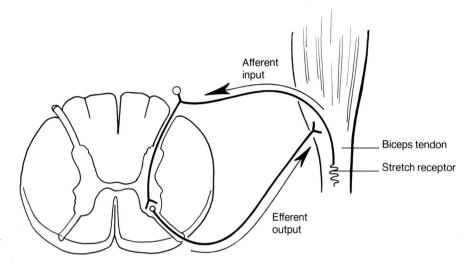

Afferent
input

Biceps tendon

Stretch receptor

Efferent
output

FIGURE 3–8. Deep tendon reflex of the biceps muscle.

biceps and brachioradialis reflexes. The three important deep tendon reflexes of the upper extremity are given in Table 3-4.

THORACIC SPINE

Inspection

The thoracic spine should first be inspected from behind. Scoliosis, a lateral curvature of the spine, may be suspected because of asymmetry of the shoulders, scapulae, waist, or skin folds (Fig. 3-9). Further inspection of the thoracic spine from behind should be done with the patient bent forward. This will permit detection of any rib cage asymmetry (Fig. 3-10). Rib prominence often accompanies scoliosis on the convex side

of the curve due to vertebral rotation. This rib prominence may be measured as the angular difference from the horizontal or as the distance from a horizontal erected from the rib prominence to the contralateral rib cage. If an unbalanced scoliosis exists, the patient may stand with a list. This list or imbalance may be measured by dropping a plumb line from the spinous process of C7 and measuring its distance to the right or left of the gluteal cleft. The patient should be asked to bend both to the right and left to determine the flexibility of any existing spinal curvature. This is further discussed in Chapter 14.

The thoracic spine should also be assessed from the side. Any increased kyphosis, such as occurs with Scheuermann's disease, ankylosing spondylitis, Paget's disease, fractures, and osteoporosis, should be noted. The clinician should

TABLE 3–3. **Grading of Deep Tendon Reflexes**

Description	Grade
Absent	0
Diminished	1
Normal	2
Increased	3
Increased with clonus	4

TABLE 3–4. **Deep Tendon Reflexes of the Upper Extremity**

Muscle	Nerve Root Innervation*
Biceps	C5, C6
Brachioradialis	C5, C6
Triceps	C7, C8

* Major innervation is underlined.

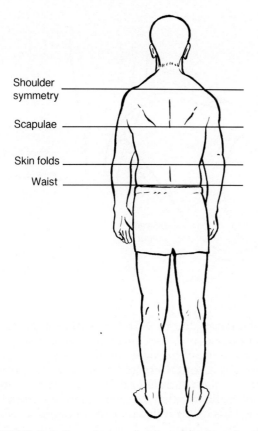

FIGURE 3–9. Posterior examination of the thoracic spine.

represents motion in the lumbar spine or hip joints. It is useful to place a thumb and index finger over two continuous spinous processes. If the distance between the two digits increases during forward flexion, it is an indication that motion is occurring at that level (Fig. 3-13).

Chest Expansion

Any disorder that affects the costovertebral joints impairs the normal motion of the chest cage. Chest excursion is measured as the increase in circumference from deep expiration to full inspiration (Fig. 3-14). A tape measure is placed around the chest at the level of the fourth intercostal space or just below the breasts in females. The patient is asked to exhale deeply and then inhale as fully as possible. Normal chest expansion is a minimum of 1 inch. An abnormally small chest expansion may be found early in the course of the disease in patients with ankylosing spondylitis.

Reflexes

Superficial reflexes depend on a simple reflex arc, with the afferent sensory neuron being stimulated by scratching or touching. After synapsing

also determine whether the increased kyphosis is over the entire thoracic spine or is an acute angular deformity limited to one or two levels (Fig. 3-11). The latter can occur with compression fractures accompanying osteoporosis (Fig. 3-12). In addition, a decreased kyphosis of the thoracic spine that may accompany scoliosis may be detected.

Range of Motion

The orientation of the thoracic facet joints allows motion in the sagittal, axial, and frontal planes. There is about 5° of both flexion-extension and lateral bending at each level. In the upper thoracic spine, there may be as much as 9° of axial rotation per level. When a patient is asked to bend forward or turn to the side, it is often difficult to determine whether the motion is coming from the thoracic spine or whether it

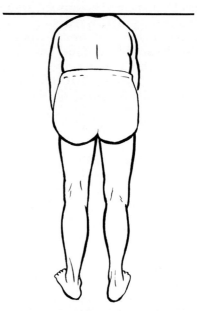

FIGURE 3–10. Detecting rib cage asymmetry.

Increased kyphosis over
entire thoracic spine

Acute angular deformity
of thoracic spine

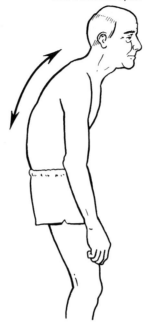 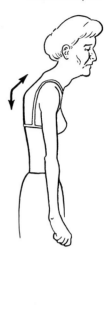

FIGURE 3–11. Thoracic kyphosis.

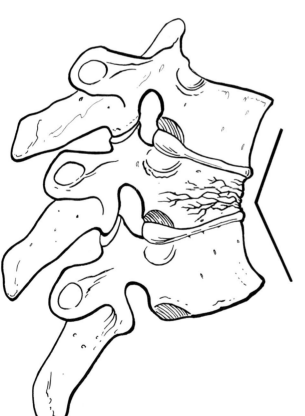

FIGURE 3–12. Compression fracture due to osteoporosis giving rise to acute kyphosis.

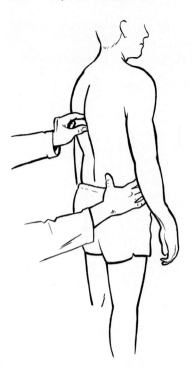
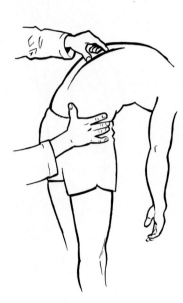

FIGURE 3–13. Measurement of motion of the thoracic spine.

at the level of the cord, there is a motor efferent neuron. Three superficial reflexes can be used to assess the thoracic nerves. These are done with the patient supine and depend on the motor efferents to the abdominal wall muscles. The *upper abdominal superficial reflex* assesses thoracic nerves 5 through 8. The skin over the lower thoracic cage is scratched from lateral to medial. A normal response is ipsilateral contraction of the muscles in the upper abdominal wall. This can often be detected by motion of the umbilicus toward the stimulated side. The *midabdominal skin reflex* assesses the 9th, 10th, and 11th thoracic nerves. The skin is stimulated at the level of the umbilicus. The 11th and 12th thoracic nerves are assessed by the *lower abdominal skin reflex*. The examiner strokes the skin from the iliac crests toward the midline (Fig. 3-15).

Sensory Examination

The dermatomal distribution of the thoracic nerves is presented in Figure 3-16. The nipple is at the T4 level. The umbilicus is at the T10 level and the iliac crests and groin are supplied by the

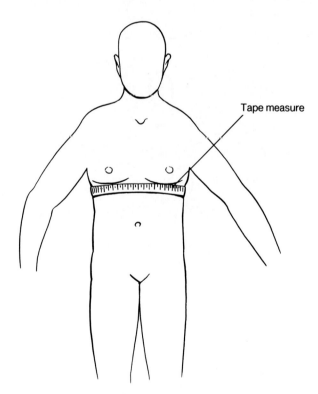

Tape measure

FIGURE 3–14. Measurement of chest expansion.

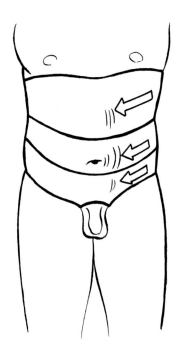

FIGURE 3–15. Abdominal superficial skin reflexes.

12th thoracic nerve. As with any evaluation of sensation, the examiner should begin by testing suspected affected areas rather than normal dermatomes. The patient is asked to compare sensation on the right and left sides in respective dermatomes. A decrease in sensation following a thoracic dermatome around the chest wall often accompanies a thoracic disc herniation.

LUMBOSACRAL SPINE

Inspection

Thorough inspection of the lumbosacral spine is a vital part of the evaluation of a patient with a spinal disorder. Underlying spinal congenital anomalies, such as spina bifida occulta, are often accompanied by cutaneous changes, including increased pigmentation or hairy patches. The patient's posture as a whole, as well as the alignment of the lumbar spine, should be evaluated. Tight hamstrings accompanying spondylolisthesis may be indicated by the patient's standing

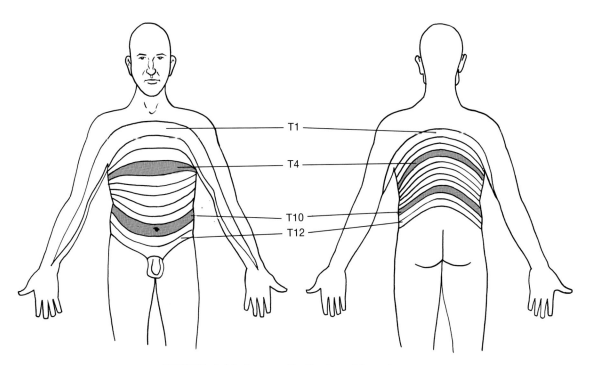

FIGURE 3–16. Sensory distribution of thoracic nerves.

with knees bent (Fig. 3-17). Lumbar muscle spasm, which may accompany sciatica, may result in the patient's standing with a list. Pelvic obliquity may result from lumbar scoliosis.

As with the thoracic spine, the patient should be evaluated from behind while standing erect, bending forward, and bending to the side (Fig. 3-18). Asymmetry in thigh skin folds or the gluteus maximus may indicate underlying scoliosis. Pelvic obliquity may be due to pathology in the spine or in the lower extremities, such as a leg-length discrepancy. This can be further evaluated by assessing the pelvis with the patient standing and sitting. The patient should also be inspected from the side. A decrease in lumbar lordosis may accompany muscle spasm; an increase in lumbar lordosis may be a manifestation of spondylolisthesis.

Range of Motion

Facet joint orientation in the lumbar spine allows primarily flexion and extension. To a lesser extent there is lateral bending, but axial rotation is normally markedly restricted. Most of the motion, particularly in the sagittal plane, occurs at the L4–L5 and lumbosacral levels. There is wide variation in the normal range of motion in the lumbar spine. In addition, it is difficult to assess lumbar spine excursion in isolation. Gross movements such as forward bending and turning to the side can be achieved almost entirely through the hip joints.

The *Schober test* is used to assess the degree of forward flexion in the lumbar spine itself (Fig. 3-19). A point is marked over the upper sacrum in the midline. A tape measure is then used to mark a spot 10 cm above this. When the patient bends forward, the distance between these two points in a normal lumbar spine should increase by at least 50%.

Particular attention should be paid to patients' complaints and symptoms while examining their range of motion. Anterior column pathology, such as discogenic disease, is often worsened by forward flexion. Facet joint symptoms are often reproduced by hyperextension.

The total range of motion of the spine and hips can be documented by measuring how close the patient's hand can be brought to the floor. In side bending, the distance measured is due only to motion of the spine (Fig. 3-20).

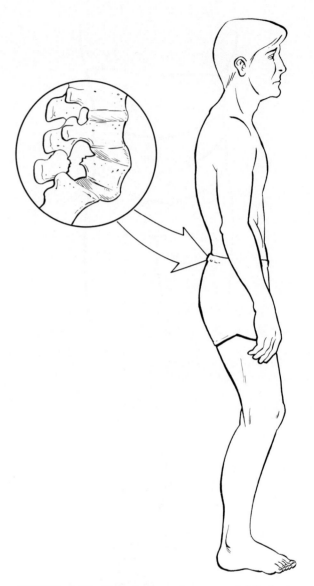

FIGURE 3–17. Altered posture due to spondylolisthesis.

Spinal rhythm refers to the smooth reversal of the normal lumbar lordosis as the patient flexes forward; that is, under normal circumstances the lumbar curve flattens as the pelvis rotates. Abnormalities in this spinal rhythm often indicate lumbar spine instability or mechanical pain (Fig. 3-21).

(text continues on page 63)

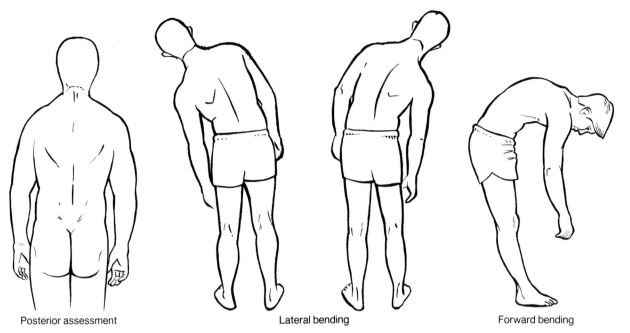

Posterior assessment   Lateral bending   Forward bending

FIGURE 3–18. Evaluation of the lumbar spine.

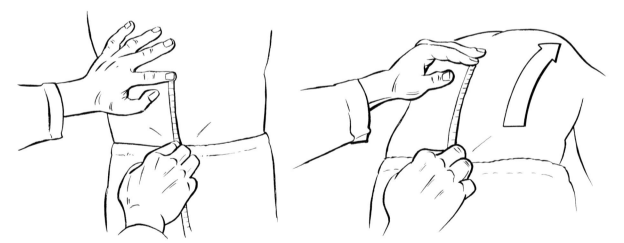

FIGURE 3–19. Schober test.

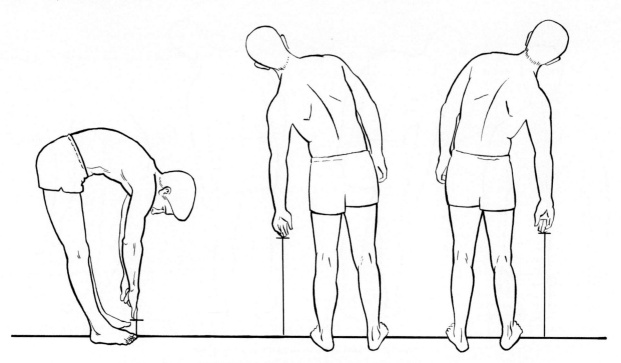

FIGURE 3–20. Measuring range of motion.

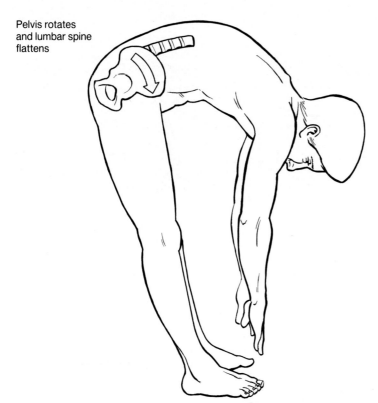

Pelvis rotates
and lumbar spine
flattens

FIGURE 3–21. Spinal rhythm.

Palpation

Palpation begins in the midline, with the examiner feeling each spinous process. A step deformity is detected if there is an underlying spondylolisthesis. Occasionally, palpation of a spinous process may elicit pain at the level of underlying symptomatic degenerative disease. The examiner should then palpate 1 or 2 cm on either side of the midline to ascertain whether there is any response to probing of the facet joints. The paravertebral muscles should be felt for spasm and point tenderness. All these structures should be palpated again while the patient is flexing and extending.

Motor Examination

The muscles of the lower extremity have either dual or triple nerve root innervation. Thus, a thorough examination is necessary to ascertain the level of a nerve root lesion. Table 3-5 lists the important muscles and their nerve root innervation. This table presents the usual situation, but the predominant motor supply may vary from person to person.

Many of the muscles of the lower extremity are more powerful than the examiner's upper body strength. This makes them difficult to examine and makes subtle weakness hard to detect. This is why it is useful to use the patient's body weight

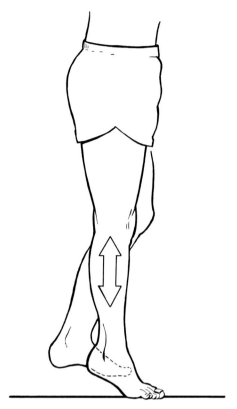

FIGURE 3–22. Determining strength of gastrocnemius and soleus muscles.

to detect motor deficits. For example, the gastrocnemius and soleus muscle group may be examined by having the patient go up and down on the toes during one-legged stance ten times per side (Fig. 3-22). The tibialis anterior may be evaluated by having the patient walk on his or her heels.

Small differences in the strength of the gluteus maximus on either side may be detected by a *delayed Trendelenburg test*. The patient is viewed from behind and the examiner places a thumb on both posterior-superior iliac spines. The patient is asked to stand on one leg for 30 seconds. If the pelvis on the unsupported side falls, it may indicate weakness of the hip abductors (Fig. 3-23).

It is occasionally difficult to distinguish between giving way and true weakness. Whenever possible, the examiner should assess the right and the left muscle groups simultaneously. This makes it difficult for a patient to consciously give way unilaterally.

TABLE 3–5. **Important Muscles and Their Nerve Root Innervation**

Muscle	Nerve Root Innervation*
Iliopsoas	L1, L2, L3
Adductors	L2, L3, L4
Quadriceps	L2, L3, L4
Tibialis anterior	L4, L5
Extensor hallucis longus	L5, S1
Hamstrings	L4, L5, S1, S2
Peroneus longus	L5, S1
Gluteus maximus	L5, S1, S2
Gastrocnemius–soleus	S1, S2

* Predominant innervation is underlined.

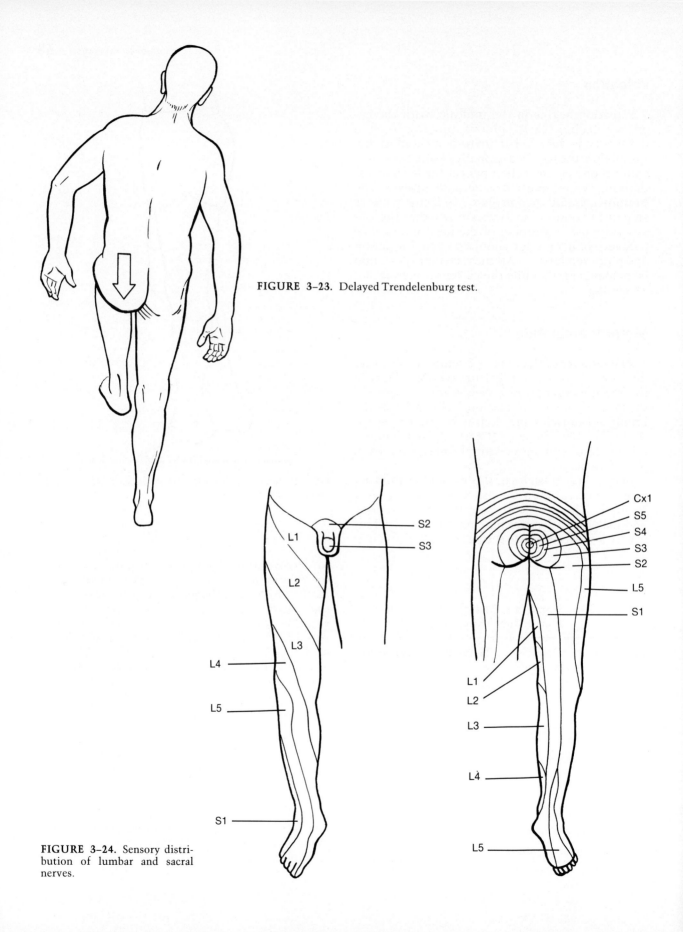

FIGURE 3–23. Delayed Trendelenburg test.

FIGURE 3–24. Sensory distribution of lumbar and sacral nerves.

Sensory Examination

The sensory dermatomes of the lower extremity are detailed in Figure 3-24. Assessment of sacral sensory integrity requires examination of the perianal area. Although dermatomal distribution may vary from patient to patient, there are fairly constant autonomous sensory zones that should be examined (Fig. 3-25).

Reflexes

There are both superficial and deep tendon reflexes mediated by the lumbosacral nerve roots. The *superficial cremasteric reflex* is the contraction of the cremaster muscle in response to stroking the medial upper thigh (Fig. 3-26). In males this results in elevation of the testicle on the ipsilateral side. The cremasteric reflex depends on the integrity of the L1 and L2 lumbar nerves. The *superficial anal reflex* is the contraction of the external and anal sphincters in response to stroking or scratching the skin in the perianal region. This reflex is mediated through the S2, S3, and S4 roots.

The deep tendon reflexes most easily elicited in the lower extremity are the quadriceps reflex or knee jerk, and the Achilles reflex or ankle jerk (Fig. 3-27 and Table 3-6). In thin patients, however, other muscle tendons are easily identified and can be used in the neurologic examination.

Although the deep tendon reflexes are a simple reflex arc, there is modulation from cortical centers via long tracts. These reflexes can be facilitated by reinforcement such as the *Jendrassik maneuver* (Fig. 3-28). The patient is asked to pull on his or her interlocked fingers while the examiner simultaneously tests a deep tendon reflex. Other reinforcement maneuvers include clench-

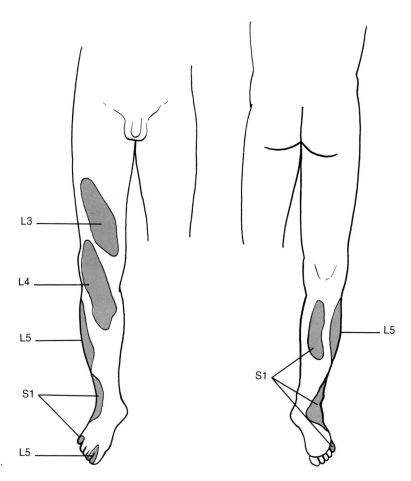

FIGURE 3–25. Autonomous sensory zones.

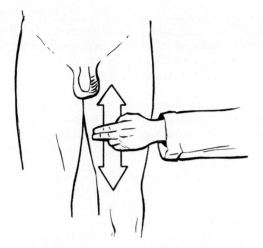

FIGURE 3–26. Superficial cremasteric reflex.

ing the fists or pulling up on the stretcher. These may be useful when reflexes are difficult to elicit, as in the elderly, diabetic, or hypothyroid patient.

Tests of Nerve Root Tension

The most common cause of sciatica, or irritation of a nerve root making up the sciatic nerve, is a disc protrusion. The tests of nerve root ten-sion elicit pain in the distribution of the affected nerve root by causing it to be drawn over the disc herniation. The classic test of nerve root tension is the *straight leg raising* examination described by Forst (Fig. 3-29). With the patient supine, the examiner gently raises the leg, placing one hand on the knee to keep it extended. This motion causes excursion of the lower lumbar and sacral nerve roots. For this test to be classified as posi-tive, it must reproduce radicular symptoms; that is, there must be pain, dysesthesia, or paresthesia down the leg in the distribution of the lower lum-bar or sacral nerve roots. Production of back pain or discomfort in the thigh due to hamstring tight-ness is not an indication of nerve root tension. A modification of this test described by Fajersztajn is often called the *foot dorsiflexion test* (Fig. 3-30). Straight leg raising is done until pain is produced. Gentle dorsiflexion of the foot is then done to ascertain whether symptoms are increased.

The *bowstring sign,* another test of nerve root tension, depends on the irritability of the nerve throughout its entire length when compressed at the level of the spinal canal (Fig. 3-31). Straight leg raising is done until symptoms are elicited. The leg is then lowered 10° and the examiner pal-pates the popliteal nerve behind the knee. This causes symptoms down the leg if there is marked compression of the L4, L5, or S1 nerve root.

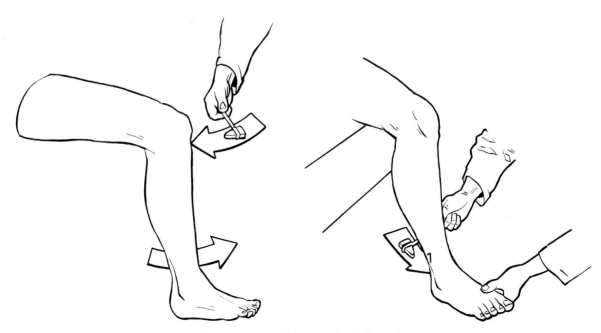

FIGURE 3–27. Quadriceps and Achilles reflexes.

TABLE 3–6. **Deep Tendon Reflexes**
of the Lower Extremity

Reflex	Nerve Root Innervation*
Adductor	<u>L2</u>, <u>L3</u>, L4
Quadriceps	L2, <u>L3</u>, <u>L4</u>
Hamstring	L4, <u>L5</u>, <u>S1</u>, S2
Achilles	<u>S1</u>, S2

* Predominant innervation is underlined.

Lasègue's sign is another test for nerve root tension (Fig. 3-32). With the patient supine, the hip and knee are gently flexed to 90°. The leg is then gradually extended while the patient is asked about reproduction of sciatica symptoms.

Cadaveric dissections have demonstrated small excursions of the lower lumbar and sacral nerve roots with movement of the contralateral lower extremity. This forms the basis of the *well-leg raising test* (Fig. 3-33). In a patient with sciatica, straight leg raising is done on the asymptomatic extremity to see if there is reproduction of pain down the affected leg. When positive, it suggests marked compression of the nerve root. It is a very specific sign for nerve compression due to a herniated nucleus pulposus, possibly by a sequestered disc.

Straight leg raising, even to 90°, does not cause movement in the upper lumbar nerve roots. These nerve roots send branches to make up the femoral nerve. The *femoral stretch test* is done with the patient prone (Fig. 3-34). The knee is gradually flexed and then the hip extended. This causes the greatest excursion in the L2, L3, and L4 nerve roots.

The *cross-over test* is an important determinant of compression of the lumbosacral roots in the midline (Fig. 3-35). The test is done by gently raising the affected leg and seeing if this produces symptoms down the asymptomatic contralateral extremity. When positive, it usually indicates a large central disc protrusion. It should not be confused with the well-leg raising test, in which lifting the unaffected leg causes symptoms down the affected extremity.

Rectal Examination

The rectal examination is a necessary part of the lumbosacral spine assessment. As the exam-

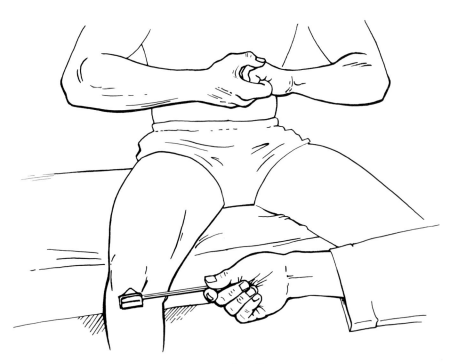

FIGURE 3–28. Jendrassik maneuver.

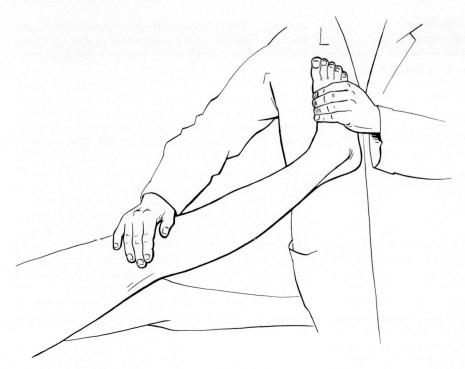

FIGURE 3–29. Straight leg raising.

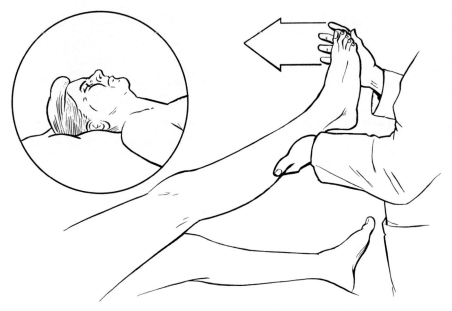

FIGURE 3–30. Foot dorsiflexion test.

iner's digit is inserted into the anus, the patient is asked about his or her sensory appreciation of the perianal area. An assessment of rectal tone is made by assessing the pressure exerted by the anal sphincter on the examining digit. Assessment of the integrity of the sacral roots is made by asking the patient to bear down, as in a Valsalva maneuver. The examiner can assess the degree to which the sphincter contracts. The anterior aspect of the sacrum and coccyx can be palpated by the examining finger. In many instances, sacral tumors will go undetected unless a rectal examination is done. Pain produced by the sacrococcygeal articulation can be elicited by pushing backward on the tip of the coccyx.

SACROILIAC JOINTS

Palpation

There are two ways in which the sacroiliac joints can be located. In thin patients, there are

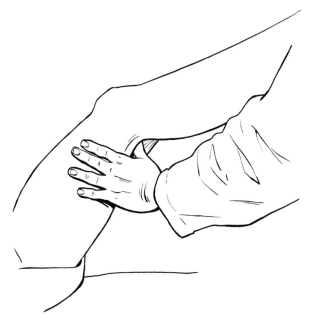

FIGURE 3–31. Bowstring sign.

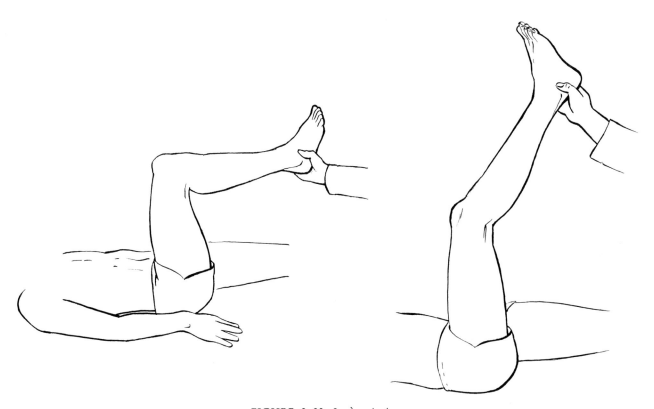

FIGURE 3–32. Lasègue's sign.

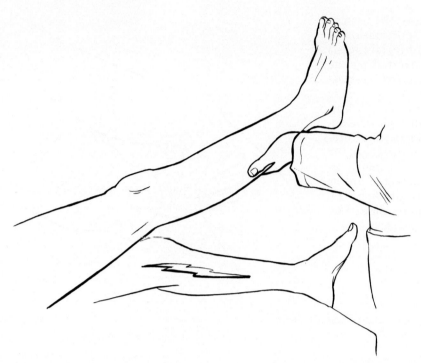

FIGURE 3–33. Well-leg raising test.

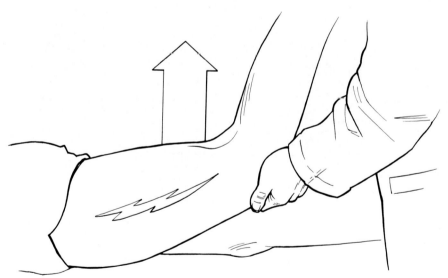

FIGURE 3–34. Femoral stretch test.

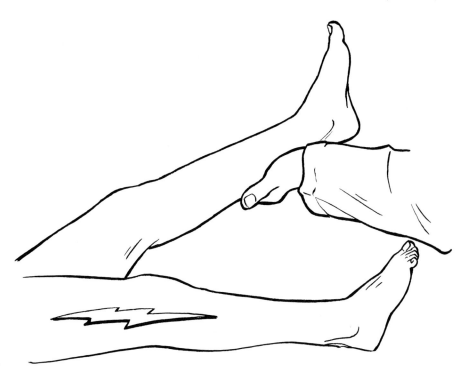

FIGURE 3–35. Crossover test.

dimples in the skin overlying the top of the joint. If these are not present, then the uppermost part of the joints should be palpated 1 cm medial to the posterior-superior iliac spine. Each joint should be palpated with the patient prone and with the patient standing. Recent studies have shown that there is motion in the sacroiliac joint of about 1 to 2 cm. Some of this motion can be brought out by flexion of the hip; therefore, the joint should be palpated while the patient either bends forward or maximally flexes the hip.

Range of Motion

Part of the normal sacroiliac joint motion involves rotation in the sagittal plane. *Gillet's maneuver* assesses this movement (Fig. 3-36). The examiner stands behind the patient and places one thumb on the posterior-superior iliac spine and the other on the sacral midline at the same level. The patient is asked to lift the leg and maximally flex the hip. This should result in a downward movement of the posterior-superior iliac spine, with an increased distance between the examiner's thumbs. Decreased or absent motion may result from inflammatory sacroiliitis, as occurs with ankylosing spondylitis; degenerative

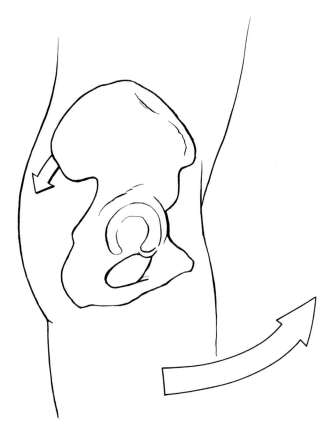

FIGURE 3–36. Sacroiliac joint motion.

joint disease, as may occur with age; or various other metabolic conditions.

Stress Test

The sacroiliac joints can be stressed in two ways. With the patient supine, the examiner places one hand around each iliac crest. Gentle force is then applied medially, tending to distract the sacroiliac joint on either side (Fig. 3-37). Stress can also be applied with the patient prone, pushing inferiorly on the posterior iliac crest and causing shear across the ipsilateral joint.

Fabere Test

The sacroiliac joint may be stressed by placing the hip in a position of flexion, abduction, and external rotation (Fig. 3-38). The test is done with the patient supine. The examiner gently places one of the patient's ankles on the opposite knee. Stress is then achieved by placing one hand on the flexed knee and the other on the contralateral iliac crest. The examiner can stress the sacroiliac joint on the side of the extended extremity by pushing down with both hands. The *Fabere test*, also referred to as Patrick's test, is an acronym for *f*lexion, *ab*duction, and *e*xternal rotation. It is of value only when the hip joints are normal.

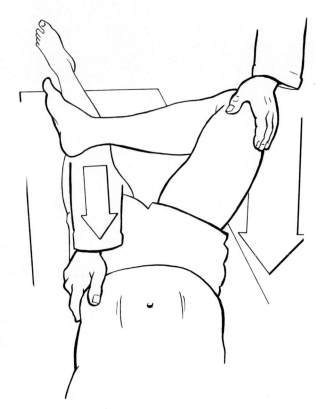

FIGURE 3–38. Fabere test.

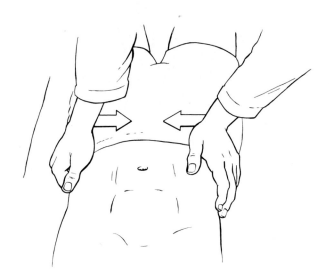

FIGURE 3–37. Stress test of the sacroiliac joints.

Gaenslen's Test

Gaenslen's test stresses the sacroiliac joint by extending the hip on one side while the other is maximally flexed (Fig. 3-39). This test, therefore, can be done with the patient either on his or her side or supine on the side of the examining table. As with Patrick's test, when this test causes pain (a positive response) the pain may be due to the sacroiliac joint or the hip joint.

MYELOPATHY

Various conditions may cause spinal cord compression. This may result in myelopathy or upper motor neuron-type neurologic dysfunction below the affected level. There may be accompanying root compression, giving signs of radiculopathy at the affected level. When neurologic examination reveals both upper and lower motor neuron findings, a disorder of the spinal cord or column should be suspected. Offending conditions include cervical spondylosis, cervical or thoracic disc herniation, meningeal tumors, cervical spine instability, or amyotrophic lateral sclerosis.

Spasticity

Spasticity is an increase in muscle tone. In the lower extremities, this may be manifest by a peculiar gait: the patient walks with the joints of the lower limb in extension and adduction. On physical examination the deep tendon reflexes can be found to be increased, sometimes to the point of *clonus*. The latter is repetitive muscle contraction produced by stretching (Fig. 3-40). This is most easily tested at the ankle. With the patient supine, the examiner places one hand under the knee, holding it in slight flexion, and the other hand under the foot. The examiner dorsiflexes the foot rapidly; when clonus is present, the foot beats up and down repeatedly. Clonus may also be elicited at the knee by rapidly pushing the patella down and detecting rhythmic contractions in the quadriceps muscle.

Plantar Response

The *plantar response* is a primitive reflex that under normal circumstances disappears as the nervous system matures. The presence of a plantar response in an adult is pathologic and can be caused by cord compression or intracranial pyramidal tract disease. The components of the plantar response include dorsiflexion of the great toe, abduction of the toes, dorsiflexion of the ankle, and flexion of the knee and hip. The plantar response may be elicited in various ways, the most popular of which is known as *Babinski's test* (Fig. 3-41). The examiner strokes the sole of the foot along its lateral border and medially along the bases of the toes. Normally, this produces plantar flexion of the toes. When positive, any or all of the plantar response is elicited. The plantar response may also be stimulated by *Chaddock's test*, in which the lateral side of the foot is scratched with a sharp point (Fig. 3-42). It may also be elicited with *Oppenheim's test*, in which

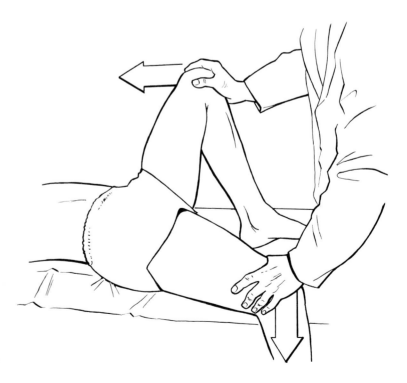

FIGURE 3–39. Gaenslen's test.

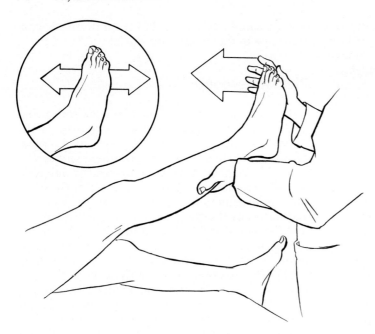

FIGURE 3–40. Ankle clonus.

the thumb and index finger are run distally along the pretibial eminence (Fig. 3-43).

Myelopathic Hand

There are two characteristic hand findings associated with cervical spinal cord damage. The *finger escape sign* is a loss of power in adduction and extension of the fourth and fifth digits (Fig. 3-44). The examiner asks the patient to extend the wrist and hold the hand with the palm facing forward. When positive, the little finger tends to drift away from the rest of the hand and cannot be held in adduction. The *grip and release test* depends on the patient's ability to carry out skilled, fine, rapid motion. The patient is asked to open and close the hand as quickly as possible while the examiner counts the number of complete cycles achieved in 10 seconds. Normally the hand can be opened and closed more than 20 times. Both the finger escape sign and the grip and release test are specific for cervical myelopathy. *Hoffmann's sign* may be positive in both cervical cord compression and intracranial central nervous system disorders. Hoffmann's sign is elicited by holding the patient's middle digit under the middle phalanx and flexing the distal interphalangeal joint (Fig. 3-45). When positive, the patient's thumb will flex and adduct.

TRAUMA

Inspection

Inspection is particularly important in the evaluation of the injured patient. Often the patient's level of consciousness is altered and he or she cannot help the examiner localize the area of injury. Careful inspection, however, can help; particular attention is paid to areas of deformity, kyphosis, bruising, or swelling.

Palpation

When evaluating the injured patient, assessment of range of motion is avoided to prevent possible further displacement of fractures or dislocations with concomitant increased neural compression. Palpation is important: the examiner may detect torn tissues, particularly interspinal and supraspinal ligaments. Occasionally a gap is palpated between two spinous processes, indicating major distraction of the posterior elements. If a step deformity is identified, it may indicate an underlying dislocation. The entire spine should be methodically evaluated, and palpation should begin at the occiput and proceed distally to the sacrum. Both midline and paramedian areas should be palpated.

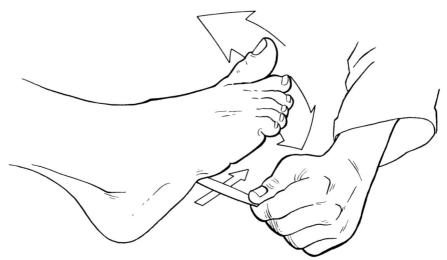

FIGURE 3–41. Positive Babinski's test.

Neurologic Evaluation

A meticulous neurologic examination is integral to the evaluation of the injured patient. Unless careful, methodical evaluation is repeated at regular intervals, the ability to make appropriate treatment decisions will be endangered.

There are a few particular syndromes associated with specific cord injuries. *Brown-Séquard syndrome* occurs when there is loss of pain and temperature sensation on one side of the body and loss of position, vibration, deep pain, light touch, and motor function on the opposite side.

This occurs because certain tracks are crossed and others are not. The syndrome results from injury to one side of the spinal cord.

If there has been trauma primarily to the posterior columns of the spinal cord, *posterior cord syndrome* exists. Clinically, this presents with sensory ataxia and some loss of pain sensation.

Anterior cord syndrome usually results from damage to the anterior spinal artery but can also occur by direct trauma to the anterior part of the spinal cord. There is usually marked weakness below the level of the injury, as well as significant loss of pain and temperature sensation. The sen-

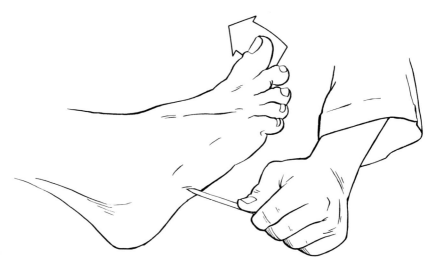

FIGURE 3–42. Chaddock's test.

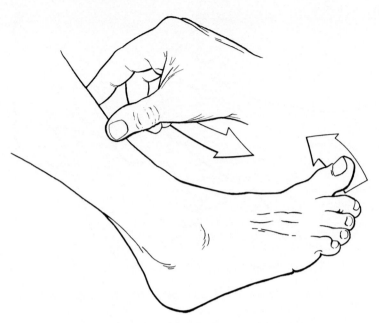

FIGURE 3-43. Oppenheim's test.

sations of position, vibration, and deep pressure are maintained, however, by means of the spared posterior columns.

Central cord syndrome occurs as a result of hematoma in the center of the cord and commonly follows hyperextension injuries to the cervical spine. There is marked weakness of the arms and weakness to a lesser degree of the legs. Bladder and sensory changes are variable.

When evaluating the injured patient, special attention must be paid to the sensory examination. Occasionally a patient presents with apparently complete loss of sensation below the level of a lesion. Closer examination, however, may reveal an area in the perianal region in which there is sparing of sensation. This sacral sparing indicates that the lesion is incomplete and offers a more favorable prognosis.

The *bulbocavernosus reflex* is used to assess whether a patient is suffering from spinal shock. In spinal shock, which can occur after major trauma, all spinal cord activity temporarily

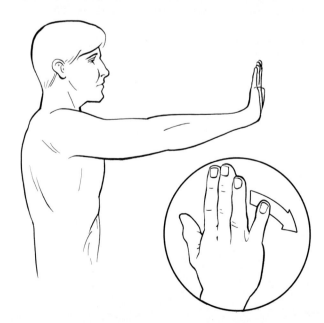

FIGURE 3-44. Finger escape sign.

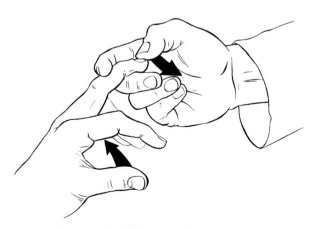

FIGURE 3-45. Positive Hoffmann's sign.

ceases. In humans, spinal shock is usually transient, lasting less than 24 hours. After major spinal trauma, a patient may be found to have complete loss of motor activity and sensation below the level of the injury. Under these circumstances, it may be difficult to determine whether the spinal cord has a complete lesion or whether the patient is suffering from spinal shock and has an incomplete lesion for which there is some potential of recovery. The bulbocavernosus reflex is a very simple cord-mediated reflex arc that is absent in the presence of spinal shock. The bulbocavernosus reflex is assessed by placing a finger in the patient's rectum. Pulling on the penis or on a urethral catheter in a female will result in contraction of the anal sphincter. When the bulbocavernosus reflex is present, spinal shock is not present. If, therefore, there is no motor or sensory activity below the level of a lesion and the bulbocavernosus reflex is present, the patient may be said to have a complete cord lesion, for which the prognosis is poor.

NONORGANIC EVALUATION

Socioeconomic factors have resulted in some patients exhibiting nonorganic signs; that is, they exhibit symptoms or demonstrate signs that have no anatomic basis. Although patients with significant physical pathology may exhibit some of these signs, multiple positive nonorganic tests may help identify patients who need further psychological assessment.

Tests for nerve root tension have already been discussed. It is worthwhile to evaluate straight leg raising with the patient seated. Being able to lift a patient's leg 90° in the seated position without eliciting pain, but having marked pain with gross limitation of straight leg raising while supine suggests nonorganic pathology. Furthermore, if straight leg raising in the supine position causes pain down the leg, it is worthwhile to flex the knee and hip. This maneuver will decrease tension on the nerve root and should relieve the discomfort. If pain is increased, it again indicates nonorganic pathology or functional overlay. The *reverse sciatic tension test* is performed by plantar-flexing rather than dorsiflexing the foot. It is positive if leg pain is elicited and is helpful in the detection of a malingerer—if plantar flexion of the foot causes leg pain, the patient may be a malingerer.

It is occasionally difficult to distinguish giving way and true muscular weakness. Muscle groups on either side of the body should be tested simultaneously. A patient complaining of weakness in one leg often cannot selectively give way unilaterally with simultaneous bilateral evaluation. *Hoover's test* similarly assesses patient compliance (Fig. 3-46). If a patient tries to lift the leg off the stretcher while supine, there is a reflex downward pressure with the opposite leg. For Hoover's test, the examiner places one hand under each of the patient's legs. The patient is instructed to lift a leg, and the examiner should feel downward pressure in the opposite extremity. If none is present, the extent to which the patient is

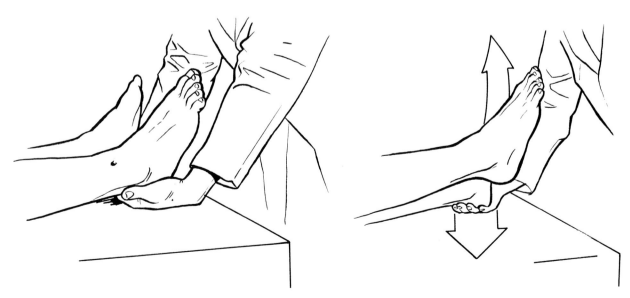

FIGURE 3-46. Hoover's test.

truly trying to raise the leg should be questioned.

Several other nonorganic physical signs have been described. Their presence must be evaluated in the context of the rest of the full patient evaluation. It has often been said, but bears repeating, that even patients with known mental illness can get physically ill, and the examiner must remember this. The presence of one or a few nonorganic physical signs does not, in and of itself, exclude major organic pathology with superimposed psychological disturbance.

KEY POINTS

1. A well-taken history is crucial to the accurate diagnosis of most spinal conditions.
2. The physical examination should be undertaken in a methodical manner. It includes an assessment not only of the spine but also of the rest of the musculoskeletal and nervous systems and may also include examination of other organ systems.
3. Although it is important to document any positive nonorganic signs, their presence does not exclude significant organic pathology.

BIBLIOGRAPHY

BOOKS

Hoppenfeld S. Orthopaedic neurology. A diagnostic guide to neurologic levels. Philadelphia: JB Lippincott, 1977.

Hoppenfeld S. Physical examination of the spine and extremities. Norwalk, CT: Appleton-Century-Crofts, 1976.

Magee DG. Orthopaedic physical examination. 2nd ed. Philadelphia: WB Saunders, 1992.

JOURNALS

Chan CW, Goldman S, Ilstrup DM, Kunselman AR, O'Neill PI. The pain drawing and Waddell's non-organic physical signs in chronic low-back pains. Spine 1993;18:1717–1722.

Gill K, Krag MH, Johnson GB, Haugh LD, Pope MH. Repeatability of four clinical methods for assessment of lumbar spinal motion. Spine 1988;13:50–53.

McCombe PF, Fairbank JC, Cockersole BC, Pynsent PB. Reproducibility of physical signs in low back pain. Spine 1989;14:908–918.

Nitta H, Tajima T, Sugiyama H, Moriyama A. Study on dermatomes by means of selective lumbar spinal nerve block. Spine 1993;18:1782–1786.

Russel AS, Maksymowych W, LeClercq S. Clinical examination of the sacroiliac joints: A prospective study. Arthritis Rheum 1981;24:1575–1577.

Smith SA, Massie JB, Chestnut R, Garfin SR. Straight leg raising: Anatomical effects on the spinal nerve root without and with fusion. Spine 1993;18:992–999.

Supik LF, Broom MJ. Sciatic tension signs and lumbar disc herniation. Spine 1994;19:1066–1069.

Thelander U, Fagerlund M, Friberg S, Larsson S. Straight leg raising test versus radiologic size, shape and position of lumbar disc hernias. Spine 1992;17:395–399.

Textbook of Spinal Disorders, by Stephen I. Esses.
J. B. Lippincott Company, Philadelphia © 1995.

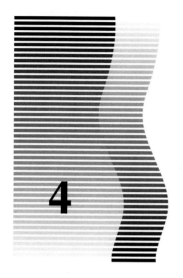

4 Spinal Imaging

RADIOGRAPHS
 Cervical Spine
 Thoracic Spine
 Lumbosacral Spine
 Special Views
TOMOGRAPHS
COMPUTED
 TOMOGRAPHY
 Cervical Spine
 Thoracic Spine
 Lumbosacral Spine

MAGNETIC
 RESONANCE
 IMAGING
 Cervical Spine
 Thoracic Spine
 Lumbar Spine
MYELOGRAPHY
RADIONUCLIDE
 SCANNING
 Technetium 99
 Gallium 67
 Indium

RADIOGRAPHS

Since the introduction of x-rays as an imaging modality, they have become the most widely used diagnostic procedure in the evaluation of spinal patients. X-rays are simply a specific type of electromagnetic radiation that has a short wavelength. The quantity of radiation from an x-ray source is measured in *roentgens* (R) after the German physicist who discovered x-rays. The amount of ionizing radiation that is absorbed is measured in *rads*. The roentgen-equivalent man (rem) is the absorbed dose, measured in rads, multiplied by a factor representing the biologic effects of that form of radiation. The factor for x-rays is one; thus, one R of radiation exposure results in one rad of absorbed dose and is equal to one rem.

Radiation exposure can have deleterious effects on living tissues. This effect is dose-related and cumulative over time. Because some tissues, such as breast, thyroid, and gonadal, are particularly sensitive to radiation, various methods have been used to reduce the radiation dose for diagnostic radiographs. With modern techniques, it is possible to decrease patient dosage significantly and effectively eliminate potential ill effects.

79

Plain radiographs are extremely important in the assessment of deformity and after trauma. There is considerable controversy about the value of plain radiographs in the investigation of low back and neck pain for two reasons: first, the incidence of radiographic abnormality is no different in patients with back pain than in those without, and second, plain radiographs rarely give critical information that influences patient treatment.

This dilemma can be resolved by considering the particular clinical scenario. Radiographs are useful in detecting tumors, infections, inflammatory diseases, fractures, and other potentially treatable entities. Thus, x-rays, when used judiciously, may be of great benefit in the assessment of the spinal patient. In cases of acute back pain of less than 1 month's duration under any of the following circumstances, radiographs are absolutely indicated: patients older than age 50, history of cancer or rest pain, history of serious trauma, unexplained weight loss, drug or alcohol abuse, treatment with steroids, fever, or neurologic deficits.

Cervical Spine

The routine radiographic views of the cervical spine are the *anteroposterior* (AP), *lateral*, *oblique*, and *through-mouth*. As can be seen in Figure 4-1, the AP x-ray clearly shows the vertebral bodies, uncovertebral joints, spinous processes, laminae, and transverse processes. In assessing the AP x-ray, the clinician should check to make sure all the spinous processes line up. Displacement from the midline of a single spinous process can indicate underlying trauma. Similarly, the distance between adjacent spinous processes should be equal. An increase in a single interspinous interval warrants further investigation.

Figure 4-2 shows the lateral radiograph of a normal cervical spine. This may be the most important film in assessing cervical trauma. Initially, one should count the cervical vertebrae that can be clearly seen on the x-ray to ensure that the C7–T1 level is included; if it is not, other x-rays should be taken. Occasionally other views, such as a swimmer's view, are necessary (see discussion later in this section).

An organized approach to looking at this x-ray begins with an examination of the prevertebral soft tissues. At the C2 level, the distance from the anterior-inferior vertebral body to the retropharynx should not exceed 7 mm. Similarly, at the inferior level of the C6 vertebral body, this interval should not exceed 22 mm. In children, the latter measurement should not exceed 14 mm. The importance of these measurements is that increases in these distances can result from bleeding and hematoma, and thus they can indicate subtle bony or soft tissue injury. The value of these measurements is reduced in children, because with crying and other Valsalva maneuvers, the distance can be temporarily increased.

After examining the soft tissues, it is worthwhile assessing vertebral body alignment. The cervical spine is normally held in lordosis. Acute muscle spasm can eliminate this. Under normal circumstances, there should be no more than 3 mm of subluxation between adjacent vertebral bodies. Alignment should be assessed, both of the anterior vertebral body borders and posterior vertebral body borders. In children, some degree of subluxation, particularly at the C2–C3 level, may be normal. This *pseudosubluxation* is due to the more horizontal orientation of the facet joint surfaces and ligamentous laxity.

Intervertebral disc spaces should be assessed for height. The C7–T1 disc is somewhat narrower than the other cervical levels. The facet joints should be carefully scrutinized on the lateral image. The anterior arch of the atlas should be examined, particularly with reference to its relation to the odontoid. The normal distance between these two structures is 3 mm in adults and 4.5 mm in children. The relation of the foramen magnum and occipital condyles to the upper cervical spine should be noted. A line drawn along the lamina of C1 should intersect the posterior foramen magnum. A line drawn up from the posterior surface of the body of the axis and dens should meet the clivus. A line drawn from the posterior margin of the hard palate to the posterior aspect of the foramen magnum should lie just below the tip of the odontoid; this is known as *Chamberlain's line* and is discussed further in the section on basilar invagination (see Chap. 13).

Oblique x-rays are used specifically to assess the neural foramina and their bony boundaries. The x-rays are taken with the x-ray beam angled 45° from the midline. With the patient's head turned to the left, the right facet joints and intervertebral foramina are seen. Conversely, when the patient's head is turned to the right, the left laminae, facet joints, and intervertebral foramina are seen (Fig. 4-3).

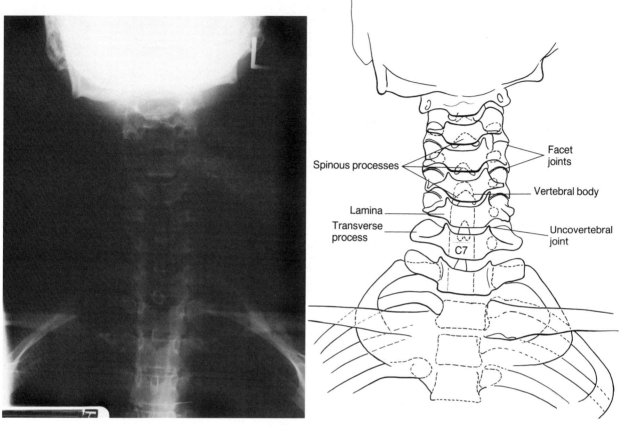

FIGURE 4–1. (*Left*) AP x-ray of the cervical spine. (*Right*) Drawing of the same view.

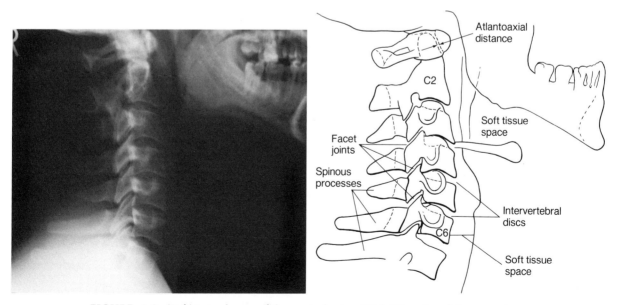

FIGURE 4–2. (*Left*) Lateral x-ray of the cervical spine. (*Right*) Drawing of the same view.

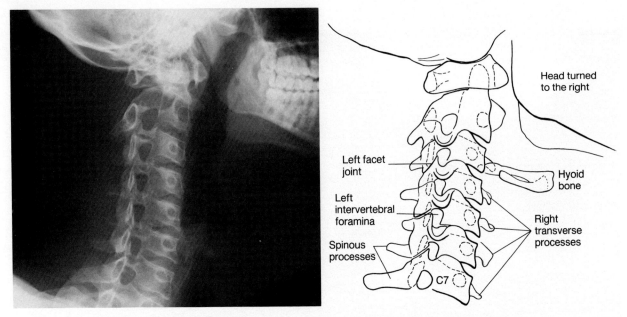

FIGURE 4–3. (*Left*) Oblique x-ray of the cervical spine. (*Right*) Drawing of the same view.

The AP x-ray does not provide an adequate image of the C1-C2 structures, so an open-mouth x-ray is taken. This x-ray provides a clear image of the odontoid process, the lateral masses of the atlas, and the atlantoaxial joints. The lateral masses of the atlas should line up perfectly with the body of C2. In addition, the distance from the odontoid to either lateral mass should be symmetric (Fig. 4-4).

Often, the lateral x-ray does not adequately show the lower cervical vertebrae or the cervico-thoracic junction. For this reason, a swimmer's

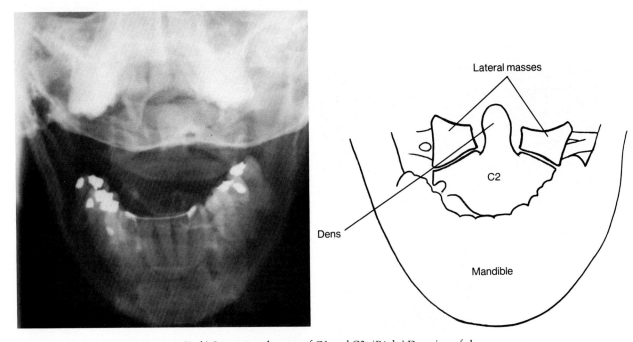

FIGURE 4–4. (*Left*) Open-mouth x-ray of C1 and C2. (*Right*) Drawing of the same area.

view is occasionally taken (Fig. 4-5). This is obtained by having the patient hold one arm above the head and angling the x-ray beam slightly cranially. Another technique that may be used to show the cervicothoracic junction involves having the patient hold weights in either arm to depress the shoulders or to have the patient's arm pulled distally while lying supine.

Pillar views can be useful in delineating abnormalities of the lateral masses or posterior arches. They are obtained by angling the x-ray beam 25° caudally and 45° to either side of midline. These are excellent views for imaging the lateral masses and laminae (Fig. 4-6).

Thoracic Spine

The routine views for assessing the thoracic spine are the AP and lateral. Figure 4-7 demonstrates the structures easily identified on the AP x-ray—the vertebral bodies, spinous processes, pedicles, ribs, transverse processes, costotransverse articulations, laminae, and intervertebral disc spaces. An organized approach to assessing this x-ray is recommended. As with the cervical spine, one should begin by assessing the soft tissue shadows. An increase in soft tissue shadows often may indicate an underlying neoplastic or infective process. Examination of the

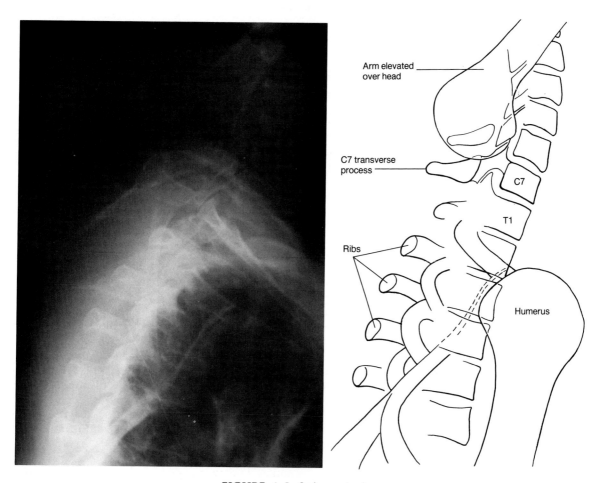

FIGURE 4–5. Swimmer's view.

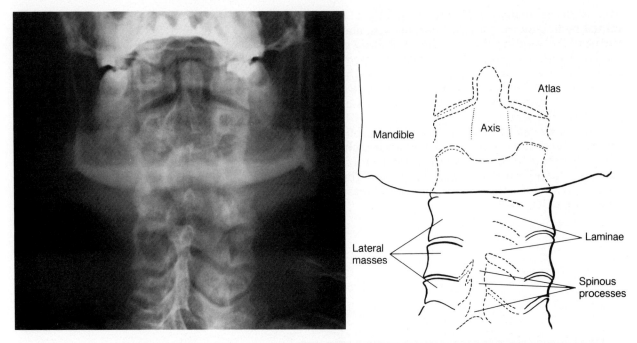

FIGURE 4–6. *(Left)* Pillar view of the cervical spine. *(Right)* Drawing of the same view.

bony column should begin by ensuring that the spinous processes are aligned. The two pedicles at each vertebral level should be identified; this is particularly important because metastatic disease often initially obscures a single pedicle. The interpedicular distance should be measured at each level. Normally, this distance increases slightly as one moves caudally. An abnormally large interpedicular distance at a single level usually indicates traumatic vertebral injury. The interspinous distance should also be assessed at each level. The configuration of each vertebral body should be examined because wedging may occur laterally.

The lateral x-ray of the thoracic spine is shown in Figure 4-8. After assessment of the soft tissues, one should ensure that the normal thoracic kyphosis exists. The vertebral bodies should be identified to rule out bony injury. The vertebral bodies are normally wedge-shaped, with a posterior vertebral body height 1 to 2 mm greater than the anterior vertebral body height. The intervertebral disc space height should be about equal at each level. The spinous processes and pedicles can be identified at each level, as well as the superior and inferior articular processes. The latter make up the facet joint, which should be assessed at each level. The intervertebral foramina should be examined for shape and size.

Lumbosacral Spine

The AP view of the lumbosacral spine should be examined using the same organized approach as for the other x-rays. The soft tissues should be assessed for symmetry. The shadow of the psoas muscle is usually well outlined on either side of the spinal column. Alignment of the bony column should be assessed, and one should ensure that the spinous processes are well aligned. The vertebral bodies should be examined for shape. The two pedicles at each level should be identified; as with the thoracic spine, obliteration of a single pedicle may indicate an underlying neoplasm. The intervertebral disc spaces should be assessed for height. Because the facet joints lie in the sagittal plane, both the superior and inferior articular processes are well delineated. Asymmetry, or *tropism*, of the facet joints should be noted. The spinous processes and the interspinous distance should be assessed. The sacrum, sacral ala, and sacroiliac joints should be identified. The superior articular processes of the sacrum can be seen as well as the first sacral foramina bilaterally (Fig. 4-9).

Figure 4-10 shows a lateral x-ray of the lumbar spine. The amount of lumbar lordosis should be *(text continues on page 87)*

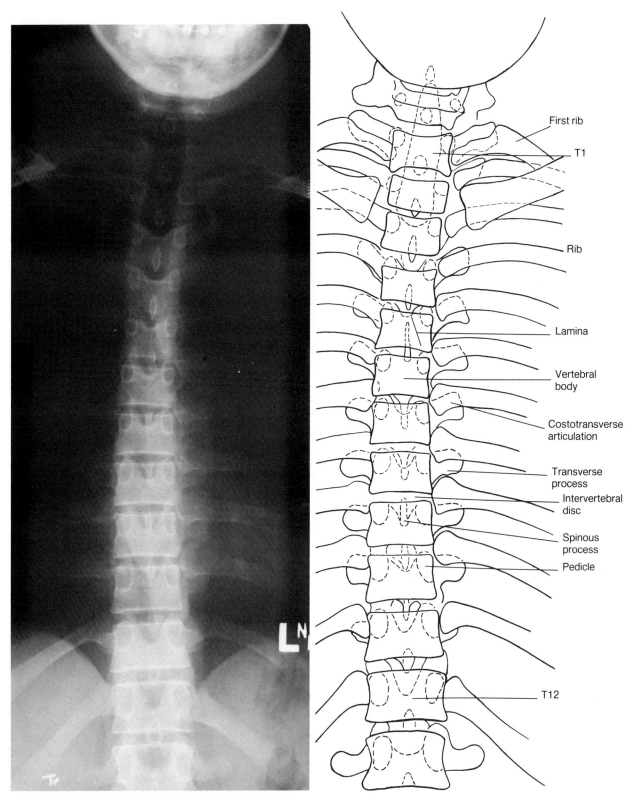

FIGURE 4–7. (*Left*) AP x-ray of the thoracic spine. (*Right*) Drawing of the same view.

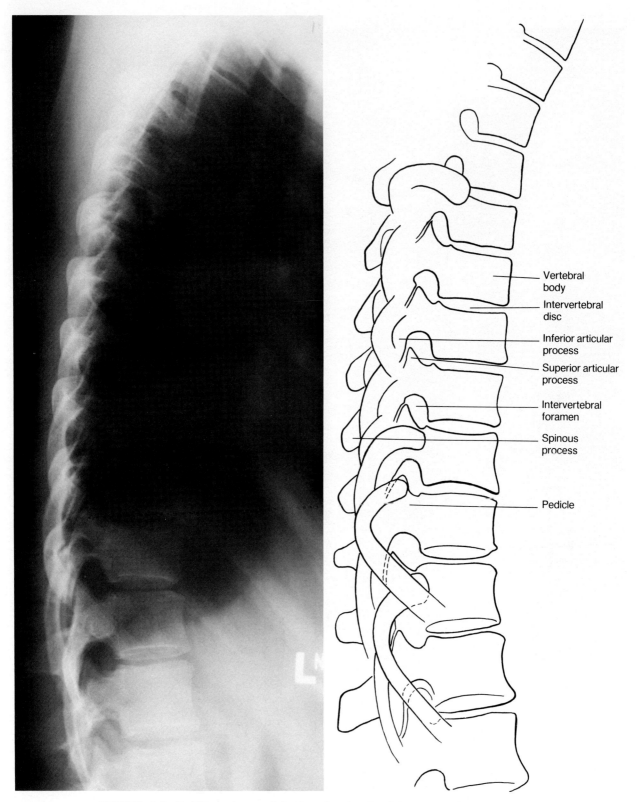

FIGURE 4–8. (*Left*) Lateral x-ray of the thoracic spine. (*Right*) Drawing of the same view.

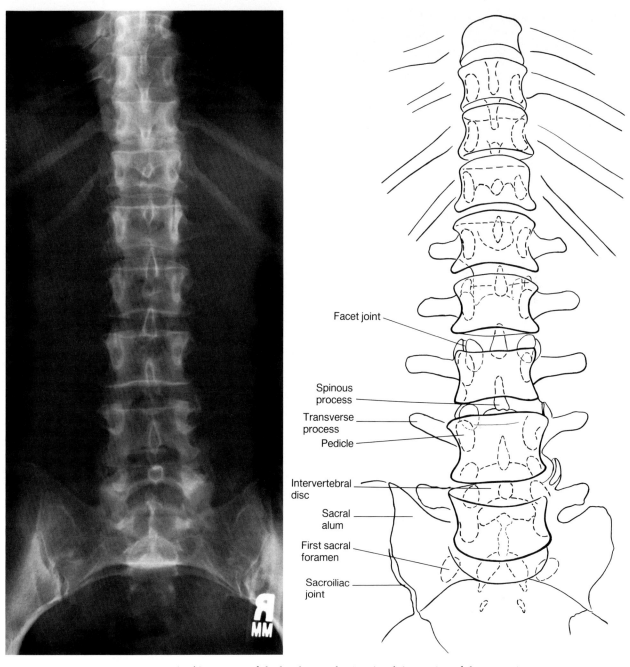

Facet joint

Spinous
process

Transverse
process

Pedicle

Intervertebral
disc

Sacral
alum

First sacral
foramen

Sacroiliac
joint

FIGURE 4–9. *(Left)* AP x-ray of the lumbosacral spine. *(Right)* Drawing of the same view.

assessed. The shape of the vertebral bodies and their alignment should be examined. Intervertebral disc space height should be noted. The pedicles, superior articular process, inferior articular process, and spinous process may be identified at each level. The sacrum, sacral promontory, and sacral canal are well seen.

The oblique x-rays of the lumbar spine are particularly useful in demonstrating the facet joints, pars interarticularis, and neural foramina (Fig. 4-11). They are taken with the x-ray tube angled 45° to the patient. With the patient turned to the right, it is possible to identify the right pedicle, right superior articular process, right pars inter-

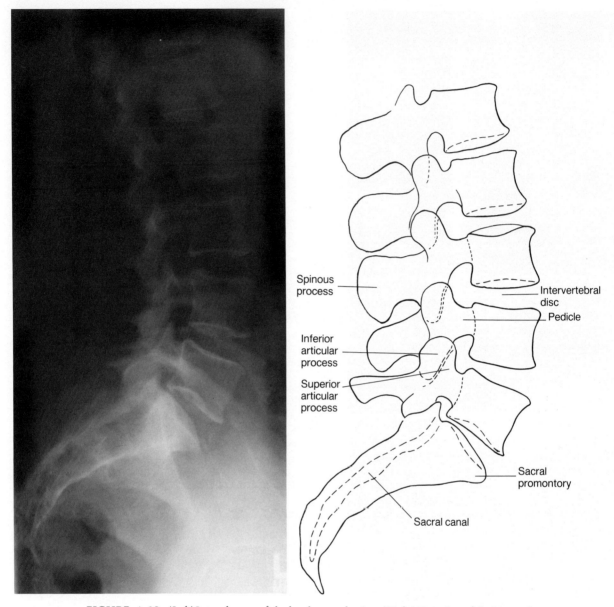

FIGURE 4–10. *(Left)* Lateral x-ray of the lumbosacral spine. *(Right)* Drawing of the same view.

articularis, right lamina, and right inferior articular process. These structures make up the so-called *"Scotty dog"* and are the head, ear, neck, body, and front foot, respectively. Each lumbar nerve root exits the spinal column under the pedicle; thus, assessment of the interpedicular distance on the oblique x-ray will give some indication as to the size of the neural foramen and room available for the exiting nerve root.

Spot x-rays, or *Hibbs' views*, of the lumbosacral articulations may be obtained to further delineate the structures in this area (Fig. 4-12).

Special Views

To assess overall body posture, the entire spinal column must be viewed on a single x-ray with the patient standing. This is usually done with the x-ray beam 36 inches (3 feet) from the patient. Both AP and lateral x-rays are taken. The former view is important in the assessment of scoliosis, the latter in the assessment of sagittal plane deformity.

Dynamic radiographs are used to show patterns of motion at various levels of the spine.

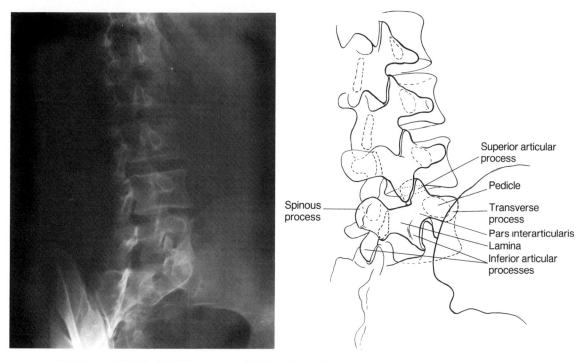

FIGURE 4–11. (*Left*) Oblique x-ray of the lumbosacral spine. (*Right*) Drawing of the same view.

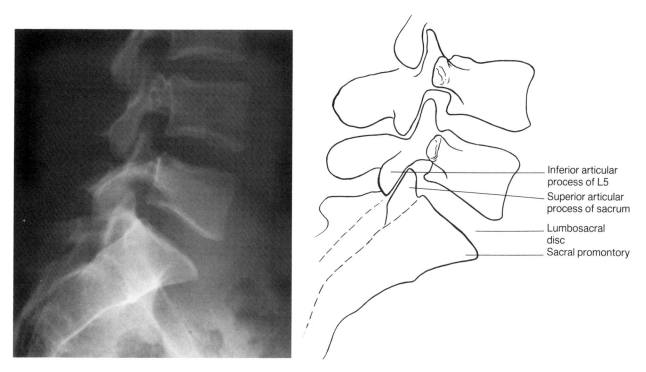

FIGURE 4–12. Hibbs' view of the lumbosacral spine.

Flexion and *extension* views are often used in both the cervical and lumbar regions. Under normal circumstances there is not more than 3 mm of motion between adjacent vertebrae. Other dynamic radiographic techniques include *traction films* and *stretch films*. The latter are particularly useful in the cervical spine. The patient is placed in a head halter and increasing increments of weight are used with sequential radiographs.

TOMOGRAPHS

A major disadvantage of plain radiographs is that all structures are superimposed on each other—that is, all structures in the frontal plane are superimposed on an AP x-ray, and all structures in the sagittal plane are superimposed on the lateral x-ray. It is impossible by looking at an AP x-ray to determine which structures are more anterior than others. Similarly, on the lateral x-ray, it is impossible to determine which struc-

tures are more medial or lateral to each other. The purpose of tomography is to x-ray specific planes and to eliminate the superimposition effect of plain radiographs. This is done by moving both the x-ray source and film in such a way that a specific plane remains clear and all structures outside that plane appear blurred. Although any plane can be chosen, the standard protocol is to take 1-cm cuts in either the AP or lateral view. On each tomogram film, there is a measurement indicating the distance of the plane in focus from the film. Lateral tomograms are normally taken with the left side down, AP tomograms with the patient supine. Thus, spatial relations can be evaluated.

With the advent of newer imaging modalities and new computer software, the indications for tomography are decreasing, although lateral tomograms of the cervical spine continue to be of great value in the assessment of the facet joints (Fig. 4-13). An example of an AP lumbar tomogram is shown in Figure 4-14.

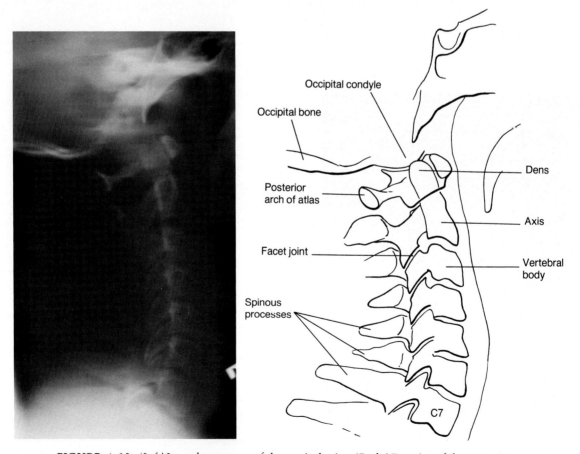

FIGURE 4–13. (*Left*) Lateral tomogram of the cervical spine. (*Right*) Drawing of the same view.

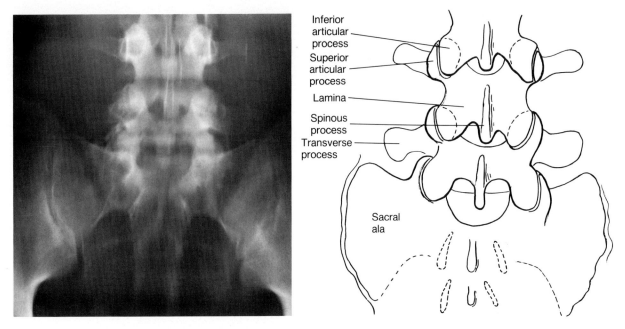

FIGURE 4–14. (*Left*) AP tomogram of the lumbar spine. (*Right*) Drawing of the same view.

COMPUTED TOMOGRAPHY

Computed tomography (CT) involves the production of a computer-generated image, usually in the transverse or axial plane. The image is produced by rotating an x-ray beam 360° around the subject. X-ray detectors determine the amount of x-ray transmission received. All the data from the detectors are processed by a computer to produce an image with a gray scale. The shade of gray is determined by the attenuation or density of the structure imaged. *Hounsfield units* are a quantification of the attenuation, with −1000 being defined as the attenuation for air, 0 for water, and +1000 for dense cortical bone. Figure 4-15 graphically represents the mechanism of CT scanning. Although the initial image is in the axial plane, computer software can produce an image in any desired plane; indeed, newer software allows for the generation of three-dimensional images that can be rotated as desired. A major disadvantage of CT scanning is the significant artifact produced by metal.

In general, CT scanning is used to provide additional detail and information about a specific level or lesion. For example, CT scanning is useful to further delineate a fracture recognized on plain radiographs. In addition, CT scanning is very helpful in looking at soft tissue structures, such as intervertebral discs, that are not seen on plain radiographs.

Cervical Spine

Figure 4-16 shows an axial CT image of the cervical spine at the level of an intervertebral disc. One can appreciate the spinal cord within the spinal canal. The uncovertebral joints and zygoapophyseal joints are seen.

Figure 4-17 is an axial CT of the cervical spine at the level of the vertebral body. The transverse process, foramen transversarium, spinal cord, and vertebral body are well shown.

As mentioned above, images can be generated in any plane. Figure 4-18 is a sagittal reformation of the cervical spine in the midline. The vertebral body, spinal cord, and spinous process are all well shown.

Thoracic Spine

CT scanning of the thoracic spine is particularly useful because overlying ribs and soft tissues make plain radiographs difficult to inter-
(*text continues on page 94*)

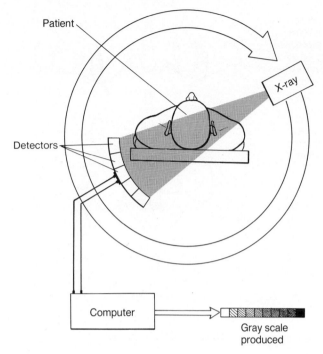

FIGURE 4–15. Mechanism of CT scanning.

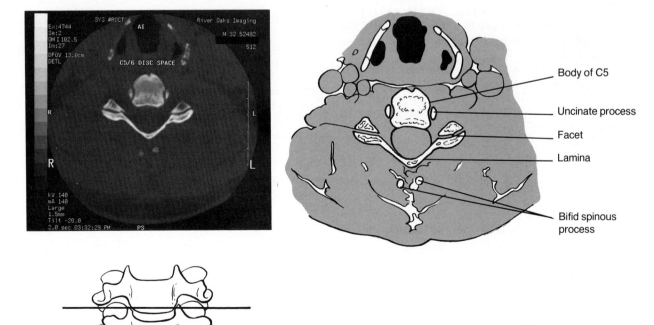

FIGURE 4–16. (*Left*) Axial CT of the cervical spine at the level of an intervertebral disc. (*Right*) Drawing of the same view.

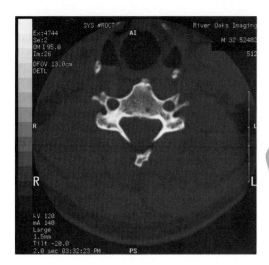

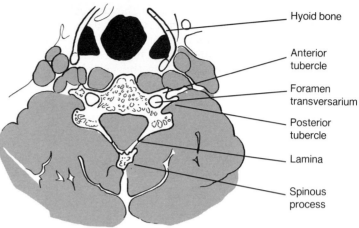

Hyoid bone

Anterior
tubercle

Foramen
transversarium

Posterior
tubercle

Lamina

Spinous
process

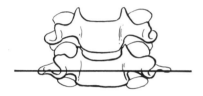

FIGURE 4–17. (*Left*) Axial CT of the cervical spine at the level of the vertebral body. (*Right*) Drawing of the same view.

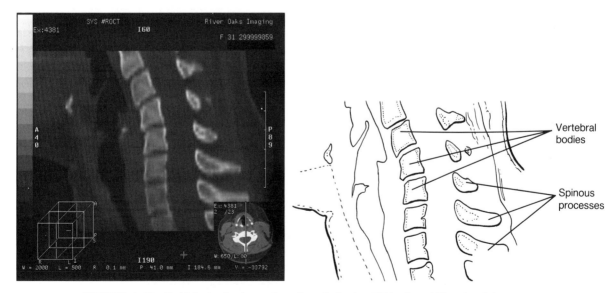

Vertebral
bodies

Spinous
processes

FIGURE 4–18. (*Left*) Sagittal reformation of cervical spine CT in the midline. (*Right*) Drawing of the same view.

pret. Figure 4-19 is an axial CT of the thoracic spine through the level of the intervertebral disc. One can appreciate the facet joints, spinal cord, and boundaries of the spinal canal. Figure 4-20 is an axial cut through the level of the vertebral body and pedicles. One can appreciate the transverse processes and their articulations with the ribs.

The sagittal reformation of the thoracic spine is very helpful in delineating any encroachment on the spinal cord. Figure 4-21 is a sagittal reformation at the level of the midline.

Lumbosacral Spine

Figure 4-22 is an axial CT at the level of a lumbar vertebral body. One can appreciate the facet joints, transverse processes, pedicles, and the boundaries of the spinal canal. The CT scan is very useful in delineating soft tissues, and the paravertebral musculature and psoas muscle are well seen. Figure 4-23 is an axial CT through the level of the upper sacrum. The promontory, ala, and sacroiliac joints can be delineated.

A sagittal reformation at the level of the neural foramina is shown in Figure 4-24. The boundaries of each nerve root foramen are well seen.

A potential problem of CT scanning is its ability to show pathology that may not have clinical relevance—that is, because it is very sensitive, the interpretation of films must be related to the patient's clinical presentation. Between 30% and 40% of young adult males with no history of back complaints will have some demonstrable abnormality on CT scan. In asymptomatic people over age 40, there is a 50% incidence of abnormal findings, including herniated disc, facet degeneration, and spinal stenosis.

(text continues on page 97)

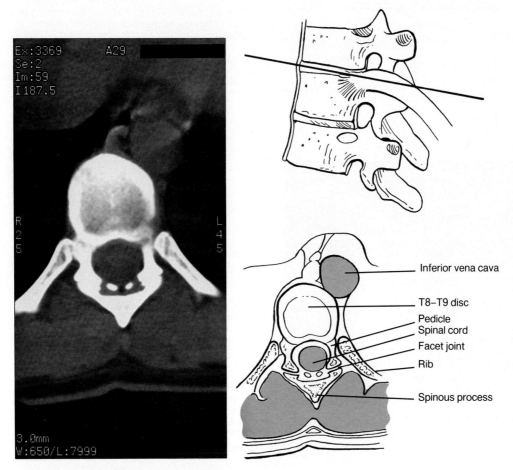

FIGURE 4–19. (*Left*) Axial CT of the thoracic spine at the level of the intervertebral disc. (*Right*) Drawing of the same view.

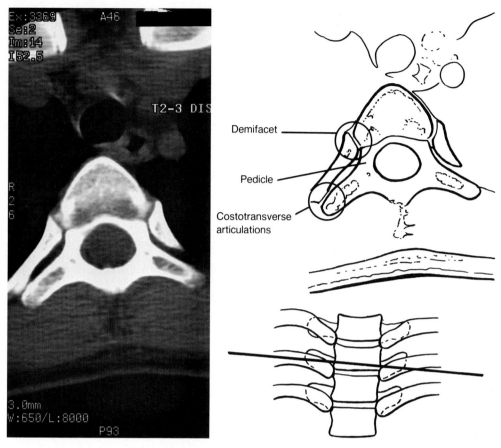

FIGURE 4–20. (*Left*) Axial CT of the thoracic spine at the level of the vertebral body and pedicles. (*Right*) Drawing of the same view.

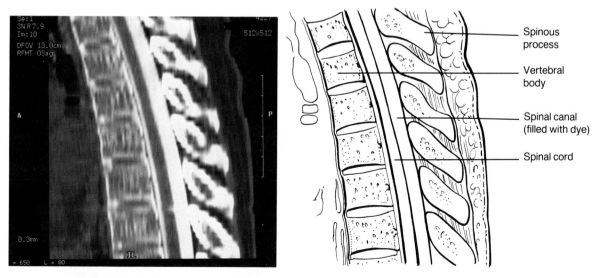

FIGURE 4–21. (*Left*) Sagittal reformation of thoracic spine CT in the midline. (*Right*) Drawing of the same view.

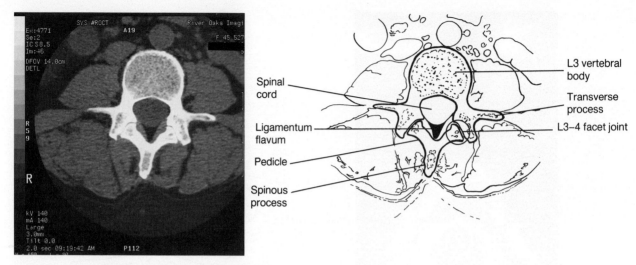

FIGURE 4–22. (*Left*) Axial CT of the lumbar spine at the level of vertebral body. (*Right*) Drawing of the same view.

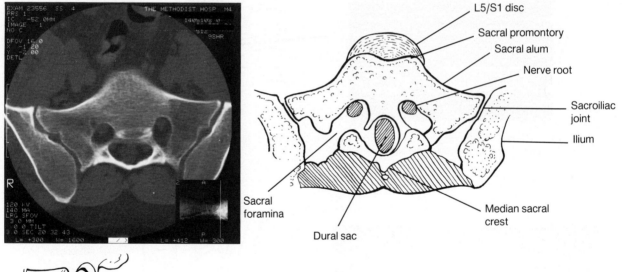

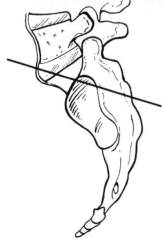

FIGURE 4–23. (*Left*) Axial CT of the lumbar spine at the level of the upper sacrum. (*Right*) Drawing of the same view.

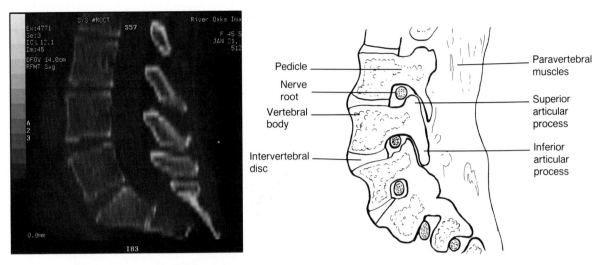

FIGURE 4-24. (*Left*) Sagittal reformation of lumbar spine CT at the level of the neural foramen. (*Right*) Drawing of the same view.

MAGNETIC RESONANCE IMAGING

Magnetic resonance imaging (MRI) is a technique by which images can be produced without ionizing radiation. To understand how an MR scan is produced, it is necessary to know that a nucleus acts like a magnet—that is, it spins on an axis. Hydrogen atoms are single charged nucleons. The hydrogen atoms in the body spin on random axes such that the total magnetic field of a person is zero. During MR scanning, the part of the patient to be imaged is placed in a strong magnet. This causes all the hydrogen atoms to line up with the same axis and thus yield a net magnetic charge. Once this has been done, a radio frequency transmitter is used to transmit into the tissue at a specific frequency. The frequency is determined by the nucleus being studied. Due to *resonance*, protons of the same precessional frequency as the pulsed waves will flip back and forth in direction, creating a radio frequency signal that is received and processed by a computer. These signals ultimately produce the MR image.

Many variables can be used to create an MR image, including not only the frequency of the pulsed radio waves but also the time that the magnet is turned on and off. The values of the *relaxation* and *excitation* times determine whether the image is *T1 weighted* or *T2 weighted*. In general, T1 images are used to study bone and bone marrow, T2 images to study water, cerebrospinal fluid (CSF), intervertebral discs, and the spinal cord. The sequence of events that produces an MR image is shown in Figure 4-25.

As with CT scanning, MR imaging is very sensitive, and not all abnormalities detected are clinically relevant. Each MR study must be interpreted in light of the patient's history, the physical examination, and other diagnostic tests.

A major disadvantage of MR scanning is the effect the magnetic field has on metallic objects. Patients who have metal fragments or implants must be carefully screened before they are allowed to enter the MR suite.

MR imaging in conjunction with the administration of paramagnetic contrast media such as gadolinium is the most sensitive and specific test to distinguish between recurrent disc and postoperative scar.

Cervical Spine

Figure 4-26 shows a sagittal T2-weighted image of the cervical spine. The CSF appears white, the spinal cord gray. Because of the high water content of the intervertebral disc, the nucleus pulposus also appears white. An axial image is shown in Figure 4-27.

(text continues on page 100)

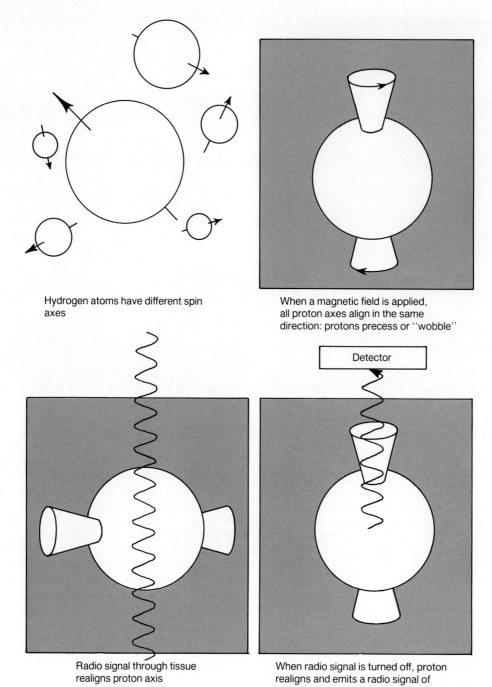

Hydrogen atoms have different spin axes

When a magnetic field is applied, all proton axes align in the same direction: protons precess or ''wobble''

Detector

Radio signal through tissue realigns proton axis

When radio signal is turned off, proton realigns and emits a radio signal of equal frequency but in opposite direction

FIGURE 4–25. Basic principle of MR imaging.

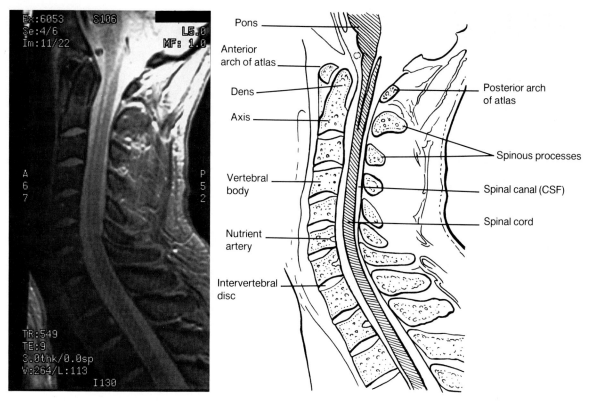

FIGURE 4–26. *(Left)* Sagittal T2-weighted MR image of the cervical spine. *(Right)* Drawing of the same view.

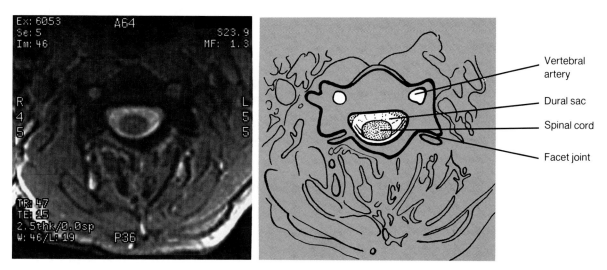

FIGURE 4–27. *(Left)* Axial T2-weighted MR image of the cervical spine. *(Right)* Drawing of the same view.

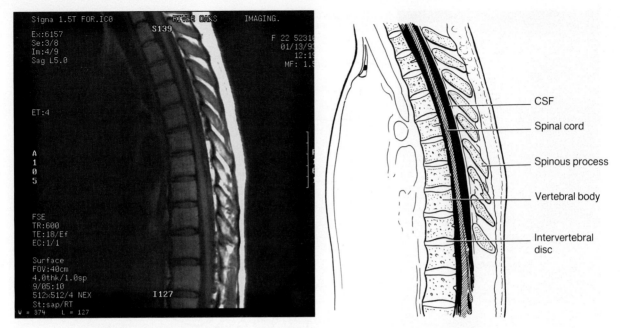

FIGURE 4–28. (*Left*) Sagittal T1-weighted MR image of the thoracic spine. (*Right*) Drawing of the same view.

Thoracic Spine

Figure 4-28 shows a T1-weighted image of the thoracic spine. With these imaging parameters, the CSF now appears black.

Lumbar Spine

Figure 4-29 is a T2-weighted image of the lumbar spine taken in the midline. Figure 4-30 is also a sagittal image but was taken in the plane of the neural foramina. It demonstrates the anatomy of the foramina and shows the exiting nerve root. Figure 4-31 is an axial image that is also T2 weighted.

MYELOGRAPHY

A *myelogram* is a plain radiograph taken with radiopaque dye in the CSF. Thus, myelography requires the placement of a needle through the skin into the subarachnoid space and the injection of contrast material. Currently, a water sol-uble dye is used; this has improved the quality of images and has decreased the incidence of complications and side effects.

With the advent of MR scanning, the indications for myelography have shrunk considerably. Indeed, as MR technology improves, myelography will probably become obsolete. Currently, some physicians think that myelography followed by CT scanning (with the dye still present) is more useful than MR imaging for evaluating bony lesions such as spinal stenosis.

Figures 4-32 and 4-33 show a cervical and lumbar myelogram, respectively. The cervical myelogram outlines the spinal cord and exiting nerve roots. The lumbar myelogram shows the cauda equina, dural sac, and lumbosacral roots. Figures 4-34 and 4-35 show a postmyelogram CT scan of the cervical and lumbar spine. Figure 4-36 shows sagittal reformation of the CT myelogram.

Because myelography is invasive, with attendant risks, it is usually not performed unless the patient's symptoms and signs are sufficiently severe to warrant surgical intervention.

(text continues on page 104)

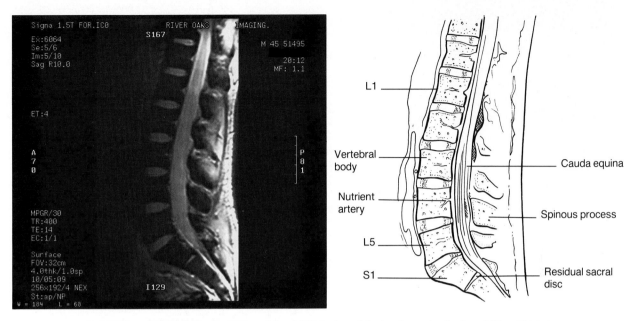

FIGURE 4–29. (*Left*) Sagittal T2-weighted MR image of the lumbar spine in the midline. (*Right*) Drawing of the same view.

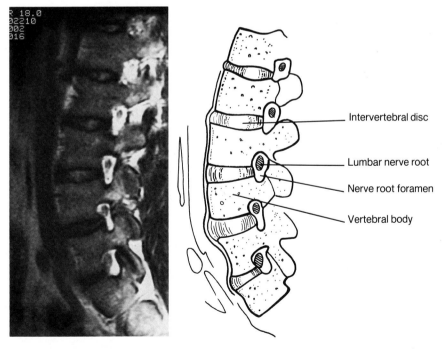

FIGURE 4–30. (*Left*) Sagittal T2-weighted MR image of the lumbar spine at the neural foramen. (*Right*) Drawing of the same view.

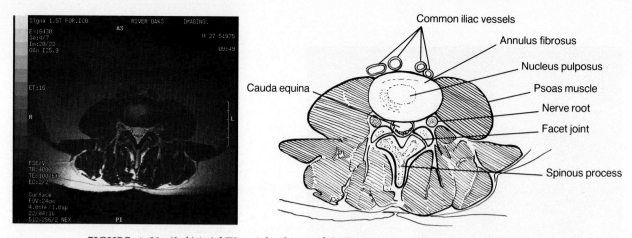

FIGURE 4–31. (*Left*) Axial T2-weighted MRI of the lumbar spine. (*Right*) Drawing of the same view.

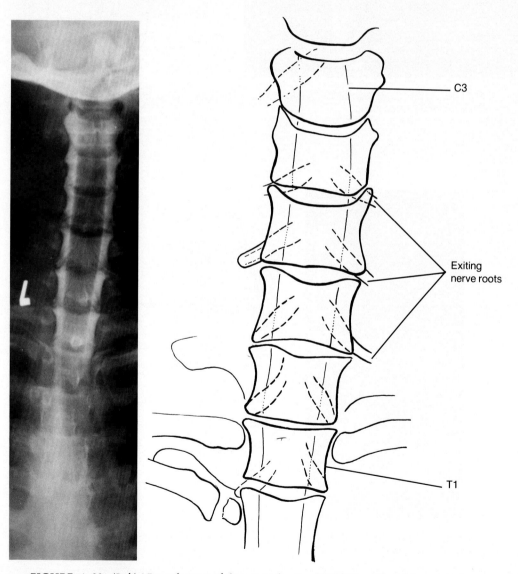

FIGURE 4–32. (*Left*) AP myelogram of the cervical spine. (*Right*) Drawing of the same view.

102

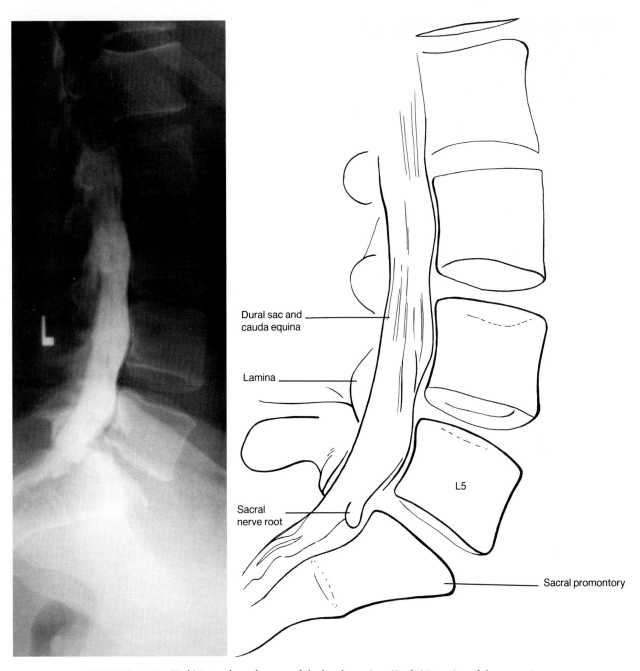

FIGURE 4–33. (*Left*) Lateral myelogram of the lumbar spine. (*Right*) Drawing of the same view.

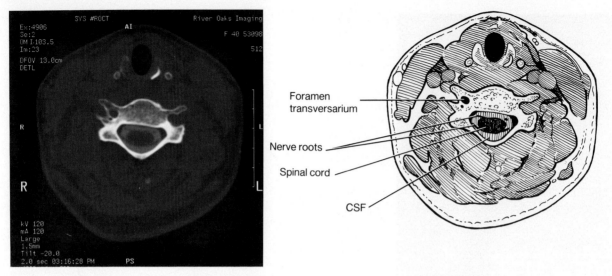

FIGURE 4–34. (*Left*) CT myelogram of the cervical spine. (*Right*) Drawing of the same view.

RADIONUCLIDE SCANNING

Technetium 99

Bone formation and resorption occur all the time, but the rate of bone turnover increases significantly when an active process (eg, tumor, infection, trauma) is present. After injection of technetium-99–labeled phosphate, the radioactive material is preferentially taken up in areas of increased bony metabolism. A bone scan image (Fig. 4-37) is a recording of the amount of radiation coming from the various areas imaged.

Gallium 67

Because gallium 67 citrate tends to accumulate within neutrophils, a gallium scan gives information as to whether any area has an increased accumulation of these cells (Fig. 4-38). Because neutrophils are an integral part of the inflammatory process, an increased uptake seen on gallium scanning usually indicates infection or inflammation.

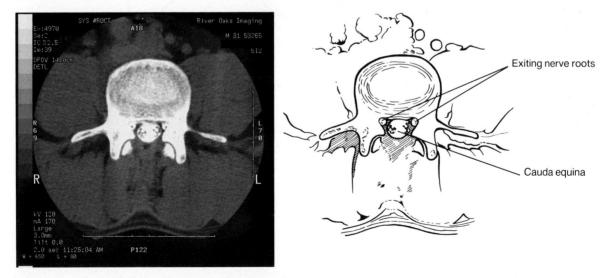

FIGURE 4–35. (*Left*) CT myelogram of the lumbar spine. (*Right*) Drawing of the same view.

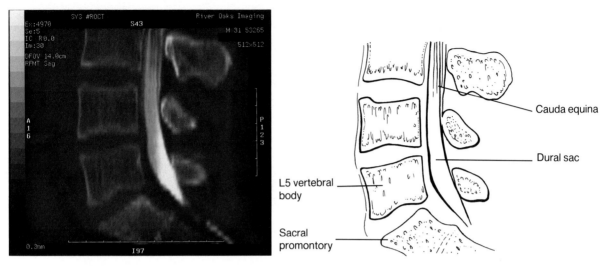

FIGURE 4–36. (*Left*) Sagittal reformation of CT myelogram. (*Right*) Drawing of the same view.

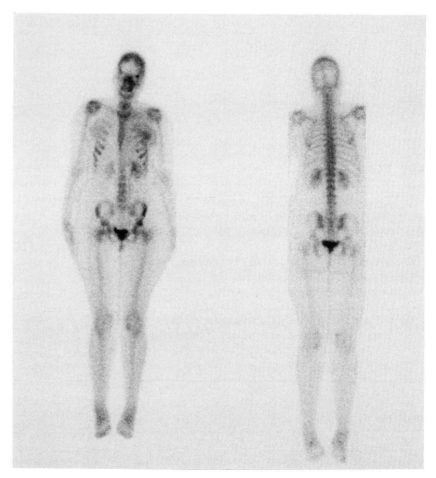

FIGURE 4–37. Technetium 99 bone scan.

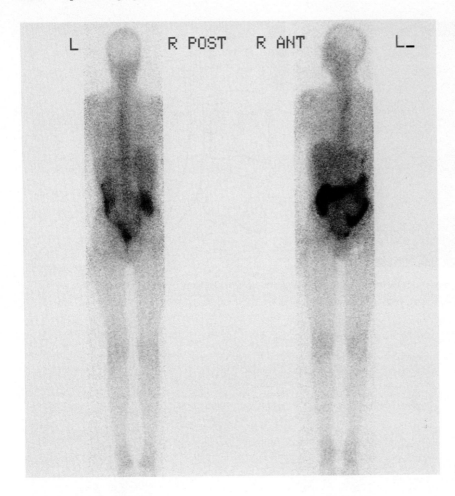

FIGURE 4–38. Gallium 67 scan.

KEY POINTS

1. An organized approach to the interpretation of plain radiographs is necessary to avoid missing abnormalities.
2. Myelography is gradually becoming supplanted by MR imaging for demonstrating the spinal cord, subarachnoid space, and nerve roots.
3. CT scanning and MR imaging are very sensitive imaging techniques. They both may show abnormalities that are not clinically relevant.

Indium

Indium scanning is very similar to gallium scanning. Its major advantage is that indium has a much more specific affinity for white blood cells than gallium. For this reason, it is more specific in detecting areas of infection.

BIBLIOGRAPHY

BOOKS

Manelfe C, ed. Imaging of the spine and spinal cord. New York: Raven Press, 1992.
Modic MT, Masaryk TJ, Ross JS. Magnetic resonance imaging of the spine. 2nd ed. Chicago: Year Book Medical Publishers, 1993
Teplick JG. Lumbar spine: CT and MRI. Philadelphia: JB Lippincott, 1992.

JOURNALS

Antti-Poika I, Soini J, Tallroth K, Yrjonen T, Konttinen YT. Clinical relevance of discography combined with CT scanning. J Bone Joint Surg [Br] 1990;72:480–485.
Boden SD, Davis DO, Dina TS, Patronas NJ, Wiesel SW. Abnormal MRI of lumbar spine in asymptomatic subjects. J Bone Joint Surg [Am] 1990;72:403–408.

Boden SD, McCowin PR, Davis DO, Dina TS, Mark AS, Wiesel S. Abnormal magnetic resonance scans of cervical spine in asymptomatic subjects. J Bone Joint Surg [Am] 1990;72: 1178–1184.

Deyo RA, Diehl AK. Lumbar spine films in primary care: Current use and effects of selective ordering criteria. J Gen Intern Med 1986;1: 20–25.

Page JE, Olliff JF, Dundas DD. Valve of anteroposterior radiography in cervical pain of non-traumatic origin. Br Med J 1989;298:1293–1294.

Parkkola R, Rytokoski U, Kormano M. Magnetic resonance imaging of the discs and trunk muscles in patients with chronic low-back pain and healthy control subjects. Spine 1993;18:830–836.

Peck WW. Current status of MRI of the cervical spine. Applied Radiology 1989;18:17–30.

Vezina JL, Fontaine S, LaPerriere J. Outpatient myelography with fine-needle technique: An appraisal. AJNR Am J Neuroradiol 1989;10:615–617.

Weinreb JC, Wolbarsht LB, Cohen JM, Brown CE, Maravilla KR. Prevalence of lumbosacral intervertebral disc abnormalities on MR images in pregnant and asymptomatic non-pregnant women. Radiology 1989;170:125–128.

Wilmink JT. CT morphology of intrathecal lumbosacral nerve-root compression. AJNR Am J Neuroradiol 1989;10:233–248.

Textbook of Spinal Disorders, by Stephen I. Esses.
J. B. Lippincott Company, Philadelphia © 1995.

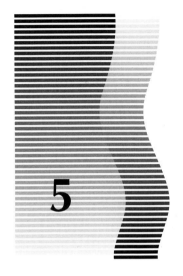

Biomechanics of the Spine

Stephen I. Esses • Brian Doherty

TERMINOLOGY
CERVICAL SPINE
  Kinematics
    Anatomic Basis of
    Kinematics
    Kinematic Properties
  Kinetics
    Spinal Ligaments
    Intervertebral Disc
  Failure Mechanisms
    Trauma
    Tumor
    Degenerative Disease
  Stabilization
    External
    Internal

THORACOLUMBAR
SPINE
  Kinematics
    Anatomic Basis of
    Kinematics
    Kinematic Properties
  Kinetics
    Vertebral Body
    Contribution of
    Abdomen and
    Muscles
    Intervertebral Disc
  Failure Mechanisms
    Trauma
    Tumor
    Degenerative Disease
  Stabilization
    External
    Internal

TERMINOLOGY

A *force* is that quantity which, when applied to a body, tends to move that body in a straight line (Fig. 5-1). A *moment* is that quantity which, when applied to a body, tends to rotate that body about a single point or axis (Fig. 5-2).

A *stress* is most easily described as a force per unit of area. This definition of stress depends on the stress being evenly distributed over the cross section of a body. This is a good assumption for cross sections that are not near points of load application (Fig. 5-3). Stress in a solid and *pressure* in a fluid are equivalent quantities. The *strain* in a body is most easily described as the overall lengthening or shortening of the body divided by the original length of the body (Fig. 5-4). Again, strain may be unevenly distributed within a body being stretched or compressed. When mechanical experiments involving application of loads to specimens are described, the terms *stress* and *strain* are often used because these quantities have had the effects of specimen size variations removed. Thus, comparisons between specimens and experiments may be more easily made.

The *stiffness* of a body is a measure of the mechanical properties of that body. In its most basic

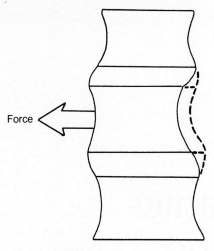

FIGURE 5–1. Force.

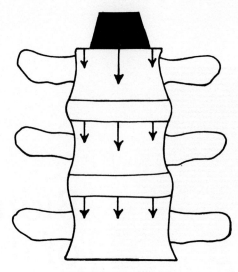

FIGURE 5–3. Stress.

form, the stiffness is defined as the force applied to the specimen divided by the resulting deflection of the specimen. If multiple loads are applied to a specimen sequentially, the resulting data may be plotted in a force–deflection diagram. The stiffness is then the slope of the resulting line (Fig. 5-5). If the data are instead converted to stress and strain, the slope of the resulting stress–strain diagram is referred to as the *modulus of elasticity* of the material (Fig. 5-6).

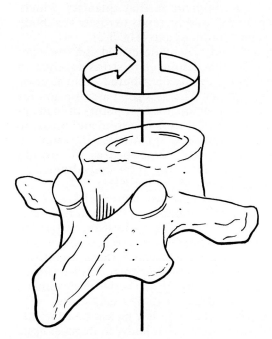

FIGURE 5–2. Moment.

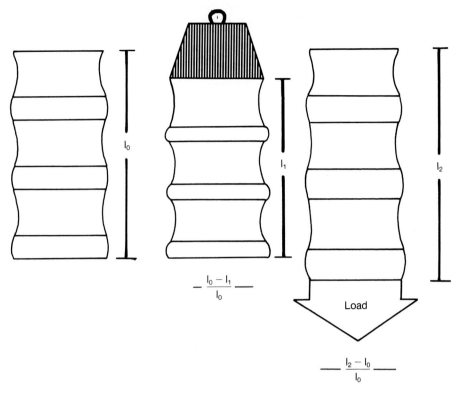

$$\frac{l_0 - l_1}{l_0}$$

Load

$$\frac{l_2 - l_0}{l_0}$$

FIGURE 5–4. Strain.

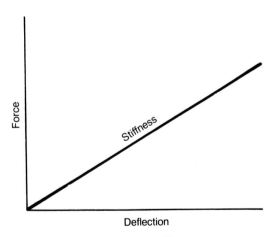

FIGURE 5–5. Stiffness.

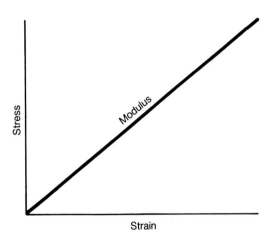

FIGURE 5–6. Modulus.

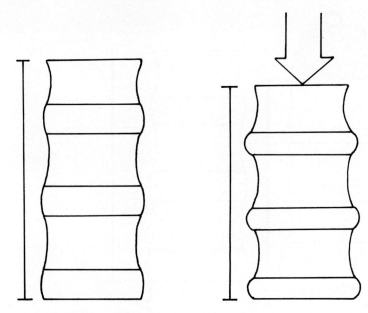

FIGURE 5–7. Axial stiffness.

For many bodies, stiffness may be defined by also referring to the direction of loading. For a slender body, the stiffness obtained when loads are applied to the long axis is referred to as the *axial stiffness* (Fig. 5-7). When a body is short, and loads are applied transversely, the stiffness is referred to as the *shear stiffness* (Fig. 5-8). If a moment is applied to a body so as to cause bending, then the slope of the bending moment plotted against the curve angle is referred to as the *bending stiffness* (Fig. 5-9). If a moment is applied to a slender body so as to cause twisting, the data may be plotted as a torque versus angle twist diagram; in this case, stiffness is referred to as *torsional stiffness* (Figs. 5-10 and 5-11).

All these terms are terms of rigidity—that is, in general, the quantity contains a load or moment divided by a resulting deflection. It is possible to define corresponding *flexibility* terms in which the displacement is divided by the load.

The *strength* of a body is different than the stiffness and flexibility properties. The strength of a body is a level of load or stress. If the body is loaded below this level, it may deform but no

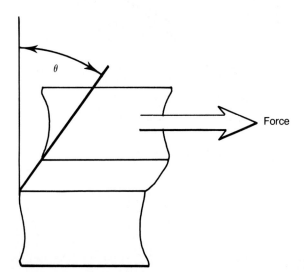

FIGURE 5–8. Shear stiffness.

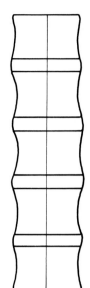
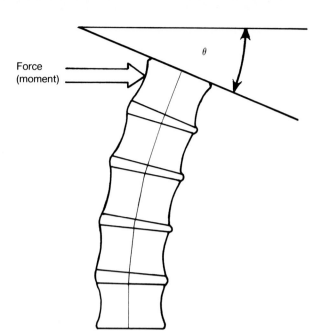

FIGURE 5–9. Bending stiffness.

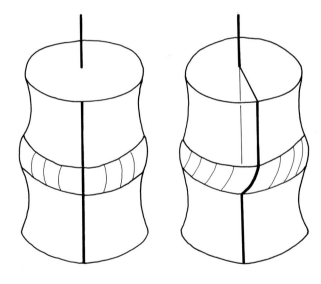

FIGURE 5–10. Torsional stiffness.

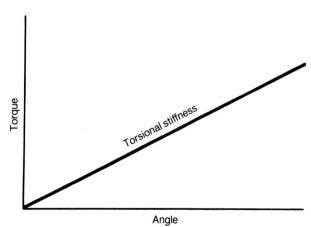

FIGURE 5–11. Torsional stiffness.

113

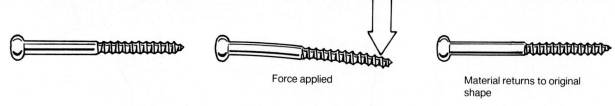

FIGURE 5–12. Elastic range.

permanent damage occurs. Removal of the load results in the body returning to its original configuration. This level of applied load is within the *elastic* range (Fig. 5-12). Loading the body above this level results in permanent, unrecoverable deformations. This level of applied load is within the *plastic* range (Fig. 5-13). A further distinction when discussing strength is yield versus fracture loads or stresses. When a body is loaded to the point of yielding, removing the load does not result in the body returning to its original configuration. However, the body can still support significant loads and is intact. When a body is loaded to the fracture or rupture point, it completely fails and cannot bear further load (Fig. 5-14). The yield strength is an important point in the clinical setting because a yielded implant no longer maintains the surgical configuration desired.

The yield and fracture strengths discussed above are defined in terms of single-cycle or low-cycle application of loads. The *fatigue* strength of a body is defined as the ability of that body to bear a repeated number of load applications. An orthopedic implant is typically expected to endure one to ten million load cycles in its lifetime. The fatigue characteristics of a material or a device are typically measured by subjecting speci-mens to various levels of load and measuring the number of cycles to failure. These data points are plotted on a stress versus number of cycles (S–N) curve (Fig. 5-15). The expected lifetime of the material or implant at a particular stress level may then be read off the curve.

All these terms are applicable to elastic bodies, meaning that the rate of application of load is not considered important. Many of the tissues of the spine have mechanical properties that vary with time, called *viscoelastic properties*. For a viscoelastic body, the rate of application of load is important. Application of a steady load to a viscoelastic body results in a slow, increasing deformation of that body, a phenomenon called *creep*. The deformation increases rapidly at first, then less rapidly, until essentially all deformation has occurred (Fig. 5-16). The time required for the deformation plateau to be reached is a characteristic of each viscoelastic material. Similarly, if a viscoelastic body is stretched and held at a certain length greater than its original length, the force required to hold this elongation reaches a maximum immediately, then falls off. For solid materials, the force falls to a plateau that is greater than zero. The time required to reach this plateau, called the *relaxation time*, is also characteristic of each viscoelastic material (Fig. 5-17).

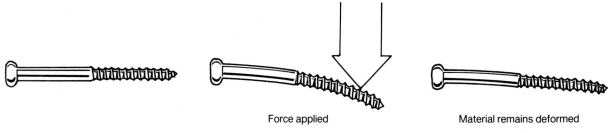

FIGURE 5–13. Plastic range.

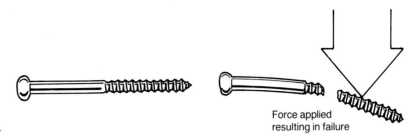

Force applied
resulting in failure

FIGURE 5–14. Loading to failure.

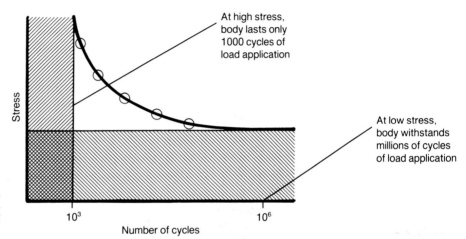

At high stress,
body lasts only
1000 cycles of
load application

At low stress,
body withstands
millions of cycles
of load application

FIGURE 5–15. Fatigue characteristics of a body: stress versus number of cycles (S–N curve).

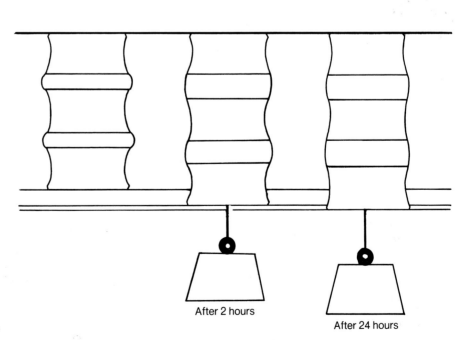

After 2 hours

After 24 hours

FIGURE 5–16. Creep.

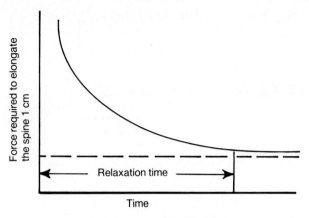

FIGURE 5–17. Relaxation time.

The spinal column consists of a series of complex joints, each known as a *functional spinal unit* (FSU). The FSU is defined as two vertebral bodies and the soft tissue joining them (Fig. 5-18). In general, these soft tissues consist of the intervertebral disc and the spinal ligaments. A single FSU can be thought of as consisting of three subjoints: the intervertebral disc and the two facet joints in the posterior column (Fig. 5-19).

Kinetics is the study of the relation between force and deformation in mechanical systems. When applied to the human spine, kinetics is the study of the mechanical function of the various parts of the spine and the mechanical characteristics of the FSU. In contrast, *kinematics* is concerned only with the description of motion without reference to the loads required to create them.

CERVICAL SPINE

Kinematics

ANATOMIC BASIS OF KINEMATICS

The cervical spine may be conceptually divided into two parts. The first part, the upper cervical spine, consists of the occiput (C0), the atlas (C1), and the axis (C2) vertebrae. This region is characterized by a large range of motion and vertebral anatomy unique in the spinal column. The second part, the subaxial cervical spine, consists of the third through seventh cervical vertebrae (C3–C7). This region is characterized by anatomy more typical of the spinal column and by

small vertebral sizes relative to the other regions of the spine (Fig. 5-20).

In the upper cervical spine, motion between C0 and C1 is generally limited by bony contact in flexion and rotation, with ligamentous structures playing a role in extension. In the joint between C1 and C2, ligamentous structures are primarily responsible for limiting motion. In the subaxial cervical spine, the intervertebral disc, particularly the annulus, limits translational motion in the sagittal and frontal planes.

KINEMATIC PROPERTIES

The neck has almost no "preferred" position, especially when the weight of the head is unsupported. Normally, in the erect position, the paravertebral muscles act to produce a gentle lordosis of the cervical spine. Most quantitative work on cervical spine kinematics has been done on spines in the passive state. The range of motion between C0 and C1 has been found to be about 25° from flexion to extension, 5° in lateral bending to each side, and 4° to 7° of axial rotation to each side. The range of motion between C1 and C2 is about 15° from flexion to extension, 7° in lateral bending, and 47° in axial rotation. In other words, about 40% to 50% of the total range of axial motion in a normal adult occurs at the C1–C2 level. In the subaxial spine, the range of motion from flexion to extension is between 12° and 23°; the angle is generally larger in the lower segments. In this region, the range of motion in

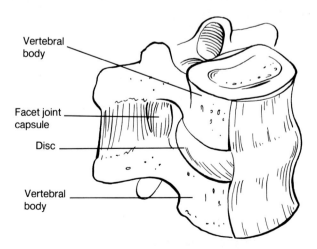

FIGURE 5–18. Functional spinal unit.

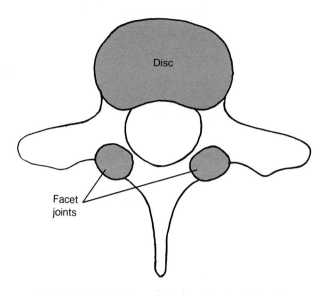

FIGURE 5–19. Joints of the functional spinal unit.

one-sided lateral bending is about 5°; there is virtually no variation along the length of the subaxial cervical spine. In axial rotation, the range of motion in the subaxial cervical spine ranges from 3° to 7° to each side; these values are generally largest at the lower levels of the cervical spine.

In addition to the primary motions, the kinematics of the cervical spine has been shown to exhibit significant coupling of motion. A coupled motion is one repeatedly associated with another motion in a different direction. For example, the most significant coupled motion in the subaxial cervical spine is axial rotation that accompanies lateral bending. The direction of this coupled motion is such that the spinous processes rotate toward the concavity of the curve. There are no significant coupled motions in the upper cervical spine.

Kinetics

SPINAL LIGAMENTS

Ligaments are mechanical structures designed to support loads in tension only. Bending, twisting, or compression generally meet with no resistance in these structures. There are several distinct ligamentous structures in the spinal column, each of which perform several functions. Figure 5-21 shows the locations of the an-

terior and posterior longitudinal ligaments, the ligamentum flavum, the facet capsular ligament, the intertransverse ligaments, and the interspinous and supraspinous ligaments. The anterior longitudinal ligament functions primarily to resist extension. The interspinous and supraspinous ligaments act primarily to resist flexion (Fig. 5-22). The capsular ligaments act to stabilize the facet joints. The posterior longitudinal ligament and ligamentum flavum, while playing roles in stabilizing the FSU in lateral bending, also act to surround and protect the spinal cord.

Spinal ligaments exhibit a nonlinear load displacement curve—that is, in the physiologic range of deformation, the ligaments are relatively easily stretched; they have relatively low stiffness. When spinal motions become larger, the ligaments become many times stiffer. This has the effect of allowing relatively easy motion in the physiologic range of spinal movements, while protecting the spine from overly large motions that could result in trauma.

INTERVERTEBRAL DISC

In contrast to the spinal ligaments, the intervertebral disc can resist forces in many different directions. The intervertebral disc is made up of

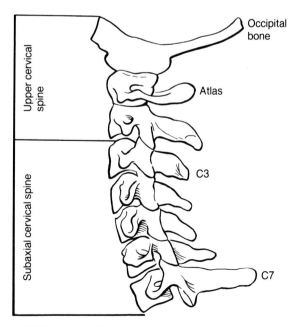

FIGURE 5–20. Kinematic regions of the cervical spine.

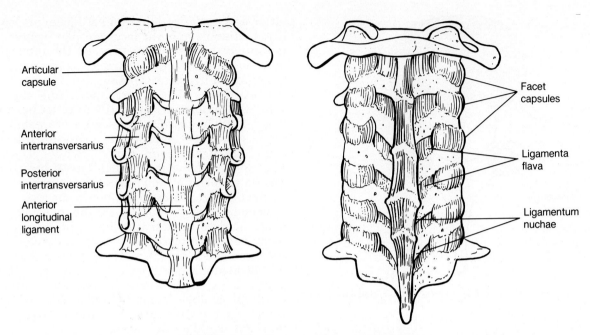

FIGURE 5–21. Ligaments of the cervical spine.

three parts: the nucleus pulposus, the annulus fibrosus, and the cartilaginous end plates (Fig. 5-23). The nucleus pulposus, a fluid-like region in the center of the disc, is surrounded by the annulus fibrosus. The annulus is composed of layers of helically wound fibers, with the direction of fibers alternating between layers. This cross-helically wound construction has been found in many cylindrical biologic structures. The combination of a fluid center and a fibrous outer structure gives the disc a soft or flexible response at low levels of load. However, when the disc is under larger loads, approaching the traumatic level, the pressurization of the fluid core creates a stiffer or less flexible response; indeed, at these levels of load, the disc can become stiffer than the

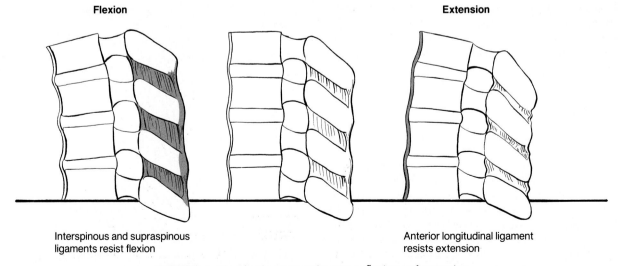

FIGURE 5–22. Ligamentous resistance to flexion and extension.

underlying bone. In addition to becoming stiffer under load, the disc is often stronger than the vertebral bone as well. The differences in stiffness between disc and bone lead to deflection of the vertebral end plates. The differences in strength explain the observation that the bone fails before disc rupture under rapidly applied large axial loads. A further discussion of the kinetics of the vertebral body is found in the section on the thoracolumbar spine.

Failure Mechanisms

Under a variety of circumstances, the cervical spine loses its ability to bear load or to move normally—that is, there is altered kinetics, kinematics, or both. When this failure occurs, the spine is considered unstable. Not all instances of instability are cause for concern, nor do they lead to clinically significant sequelae. However, when the instability pattern is symptomatic or potentially so, we call this *clinical instability*. As discussed above, this refers to a failure of the normal kinematics, kinetics, or both such that there is neurologic deficit, deformity, or pain. In addition, clinical instability exists when continued physiologic loading of the spine would result in one or all of these complications.

TRAUMA

After trauma to the cervical spine, an assessment must be made as to whether the neck has been rendered unstable. If so, the examiner must further assess whether there is clinical instability and whether the patient's health is endangered. This assessment begins with a thorough history and physical examination. A patient's recollection that he or she experienced transient paresis or paresthesia at the time of the trauma, or the finding of a neurologic deficit on physical examination, means there was clinical instability at the time of injury. The examiner must further assess whether clinical instability continues to exist. This usually requires radiologic examination.

The upper cervical spine is particularly prone to injury. A fracture of the atlas, known as a Jefferson fracture, is not necessarily unstable. When there is splaying of the lateral masses greater than 7 mm, however, there has been a concomitant rupture of the transverse ligament; this situation is unstable (Fig. 5-24). As discussed in Chapter 4, the distance from the posterior portion of the anterior ring of C1 to the anterior as-

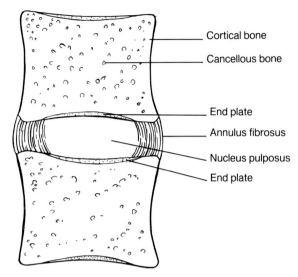

FIGURE 5–23. Intervertebral disc.

pect of the dens should not measure more than 3 mm; this is called the A–A distance (Fig. 5-25). An increase in this interval suggests underlying instability.

Flexion-extension x-rays are very useful in further assessing motion between C1 and C2 (Fig. 5-26). In the middle and lower cervical spine, displacement of one vertebra greater than 3.5 mm or angulation more than 11° compared with adjacent levels suggests instability. The usual way these measurements are made is shown in Figures 5-27 and 5-28. Abnormalities in these measurements may be identified only on flexion-extension x-rays. These x-rays should be done only on awake, alert patients. They may not be valid in acute trauma situations where spasm and pain may prevent adequate motion.

White and Panjabi have developed a checklist for the diagnosis of clinical instability in the middle and lower cervical spine (Table 5-1). The diagnosis of clinical instability is multifactorial—that is, it is based not only on radiographic criteria but also on neurologic status and the patient's activities.

TUMOR

Both primary and secondary tumors affecting the cervical spine can alter the structural integrity of the spinal column. This may make it prone to catastrophic failure. Furthermore, these tumor deposits may cause direct compression of

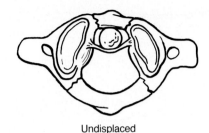

Undisplaced

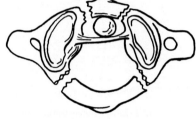

Displaced but stable

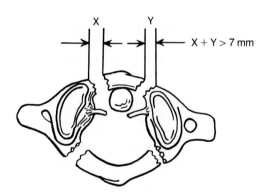

X + Y > 7 mm

Displaced and unstable

FIGURE 5-24. Jefferson fracture.

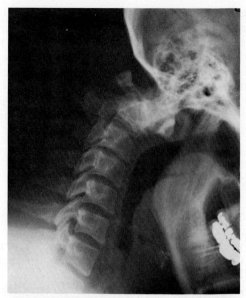

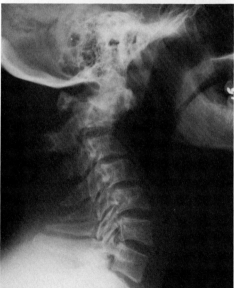

FIGURE 5-26. Flexion-extension x-rays.

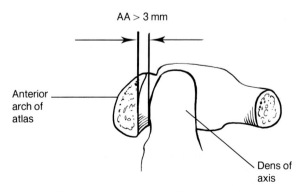

FIGURE 5-25. Atlantoaxial (A–A) distance.

the spinal cord or nerve roots, resulting in neurologic deficits. The normal cervical lordosis results in some axial compression of the posterior elements and some tensile force on the anterior cervical spinal column. As the neck flexes forward, these forces change, resulting in tension on the posterior elements and compression or bending moments on the anterior column. The clinician must determine when enough bony destruction has occurred to cause the spine to be prone to failure. When neural compression mandates

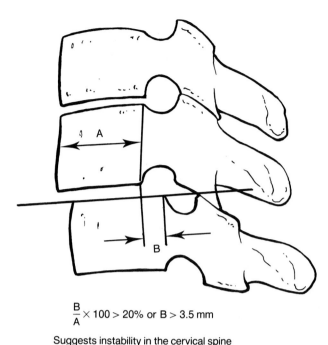

$$\frac{B}{A} \times 100 > 20\% \text{ or } B > 3.5 \text{ mm}$$

Suggests instability in the cervical spine

FIGURE 5-27. Measurement of cervical displacement (after White and Panjabi).

surgical decompression, the clinician must determine whether this decompression will result in iatrogenic instability.

When a vertebral body has been affected by a neoplastic deposit, the status of the posterior vertebral cortex should be carefully assessed. This may require computed tomography (CT) or magnetic resonance (MR) scanning. If the posterior vertebral cortex has been breached, then instability is probable because the vertebra will no longer be able to resist load in bending. If the neoplasm has affected the posterior elements of the vertebra, then the facet joints on either side must be carefully assessed. If both facet joints have lost their structural integrity, the spine will be unlikely to resist the tensile forces accompanying forward flexion, and instability probably exists. In either of these circumstances, some intervention is warranted.

DEGENERATIVE DISEASE

Normally, the spinal cord lengthens and shortens with cervical flexion and extension. These

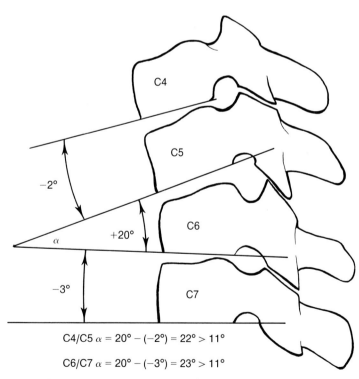

C4/C5 $\alpha = 20° - (-2°) = 22° > 11°$

C6/C7 $\alpha = 20° - (-3°) = 23° > 11°$

If angulation (α) is greater than 11° compared to either adjacent interspace angle, this is considered abnormal angulation

FIGURE 5-28. Measurement of cervical angulation (after White and Panjabi).

changes are not accompanied by any alterations in the stresses or forces on the spinal cord. As noted in Chapter 1, there are three main joint complexes in the cervical spine: the intervertebral disc, uncovertebral joints, and zygoapophyseal joints. Degenerative changes in any or all of these joints can result in osteophyte formation, decreased intervertebral disc height, disc bulging, buckling of the ligamentum flavum, and narrowing of the spinal canal. Under these circumstances, compression of the spinal cord may result, and this compression may be accentuated by flexion or extension. The main goal of treatment in this case is to reduce the compressive stresses on the spinal cord. Biomechanical studies have shown that the most effective method of decreasing anterior compressive forces is by anterior decompression. Similarly, posterior compressive lesions are best treated by posterior decompression. If this is to be done, a careful analysis of the extent of decompression necessary is essential in determining whether instability may result. The guidelines given above regarding the vertebral body and facet joints are useful in this assessment.

Stabilization

EXTERNAL

Four groups of external immobilization devices are used for the cervical spine: halo devices, cervicothoracic orthoses, poster orthoses, and collars.

Halo devices consist of a metal ring that is screwed to the skull and attached to the thorax by means of a vest or plaster cast. Overall, halo devices reduce flexion-extension and rotation by 70%, but they are not particularly effective in reducing compression and distractive motions. Thus, in assessing whether a halo device is effective for a particular patient, x-rays should be taken supine and upright. Halo devices are not good if constant distraction or compression must be maintained. The effectiveness of a halo depends on good pin placement. The optimal site for anterior pin placement is just above the eyebrow at the junction of its middle and lateral thirds. It is in this area that the skull table is thickest.

Cervicothoracic orthoses attach the head and neck to the thorax by posts. One example is a Somi, an acronym for *s*ternal *o*ccipital *m*andibular *i*mmobilization. The cervicothoracic orthoses and poster orthoses are useful in reducing flexion

TABLE 5–1. Checklist for the Diagnosis of Clinical Instability in the Middle and Lower Cervical Spine

Element	Point Value
Anterior elements destroyed or unable to function	2
Posterior elements destroyed or unable to function	2
Positive stretch test	2
Radiographic criteria	4
1. Sagittal plane translation >3.55 mm	2
2. Sagittal plane rotation >20°	2
Abnormal disc narrowing	1
Spinal cord damage	2
Nerve root damage	1
Dangerous loading anticipated	1
Total of 5 or more = Unstable	

and extension but do not significantly reduce rotation or lateral bending.

Collars can be either soft or hard; an example of the latter is a Philadelphia collar. Hard collars such as the Philadelphia can reduce flexion, but soft collars are not particularly useful in controlling any motion.

When deciding to place a patient in an external brace for a cervical problem, the clinician must assess what particular motion is to be controlled and at what level. In this way, the appropriate orthosis can be selected for each individual case.

INTERNAL

Four basic biomechanical principles are used in stabilization of the cervical spine: tension banding, compression, buttressing, and distraction.

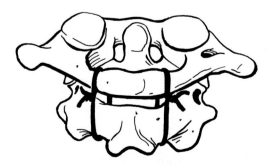

FIGURE 5–29. Posterior C1–C2 wiring.

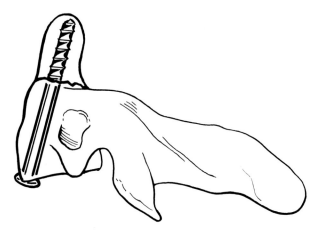

FIGURE 5–30. Lag screw fixation of an odontoid fracture.

Tension banding is a technique by which tensile forces are converted into axial compressive forces. An example of this is posterior C1–C2 wiring in cases of posterior ligament complex rupture (Fig. 5-29). An example of compression fixation is lag screw fixation for odontoid fractures (Fig. 5-30). The lag screw results in compression and impaction at the fracture site. Buttressing is usually done with plates placed anteriorly. The plate prevents the bone graft from collapsing and helps to resist load in forward flexion (Fig. 5-31). Occasionally, plates are

used for distraction. Because distraction is not the ideal environment for bone graft to incorporate, the implant is most commonly used to effect distraction, after which bone graft is inserted under compression. This reduces the forces on the implant and helps prevent implant failure.

Three types of implants are used to stabilize the cervical spine posteriorly: wires, screws, and hooks. Wires can be placed around or through the spinous process or under the lamina (Fig. 5-32). Screws are usually placed in the lateral masses (Fig. 5-33). Hooks are most commonly placed around the laminae (Fig. 5-34). Several biomechanical studies have been undertaken to evaluate and compare these implant systems. Under conditions of single-level posterior instability, there are no major differences between these implants. When there is circumferential instability at a single level of the lower cervical spine, anterior cervical plating and screw fixation provide the least amount of stability. Anterior cervical plate stabilization alone is insufficient, and a posterior cervical stabilization procedure is also required. When multiple-level posterior instability exits, techniques that allow segmental instrumentation are optimal.

Anteriorly, plates are the most common implants used. Biomechanically, plates are useful when there is isolated anterior instability. Clinically, there has always been the realistic concern that if screws loosened or backed out of the plate, esophageal erosion or perforation could

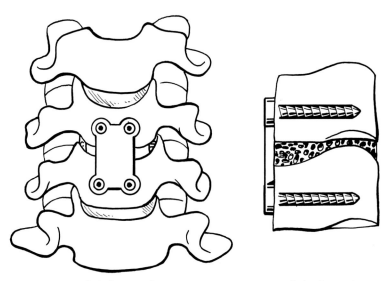

FIGURE 5–31. Anterior plating of the cervical spine.

Anterior aspect   Lateral aspect

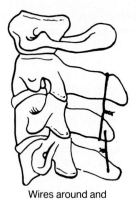

Wires around and
through spinous
processes

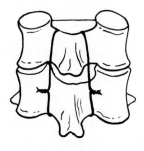

Wires around laminae

FIGURE 5–32. Wiring of the cervical spine.

occur. Newer systems allow for locking of these screws to the plate to prevent this disastrous complication.

THORACOLUMBAR SPINE

Kinematics

ANATOMIC BASIS OF KINEMATICS

The thoracolumbar spine may be conceptually divided into two parts (Fig. 5-35). The first part, the lower thoracic spine, consists of the first through the 12th thoracic vertebral levels. This region is characterized anatomically by a relatively small lateral dimension and spinous processes sharply angled with respect to the long axis of the spine. The second part, the lumbar spine, consists of the first through fifth lumbar vertebral levels. This region is characterized by prominent transverse processes and large vertebral bodies. Spinous processes are semicircular in sagittal plane appearance and do not overlap.

In the thoracic spine, the posterior elements play a role in limiting both extension and axial rotation (Fig. 5-36). The facet joints, whose alignment is more like that of the cervical spine than that of the lumbar spine, play a role that has not yet been fully determined. In the lumbar spine, the facet joints and other posterior elements function primarily to limit axial rotation (Fig. 5-37). Some studies have shown that these facet joints also limit anterior translation of lumbar vertebral bodies. At these levels, the intervertebral disc provides the main resistance to axial translation and frontal and sagittal plane rotation.

KINEMATIC PROPERTIES

The kinematics of the lower thoracic spine is influenced by the fact that it is a transitional region of the spinal column. The term *transitional* here means that the kinematic properties in this region gradually change from those typical of the cervical spine to those observed in the lumbar spine. For example, in flexion-extension motion, the upper thoracic spine has a limited range of motion (about 4°). In the lumbar spine, this motion ranges from 12° to 16°. The lower thoracic spine exhibits a flexion-extension range of motion of 6° to 12°, increasing as the level becomes more caudad. In axial rotation, however, this pattern is reversed. The upper thoracic spine has a larger range of motion (7° to 9°) than the lumbar spine (about 2°). The lower thoracic spine has been found to have range of motion in axial

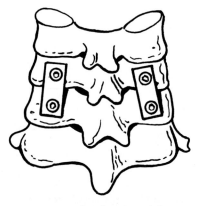

FIGURE 5–33. Screw-plate fixation of the cervical spine.

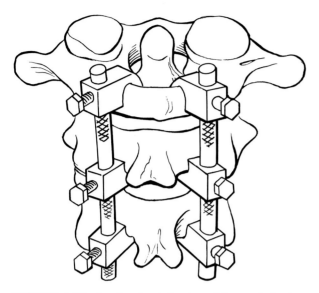

FIGURE 5-34. Laminar hook fixation of the cervical spine.

cortical bone. Some studies have shown that vertebral resistance to compression is increasingly provided by the cortical shell with advancing age and with progressive degeneration of the intervertebral disc. Disc degeneration affects the way the vertebral body carries the load because the distribution of load changes: in a disc with a

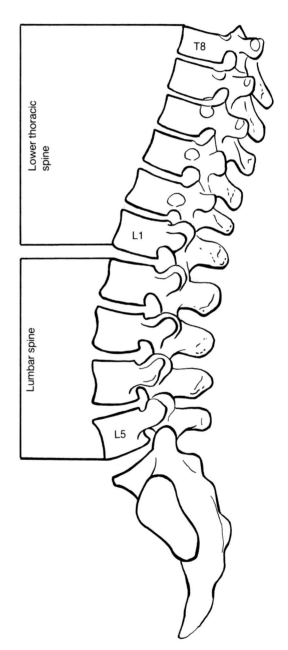

FIGURE 5-35. Kinematic regions of the thoracolumbar spine.

rotation of between 2° and 6°. In other words, as one moves down the spinal column, flexion-extension range of motion increases, while axial rotation range of motion steadily decreases. The range of motion for lateral bending is relatively constant at about 60° from the lower thoracic to the lumbar spine.

In addition to the anatomic characteristics described above, the patterns of coupled motion are important in the evaluation of spinal deformity. In the thoracic spine, lateral bending is coupled with axial rotation in such a way that the posterior elements move toward the convexity of the lateral curve. This is the mechanism by which a rib hump is produced in thoracic scoliosis.

Kinetics

VERTEBRAL BODY

The following description of the load-bearing capabilities of vertebral bodies applies to the whole spinal column, but the experimental work it is derived from was performed primarily on vertebrae from the lumbar spine.

The vertebral body is made up of both cortical and cancellous bone (see Fig. 5-23). Unlike the long bones, the vertebral bodies have only a thin outer layer of cortical (or compact) bone. It is not yet clear what proportion of the total load-bearing capacity of a vertebra is carried by the

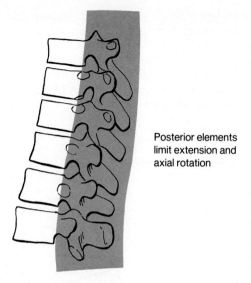

FIGURE 5–36. Kinematics of the lower thoracic spine.

Posterior elements limit extension and axial rotation

like array of fine bony plates and rods collectively known as trabeculae. Marrow and other fluids are found in the spaces between the trabeculae. The strength of this cancellous bone comes not only from the inherent strength of the bone itself but also from the resistance to the flow of the intertrabecular fluid created by the size of the trabecular spacing. Noninvasive methods of measuring bone density generally measure properties of the bone itself and do not take into account the contribution of this fluid resistance to the actual strength.

Overall, the stiffness and strength of the vertebral body are made up of contributions from both cortical and cancellous bone. Like the nonlinear responses in tension observed in the spinal ligaments, the FSU acts to create a mechanical unit that is initially flexible but becomes much less so as the imposed loads approach injurious levels. Under conditions of low load, the intervertebral disc is easily deformed (Fig. 5-38). As loads increase, the normal disc becomes pressurized and almost rigid. This places the annulus under tension, greatly reducing the flexibility of the FSU. Under these conditions, the bone underlying the nucleus actually deforms. In the presence of repetitive low-level loads, this bone can fail in certain locations due to the stresses imposed on it

healthy nucleus it is distributed centrally, whereas in a disc with a degenerated nucleus it is distributed peripherally.

The core of the vertebral body is made up of cancellous (or spongy) bone. This form of bone is so named because it is made up of a honeycomb-

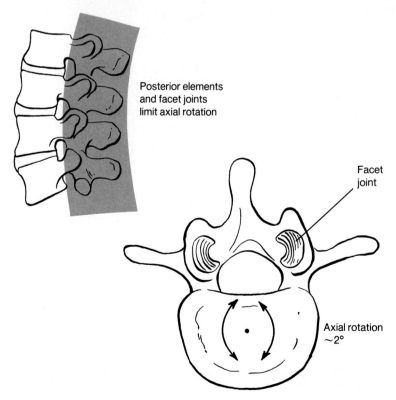

Posterior elements and facet joints limit axial rotation

Facet joint

Axial rotation ~2°

FIGURE 5–37. Kinematics of the lumbar spine.

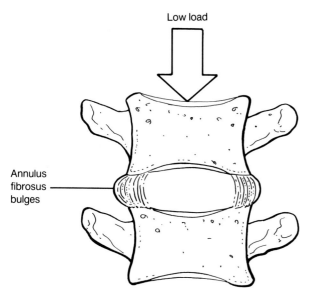

Low load

Annulus
fibrosus
bulges

FIGURE 5–38. Low loading of an intervertebral disc.

by the disc. A condition known as Schmorl's nodes can occur (Fig. 5-39). When the disc passes sudden large loads to the bone, such as in a fall from a height, the vertebra can fail. This can lead to end plate fractures and burst fractures.

CONTRIBUTION OF ABDOMEN AND MUSCLES

The strength of the back is only partially made up of the strength of the spine itself. There are also significant contributions from muscle contraction and from pressurization of the abdomen. These effects are difficult to measure in patients. Some information is available, however, from studies of the load on the lumbar spine during typical work activities.

The isometric strength of the trunk extensors is much greater than that of the flexors. Trunk strength usually decreases with age, beginning in the fourth decade of life. Estimates of the compressive load on the lumbar spine are available from several sources. Because it is impossible to measure the loads on the spine in vivo, most investigations depend on a semi-empirical approach that combines theoretic postulates and practical observations. Typically, the result is a mathematical model of the body that can predict loads on the spine. This model is correlated with actual measurements of such variables as the load being lifted, reaction forces at the foot–

ground interface, and muscle activity. This correlation has the effect of increasing the physician's confidence in the load predictions of the model, giving it more clinical utility.

An estimate of the load on the lumbar spine based on a typical lifting load and the differences between the moment of the arms and the posterior musculature of the lumbar spine resulted in an estimate of 1600 pounds. Intra-abdominal pressure, although an important factor, probably reduces this estimate by only a few hundred pounds. Calculations of lumbar loads have also been made based on in vivo pressure measurements. Several in vivo studies of pressure increases in the lumbar intervertebral discs have included correlations with external loads.

Several studies have been done on the compressive loads on the lumbar spine during maximal lifts. Using a mathematical model in concert with electromyographic measurements on human volunteers, one study determined the load on the lumbosacral joint during lifting of boxes of various sizes and weights. The volunteers were allowed to determine the maximum box load they were comfortable with, resulting in a range of 50 to 150 pounds. The calculated lumbar loads resulting from these lifts were in the range of 1500 to 2000 pounds. The key determinants of lumbar spine compression forces that occur during lifting are the moments acting on

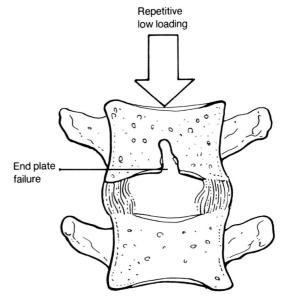

Repetitive
low loading

End plate
failure

FIGURE 5–39. Repetitive low loading of an intervertebral disc.

the spine. The key determinants of the load moments are the load magnitude, load location, and speed of the lift. Although trunk muscle strength and intra-abdominal pressure have some effect on compression forces, they are very small.

INTERVERTEBRAL DISC

Intradiscal pressures have been measured in vivo in different body positions. In the mid-lumbar spine, the load on the intervertebral disc while standing is about body weight. It decreases by about 50% in the supine position and increases by 50% during sitting.

Failure Mechanisms

The above discussion on kinematics and kinetics of the thoracolumbar spine is useful in understanding the biomechanical attributes of this part of the spinal column. However, there must be a logical approach to assessing the stability of the thoracolumbar spine under a variety of pathologic conditions. One way of doing this is to think of the thoracolumbar spine as having three columns (Fig. 5-40). The *anterior column* is composed of the anterior longitudinal ligament, the anterior annulus fibrosus, and the anterior part of the vertebral body. The *middle column* consists of the posterior longitudinal ligament, the posterior annulus fibrosus, and the posterior wall of the vertebral body. The *posterior column* is formed by the posterior bony arch and posterior ligamentous complex. In general, instability exists when two or more of these columns lose their integrity.

TRAUMA

Although the three-column concept has furthered our understanding of the mechanical sequelae of traumatic injuries, it cannot, by itself, be used to characterize thoracolumbar injuries. This is because it is exclusively a mechanical model and does not consider concomitant neurologic damage. Neurologic damage can occur without bony injury to the spinal column. Soft tissue injury is often hard to diagnose and may be recognized only by the presence of a neurologic deficit.

Apart from analyzing the three columns of a fractured vertebra, it is also important to consider the level of injury. Fractures between T1 and T9 have greater inherent stability due to the

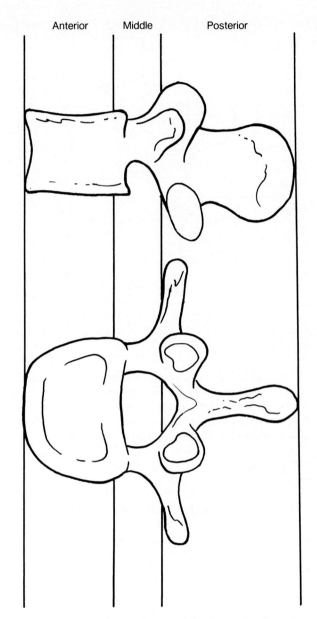

FIGURE 5-40. Three columns of the thoracolumbar spine.

rib cage and sternum. Conversely, the thoracolumbar junction is inherently unstable. It represents a transition between the thoracic kyphosis and lumbar lordosis; there is also a change in the orientation of the facet joints at this level. Therefore, before a decision is made concerning treatment of a thoracolumbar fracture, it is necessary to consider the damage to the three columns of the spine, the level of the injury, the presence of neurologic injury, and associated soft tissue injury.

TUMOR

As mentioned, an assessment of instability requires not only an analysis of structural damage to the spinal column but also attention to clinical factors. This is particularly relevant to cases in which there is neoplastic involvement of the thoracolumbar spine. White and Panjabi's checklist for the diagnosis of clinical instability in the lumbar spine (Table 5-2) is very useful in determining whether therapeutic intervention is warranted in tumor cases.

DEGENERATIVE DISEASE

The kinematics of the normal thoracolumbar spine has already been discussed. With degenerative disease, abnormal motion can occur, either increased or decreased motion at specific levels. The abnormal motion can be translational or rotational. Because there are three planes, there can be six abnormal movement patterns (Fig. 5-41). Abnormal translation or rotation in the frontal plane results in lateral listhesis or scoliosis, respectively. In the axial plane, translational motion results in decreased disc space height. Axial rotation of a vertebra results in asymmetric facet joint loading and torsion of the adjacent intervertebral discs. In the sagittal plane, increased translation results in spondylolisthesis, and increased rotation results in kyphosis.

These instability patterns can sometimes be detected on plain x-rays. Sagittal plane displacement of greater than 4.5 mm or 15% is abnormal. Relative sagittal plane angulation of more than 22° is also abnormal. The technique for making these measurements is shown in Figures 5-42 and 5-43. Occasionally, dynamic imaging is needed to detect instability; flexion-extension x-rays are useful in this regard (Fig. 5-44). Most pain receptors in the lumbar spine respond to changes in tension. When there is abnormal motion, there can be accompanying excessive stretch, and thus there may be pain. In addition, these abnormal motions may place neurologic tissue under excessive stretch or compression, resulting in neurologic symptoms.

Stabilization

EXTERNAL

Four main types of orthoses are used for the thoracolumbar and lumbosacral spine: hyperex-

tension braces, molded jackets, rigid braces, and corsets. Hyperextension braces use the three-point fixation concept to prevent flexion. There are two anterior pads, one over the sternum and one over the pubis, and a single posterior pad at the lower thoracic spine (Fig. 5-45). Molded jackets are usually constructed from plastic and can be individually contoured. They may only have a posterior shell with a canvas front or may be designed with a plastic anterior shell. Rigid braces are designed to immobilize the lumbar spine. There are rigid upright posts both laterally and posteriorly. The chair-back brace is an example of this kind of orthosis (Fig. 5-46). Corsets are made of canvas or similar material and may or may not have longitudinal stays. They may wrap around the lumbar spine only or both the thoracic and lumbar areas.

These orthoses have three main purposes. The first is to correct or prevent deformity. For example, after a wedge compression fracture, a hyperextension brace may be prescribed. The second purpose is to immobilize the spinal column. For example, a molded jacket or rigid brace may be prescribed after a lumbar fusion procedure while the bone graft is incorporating. Third, these orthoses can be used to compress the abdomen so as to increase the intra-abdominal pressure and decrease loading on the spinal column. A corset *(text continues on page 133)*

TABLE 5-2. Checklist for the Diagnosis of Clinical Instability in the Lumbar Spine

Element	Point Value
Anterior elements destroyed or unable to function	2
Posterior elements destroyed or unable to function	2
Radiographic criteria	4
Flexion-extension x-rays	
1. Sagittal plane translation >4.5 mm or 15%	2
2. Sagittal plane rotation >15° at L1–L2, L2–L3, and L3–L4 >20° at L4–L5 >25° at L5–S1	2
Cauda equina damage	3
Dangerous loading anticipated	1
Total of 5 or more = Unstable	

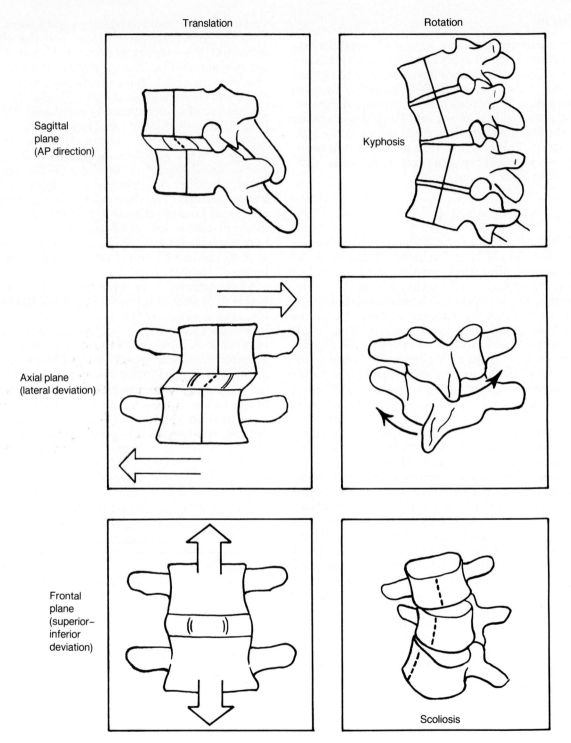

Translation

Rotation

Sagittal plane (AP direction)

Kyphosis

Axial plane (lateral deviation)

Frontal plane (superior–inferior deviation)

Scoliosis

FIGURE 5–41. Abnormal movement patterns.

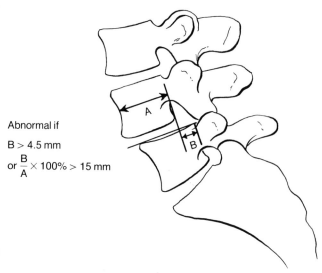

Abnormal if

$B > 4.5 \text{ mm}$

or $\dfrac{B}{A} \times 100\% > 15 \text{ mm}$

FIGURE 5–42. Measurement of lumbar displacement (after White and Panjabi).

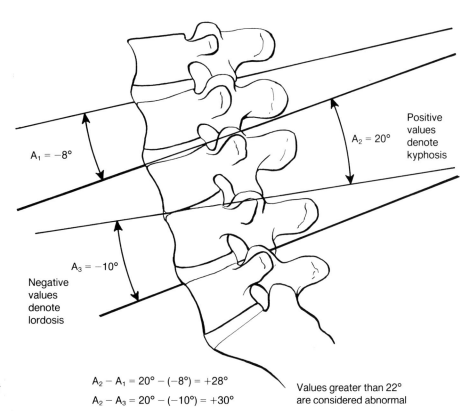

$A_1 = -8°$

$A_2 = 20°$

Positive values denote kyphosis

$A_3 = -10°$

Negative values denote lordosis

FIGURE 5–43. Measurement of lumbar angulation (after White and Panjabi).

$A_2 - A_1 = 20° - (-8°) = +28°$

$A_2 - A_3 = 20° - (-10°) = +30°$

Values greater than 22° are considered abnormal

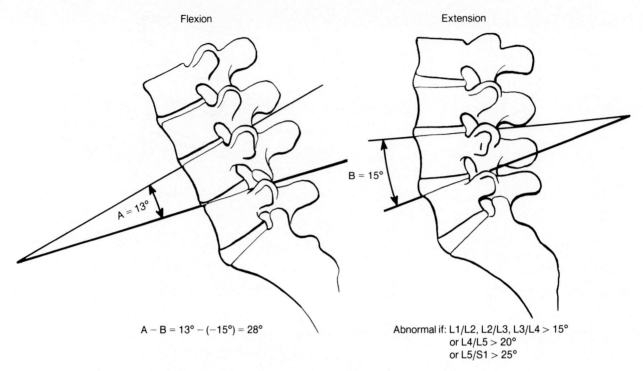

Flexion

Extension

$A = 13°$

$B = 15°$

$A − B = 13° − (−15°) = 28°$

Abnormal if: L1/L2, L2/L3, L3/L4 > 15°
or L4/L5 > 20°
or L5/S1 > 25°

FIGURE 5–44. Measurement of angulation on flexion-extension x-rays.

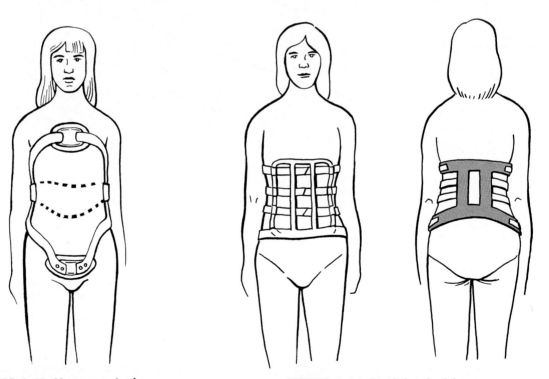

FIGURE 5–45. Hyperextension brace.

FIGURE 5–46. Rigid chair-back brace.

may be prescribed, for example, to a patient with low back pain who has moderate obesity or weak abdominal muscles.

Although these orthoses are commonly prescribed, there is little scientific validity for their use. The experimental data concerning their ability to restrict motion are controversial. Although some of these braces may decrease flexion and extension in the lumbar spine, they may actually increase motion at the thoracolumbar and lumbosacral junctions. The custom-molded thoracolumbosacral orthosis that includes the thigh is the most effective brace for restricting lumbar spine motion from L1–L5. Recent investigations have shown little, if any, increase in intraabdominal pressures using these orthoses.

The most common goal in prescribing an orthosis is to relieve pain. Notwithstanding the above information concerning experimental investigations, a significant number of patients do experience pain relief from these orthoses. The mechanism by which this is achieved will require further study, but it is probably through the provision of proprioceptive feedback.

INTERNAL

Instrumentation of the thoracolumbar spine can be divided into implants used posteriorly and those used anteriorly. Posterior implants include screws, wires, hooks, plates, and rods. In addition to the biomechanical principles described above for cervical implants, many thoracolumbar implants are placed for the purposes of neutralization. In other words, they are inserted without prestressing and are used simply to immobilize levels of the spine that the surgeon chooses to fuse. It is hoped that this rigid internal immobilization will increase the fusion rate. Surprisingly, few scientific data substantiate this approach. Nevertheless, there has been an increase in popularity of many of these implants. In particular, implant systems that incorporate screws placed down the pedicle into the vertebral bodies are becoming increasingly used. One reason for this is that these systems tend to be more rigid than hook or wire systems. Another reason is the fact that a screw has multidirectional stability, in distinct contrast to a hook, which is stable only when loaded in one direction (Fig. 5-47).

Anterior fixation devices are not as popular as posterior systems for various reasons. They are perhaps more technically difficult to insert. They are placed close to major vascular structures and have the potential for causing injury to them.

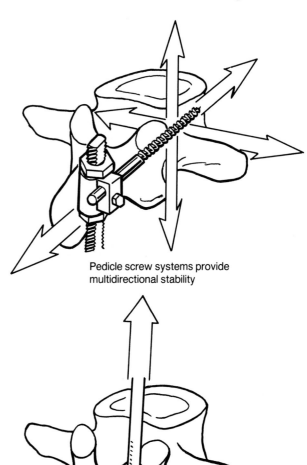

Pedicle screw systems provide multidirectional stability

Hooks provide stability when loaded in only one direction

FIGURE 5–47. Pedicle screw versus hook systems.

This can occur either at the time of implantation or later due to erosion. Biomechanical investigations have supported the rationale for the use of these anterior devices. When there is anterior instability, as with a vertebrectomy, supplementing a graft with instrumentation enhances the stability of the spine. All the anterior devices do well with axial and flexion loading, but with torsional loading, plates and linked rods are superior to single or unlinked rod systems.

KEY POINTS

1. The complex anatomy of the spine results in coupled motion.
2. The mechanical behavior of the spine is nonlinear.
3. Spinal kinetics and kinematics depend on abdominal and paravertebral musculature, and these effects have not been well studied.
4. There are radiographic guidelines for instability both in the cervical and lumbar spines. They do not always correlate with clinical symptoms.
5. Orthoses and internal fixation provide only temporary stabilization of the spine while healing or fusion occurs.

BIBLIOGRAPHY

BOOKS

Groel VK, Weinstein JN. Biomechanics of the spine: Clinical and surgical perspective. Boca Raton, FL: CRC Press, 1990.
White AA, Panjabi MM. Clinical biomechanics of the spine. 2nd ed. Philadelphia: JB Lippincott, 1990.

JOURNALS

Avramov AI, Cavanaugh JM, Ozaktay CA, Getchell TV, King AI. In vitro study of controlled loading on afferent units from lumbar facet joint. J Bone Joint Surg [Am] 1992;74: 1464–1471.
Asano S, Kaneda K, Umehara S, Tadano S. The mechanical properties of the human L4–5 functional spine unit during cycle loading: The structural efforts of the posterior elements. Spine 1992;17:1343–1352.
Axelsson P, Johnsson R, Stromqvist B. Effect of lumbar orthosis on intervertebral mobility: A roentgen stereophotogrammetric analysis. Spine 1992;17:678–681.
Cunningham BW, Sefter JC, Shono Y, McAfee PC. Static and cyclical biomechanical analysis of pedicle screw spinal constructs. Spine 1993;18:1677–1688.
Goel VK, Kong W, Han JS, Weinstein JN, Gilbertson LG. A combined finite element and optimization investigation of lumbar spine mechanics with and without muscles. Spine 1993;18:1531–1541.
Mayer T, Brady S, Bovasso E, Pope P, Gatchel RJ. Noninvasive measurement of cervical tri-planar motion in normal subjects. Spine 1993;18:2191–2195.
Nowinski GP, Visarius H, Nolte LP, Herkowitz HN. A biomechanical comparison of cervical laminaplasty and cervical laminectomy with progressive facetectomy. Spine 1993;18:1995–2004.
Smith MD, Cody DD. Load-bearing capacity of cortico-cancellous bone grafts in the spine. J Bone Joint Surg [Am] 1993;75:1206–1213.
Zdeblick TA, Warden KE, Zou D, McAfee PC, Abitbol JJ. Anterior spinal fixators: A biomechanical in vitro study. Spine 1993;18:513–517.
Zdeblick TA, Abitbol JJ, Kunz DN, McCabe RP, Garfin S. Cervical stability after sequential capsule resection. Spine 1993;18:2005–2008.

Textbook of Spinal Disorders, by Stephen I. Esses.
J. B. Lippincott Company, Philadelphia © 1995.

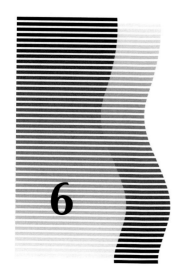

Nonoperative Care of the Spine

6

Stephen I. Esses • Charles Reitman

BED REST
EXERCISE
HEAT
  Phonophoresis
CRYOTHERAPY
ELECTROTHERAPY
  Transcutaneous
   Electrical Nerve
   Stimulation
  Iontophoresis
MANUAL THERAPY
  Chiropractic
  Osteopathy
  Physical Therapy
  Other Techniques

TRACTION
BIOFEEDBACK
ORTHOSES
BACK SCHOOL
MEDICATIONS
  Analgesics
  Nonsteroidal Anti-
   Inflammatory Agents
  Muscle Relaxants

Successful treatment of back disorders begins with a precise diagnosis. Once the cause of the spinal disorder has been identified, appropriate treatment may then be selected. All too often, nonoperative treatments for spinal dysfunction are lumped together, and this often results in unguided or misdirected management. There are myriad nonoperative measures undertaken to treat back pain. Many of them have strong empirical evidence for effectiveness, but truly objective support of their efficacy is often lacking.

BED REST

Bed rest is a frequently implemented form of advice and treatment. There are two theoretical reasons for recommending bed rest: first, intradiscal pressures are reduced in the supine position, and second, many spinal disorders are made worse by activity. Studies have evaluated the role of bed rest for acute back pain, and it appears that bed rest does not alter the natural history of back pain; in fact, it can be detrimental to optimal recovery and to minimizing the time required to return to work. This is particularly true for patients who are not neurologically impaired. If instituted at all, bed rest is rarely indicated for longer than 2 days. Beyond this time, there is the increasing probability that bed rest will result in neuromuscular and cardiopulmonary deconditioning.

EXERCISE

Exercise is bodily or mental exertion, particularly with the aim of training or improvement. Exercise may be active, passive, or resistive. The rationale for exercise is that movement is beneficial to the nutrition of the intervertebral disc, influences the neurophysiologic perception of pain in part through the release of endorphins, and may decrease spinal column loading by strengthening the paravertebral and abdominal muscle groups.

Various exercise programs have been advocated, and clearly the success of the treatment program depends on the selection of the most suitable form of exercise for each patient. Williams introduced flexion exercises consisting of partial sit-ups, pelvic tilts, and stretching of the hip flexors (Fig. 6-1). The reasoning for these exercises is that flexing the lumbar spine opens the intervertebral foramina and facet joints, thereby reducing nerve compression. The theoretical risk of this exercise program is that because it results in increased intradiscal pressures, disc herniation can potentially result.

Extension exercises are aimed at strengthening the back extensor muscles, increasing the range of motion, and shifting the nucleus pulposus of the intervertebral disc anteriorly (Fig. 6-2). Extension exercises are not the same as McKenzie exercises. McKenzie popularized the use of extension exercises in treating the spine, but his prescription of exercise is certainly not limited to extension.

Some exercises are directed at increasing proprioceptive awareness of the spine and strengthening paravertebral muscles. Theoretically, this helps stabilize symptomatic segments of the spine and decreases susceptibility to injury, but there is no scientific documentation that this occurs.

Aerobic exercises are used to improve cardiovascular and general fitness. There is good evidence that people with increased general fitness and endurance of the spine are less prone to back problems.

Exercise is not a panacea for all back conditions. Caution must be used with both passive and active exercises that can load the interverte-

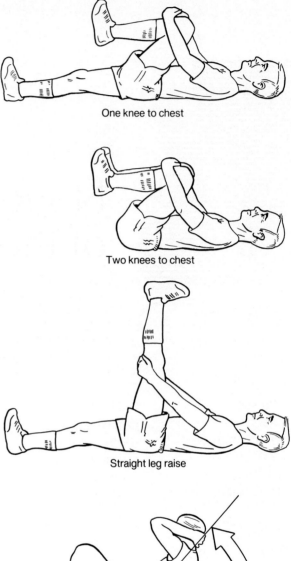

One knee to chest

Two knees to chest

Straight leg raise

FIGURE 6–1. Flexion exercises.

bral disc and facet joints. Exercise may be contraindicated in acute disc prolapse, the multioperated back, spinal stenosis, malignancy, infection, and spondylolisthesis. The use of standardized exercise regimens that essentially assume all

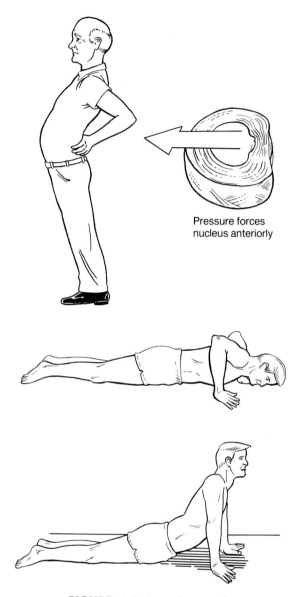

Pressure forces
nucleus anteriorly

FIGURE 6–2. Extension exercises.

back disorders to be the same should be discouraged. Support has been shown for conditioning, strengthening, and flexibility exercises, but there is no indication that one specific type of exercise program is consistently better than another. Success depends on selectivity and progression of exercise based on an ongoing, thorough clinical evaluation.

HEAT

The major effect of heat treatment is local vasodilation, which leads to increased blood flow. This results in an increased metabolic rate, increased clearing of local metabolites, and accelerated soft tissue repair. It is also intended to decrease muscle spasm, improve soft tissue extensibility, assist in resolution of subacute inflammation, decrease pain, and induce a feeling of relaxation and well-being. Contraindications include an anesthetic area, an obtunded patient, areas of poor vascular supply, hemorrhagic diathesis, and malignancy. Heat should not be applied over the gonads or a fetus. Because the effects of heat mimic the inflammatory response, it should not be used for acute conditions.

Heat can be delivered in various forms (Fig. 6-3). The most commonly used are electrically controlled heating pads and heat-retaining chemical packs that are stored in hot water. The duration of application is generally 15 to 20 minutes. These heating systems provide only superficial heat and do not penetrate deeper than the subcutaneous tissues.

Ultrasound is energy produced by a crystal in a sound head that is exposed to an electric current. It delivers heat deeply and can penetrate up to 5 cm through soft tissue. It seems to selectively heat large nerve trunks, scar tissue, tendons, and synovial sheaths over muscle and is particularly effective at heating interfaces between soft tissue and bone. Ultrasound must be administered under the supervision of a health-care practitioner and therefore requires a medical prescription.

There is little scientific documentation supporting the use of heat alone delivered in any form for the treatment of spinal problems. If heat is to be used, it should be combined with exercise.

Phonophoresis

Phonophoresis is the use of ultrasound to transmit topically applied medication, usually steroids, past the epithelium into the soft tissues below. The purpose is to achieve local anti-inflammatory effects noninvasively. Several studies have shown that medication does penetrate into the subcutaneous tissues, but there has been no good determination of the depth of penetration or of medication concentration. No randomized, prospective, controlled studies have

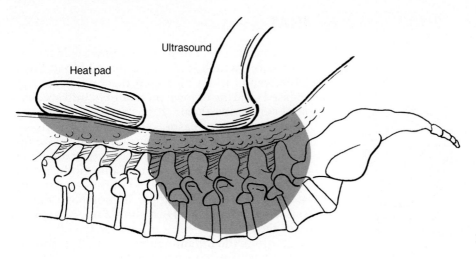

FIGURE 6–3. Heat delivery.

been done on the use and efficacy of phonophoresis in the treatment of spinal disorders. Therefore, despite some data that anti-inflammatory agents can be transmitted to underlying tissues, the relative outcome of such treatment is unknown.

CRYOTHERAPY

The effects of cold treatment are mediated primarily through the vasoconstriction that it causes. This results in decreasing edema, inflammation, and muscle spasm. Cold also slows nerve conduction and thus can decrease pain. It is primarily recommended for acute conditions. Contraindications include hypersensitivity reactions and Raynaud's phenomenon.

Cryotherapy can be applied in several forms, including ice massage, commercial ice packs, ice baths, and ethyl chloride spray. Ice packs are usually applied for 10 minutes, and ice massage is usually applied for 3 to 7 minutes, depending on the area. The patient usually experiences an initial cold sensation, followed shortly afterward by a relatively painful or paradoxical burning sensation that lasts for many minutes. This is followed by a numb sensation, at which time the application duration is at full effectiveness.

When used alone, cryotherapy has no documented efficacy in the treatment of spinal dysfunction. Its primary role is probably the control of treatment-related pain and edema, which facilitates exercise.

ELECTROTHERAPY

The variety in the forms of electrotherapy stems from differences in electric properties and characteristics, each of which is supposed to provide an advantage over another in terms of influencing the physiology of the underlying tissue. In general, electrotherapy is accomplished by applying electrodes to a particular site or sites based on pathology, trigger points, and acupuncture points. The machines are portable but generally require professional personnel for their setup (Fig. 6-4). Although the patient is aware of an electric-type sensation, it is usually not painful. Each treatment usually lasts 15 to 20 minutes.

High-voltage galvanic stimulation has a characteristic monopolar twin-peak wave form (Fig. 6-5). The high voltage produces spontaneous breakdown in skin resistance, thereby allowing more current to pass to the deeper tissues with fewer cutaneous effects. The rationale for its use is to provide direct stimulation of nerve fibers, which indirectly alters blood flow. It is intended to promote wound healing, decrease edema, modulate pain, and stimulate the neuromuscular system. There are no controlled prospective studies to substantiate its efficacy.

Interferential current is a medium-frequency current. Its purported advantage is the development of a stronger, summated current at the point of crossing of two perpendicular currents of slightly dissimilar frequencies (Fig. 6-6). This allows for greater depth of stimulation and per-

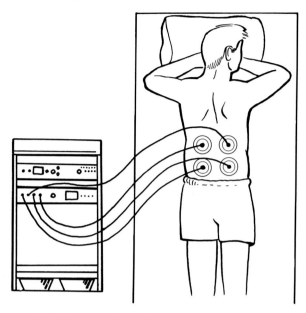

FIGURE 6-4. Electrotherapy machine and setup.

fusion of a larger volume of tissue than does current from bipolar leads. Its proposed effects are the same as those of high-voltage galvanic stimulation. Again, there are no studies proving its efficacy.

Transcutaneous Electrical Nerve Stimulation

Transcutaneous electrical nerve stimulation (TENS) is low-voltage electric stimulation applied with varying frequencies and wave forms.

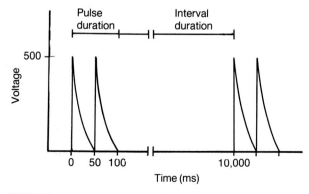

FIGURE 6-5. Wave pattern of high-voltage galvanic stimulation.

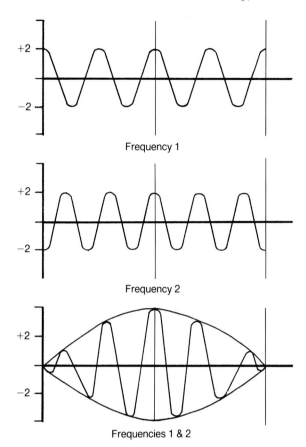

FIGURE 6-6. Wave pattern of interferential current.

Its main effect is derived through interaction with the sensory nervous system. Proposed mechanisms of action include altered sensitivity of peripheral receptors, the gate theory, alteration of internal levels of glucocorticoids, enkephalins, or endorphins, and central biasing in the midbrain. None of these theories have been specifically proven. The frequency and placement of electrodes are crucial to the success of TENS; therefore, skill in application and patient education play a critical role in outcome (Fig. 6-7).

Contraindications to TENS are few. It should not be used in the presence of a pacemaker, nor should it be placed over the carotid sinus, due to potential production of a vasovagal response. There are no data to confirm its safety during pregnancy. The primary problem with TENS arises from skin sensitivity to the electrodes or tape.

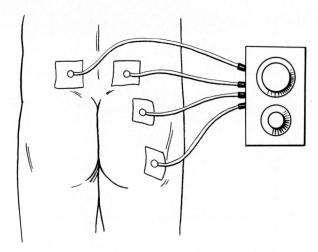

FIGURE 6–7. Transcutaneous electrical stimulation for low back pain.

TENS has been shown to be more effective than placebo at decreasing subjective symptoms of pain, but it has not been shown to accelerate return to work or to a usual level of function. TENS appears to be an effective modality to decrease pain. It is probably best used to facilitate exercise training and return to function.

Iontophoresis

Iontophoresis is the use of electrotherapy in driving topically applied medication into subcutaneous tissues. It involves the transport of ionic molecules by means of direct current using appropriate electrode polarity. The purpose is to achieve specific, local anti-inflammatory effects noninvasively. There is considerable debate as to whether iontophoresis is an effective means of medicinal transmission. There is no scientifically sound study to validate its use.

MANUAL THERAPY

Manual therapy refers to any treatment in which the therapist uses his or her body to treat the patient directly. Thus, manual therapy includes mobilization, manipulation, and massage. Mobilization involves the movement of a joint through its physiologic range. The therapist can use various combinations of amplitude, frequency, duration, rhythm, and direction of movement. Manipulation involves a sudden thrust of the joint complex beyond the normal physiologic range without exceeding the boundaries of anatomic integrity (Fig. 6-8). It is sometimes accompanied by an audible pop. Mobilization and manipulation are proposed to produce their effects in similar fashions: alteration of the neurophysiologic perception of pain, release of entrapped synovial folds, stretch of segmental muscles, initiating spindle-mediated reflexes that relieve the state of hypertonicity, reduction of a subluxation, and breaking of intra-articular adhesions. The goal of manual therapy is to decrease pain as well as to increase proprioceptive input to the spine and improve function. Spinal manipulation has been subjected to well-

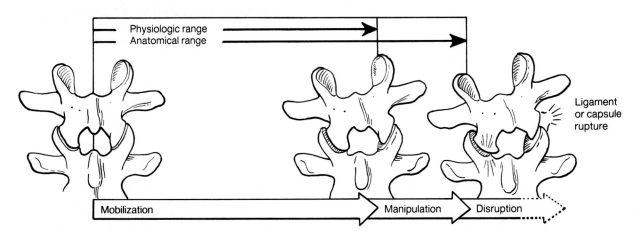

FIGURE 6–8. Manual therapy of the spine.

controlled prospective clinical studies. These indicate a beneficial effect for the first few weeks after onset of low back pain. There is no documentation that manipulation provides any long-term benefit.

Massage is a group of systematic maneuvers of body tissues, usually performed with the hands. The intent is to improve circulation, encourage relaxation, and decrease pain through interaction with the nervous system. Studies have suggested that although massage seems to effect temporary pain relief in many conditions, it does not necessarily contribute to long-term pain control or outcome. Massage may be useful as an ancillary treatment to help facilitate exercise.

Chiropractic

Chiropractic is a school of thought that postulates that many pathologic conditions, both spinal and nonspinal, are due to malalignment or subluxation in the vertebral column or pelvis. Treatment of these conditions, therefore, is directed toward correcting the supposedly abnormal structural relations. Chiropractic philosophy has changed significantly in the last few decades, and most chiropractors do not now use manipulation to treat conditions such as diabetes mellitus or hypertension. For the most part, chiropractors treat back and neck pain. The major argument against the use of chiropractic treatment is the lack of scientific documentation that these malalignments exist, and the fact that major vertebral malalignments, such as spondylolisthesis, can exist without untoward bodily effects.

Osteopathy

Osteopathy postulates that abnormalities in structure and mechanics adversely affect the harmony and efficiency of the body. The primary goal of osteopathic treatment is to restore function and minimize mechanical stresses. The basic difference from chiropractic is that emphasis is placed on dynamic mechanics rather than positional relationships. The basic osteopathic spinal lesion is a condition of impaired intervertebral joint mobility, and treatment is thus aimed at restoring this mobility. Soft tissue and joint function are assessed. Manipulation is a primary form of treatment when movement is indicated.

Physical Therapy

The physical therapist is an allied health professional. Patients are referred to physical therapists through medical prescriptions. These therapists are trained in the treatment of neuromuscular and skeletal dysfunction. They can use any or all of the modalities included in this chapter. The physician guiding patient care should be aware of the various modalities being used. It is important that the physician accurately diagnose the problem and convey any specific contraindications to the physical therapist. By and large, physical therapists are specialists in exercise training but use other techniques as well to facilitate rehabilitation and recovery.

Other Techniques

There are many alternate forms of manual therapeutic techniques. Although they are not as common as chiropractic, physical therapy, or osteopathy, it is not unusual for a medical practitioner to be exposed to these philosophies, particularly when caring for chronic back pain patients who are searching for a cure.

The *Alexander technique* promotes improved use of the body during all activities by enhancing balance, ease and efficiency of movement, and function. Its goals are to recognize and correct detrimental postural habits, eliminate excessive muscle tension, and align the entire musculoskeletal system. This is done through verbal instruction and gentle guidance, and is thus more a process of thinking than a manual treatment regimen.

Shiatsu has evolved from the philosophies of Eastern medicine. It is based on dynamic networks of energy throughout the body called *meridians* and is dedicated to maintaining homeostasis through manual means. Practitioners use pressure along these meridians to treat disorders of the spine and also to maintain general well-being.

The *Traeger approach* is based on learning or relearning ways to allow enhancement of movement. This is attained by gentle manual movements and stimulation.

Craniosacral therapy is based on the hypothesis that there is rhythmic mobile activity of the craniosacral system that is composed of the meningeal membranes, cranial sutures, cerebrospinal fluid (CSF), and the structures that produce

CSF. Changes in the symmetry, quantity, or quality of this movement are thought to result in bodily disorders, including neck and back pain. Abnormalities in the craniosacral system are reported to be restored through gentle manual guidance and pressure.

Structural integration is also called *Rolfing*, after its founder, Ida Rolf. Her studies led to the belief that structure encompasses myofascial relationships of balance, symmetry, and energy flow as well as the psychological characteristics of behavior, attitudes, and capacities. Imbalances supposedly cause compensation, deformity, and strain as soft tissues and joints seek new but less efficient positions to acquire a more appropriate equilibrium. Rolfing involves a 10-hour cycle of deep, manual soft tissue mobilization of the entire body. The pelvis and spine are especially important in the treatment scheme.

TRACTION

Traction is a distractive force applied to the vertebral column. Its intended purposes include mobilization of soft tissues or joints, nerve root decompression, unloading of the disc or facet joints, and reduction of a herniated disc. Traction can be accomplished in many ways, and the type, intensity, and duration of traction should be based on a thorough assessment of each patient (Fig. 6-9).

Traction can be applied manually or on a traction table using a harness attached to weights or a calibrated motor. In inversion traction, the subject wears boots that hook over a fixed bar. In the inverted position, the weight of the body and gravity provide the traction force. Cotrell traction uses a portable frame with a pulley system attached to an overhead crossbar. Patients apply a harness to the pelvic area and position themselves supine in about 90° of hip and knee flexion. The pulley system is fastened to the harness and controls the amount of traction applied. Traction can be applied in three dimensions using special frames, such as that developed by Lind, and is commonly called autotraction.

Several controlled prospective studies have failed to demonstrate the efficacy of traction for the treatment of vertebral column disorders. Contraindications include malignancy, sepsis, vascular compromise, and any condition in which movement is potentially dangerous. In addition, precautions should be taken in the presence of inflammatory spondylitis, aortic aneu-

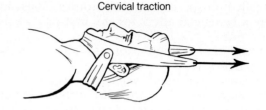

Cervical traction

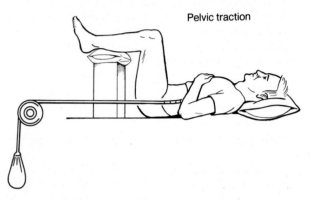

Pelvic traction

FIGURE 6–9. Cervical and pelvic traction.

rysm, vertigo, pregnancy, and hiatal hernia. Inversion traction should be used with medical supervision because of the risk of periorbital and pharyngeal petechiae, headache, and blurring of vision. For the individual who experiences temporary relief with traction, the use of this technique concurrent with exercise may allow earlier, active, more vigorous training and facilitate recovery.

BIOFEEDBACK

Biofeedback is the use of equipment that reflects the state of internal physiology, both normal and abnormal, in the form of auditory or visual signals. The patient is made aware of his or her physiologic state, and the goal is to alter these neuromuscular signals for symptomatic improvement. This includes relief of both autonomic and somatic symptoms.

Initially, biofeedback requires the use of equipment of varying portability and sophistication. Use of the equipment is relatively straightforward. The learning begins in a controlled environment to optimize the patient's ease of increasing conscious awareness of the physiologic state. Over time, it is hoped that patients can transfer their learning to the setting of their usual activities.

It is unclear whether neuromuscular feedback is related to symptoms. For example, although it may be possible for a patient to decrease paraspinal electromyographic activity, this may not result in any decrease in pain.

Biofeedback takes time to learn and thus is indicated only in well-motivated patients. Although there is some empiric evidence that it can result in pain relief, there is no specific study to support its efficacy in the treatment of spinal disorders.

ORTHOSES

The major use of cervical orthoses has been for traumatic conditions. The various types of cervical orthoses are discussed in Chapter 5. Thoracolumbar braces have their major role in the treatment of deformity such as scoliosis and Scheuermann's disease and are discussed in Chapter 14.

Despite the paucity of scientific evidence documenting the benefit of lumbosacral braces, they are one of the most common forms of treatment for low back pain. There are two theoretical reasons for using these braces. A tightly applied brace can increase intra-abdominal pressure; this decreases the force of contraction of the iliopsoas and thus reduces the compressive force on the lumbar spine. The second reason for using these braces is to reduce motion of the lumbar spine, particularly in patients who have multilevel degenerative disease. Interestingly, there is good scientific documentation that these braces paradoxically increase lumbar spine motion rather than reducing it. The disadvantages of bracing most often cited are the potential deconditioning and laxity of the abdominal musculature with prolonged use.

BACK SCHOOL

Some have proposed that educating patients about neck and low back pain would result in an improved ability to manage their symptoms. Among the specific goals of such back schools are increasing patient self-confidence, avoiding unnecessary and potentially harmful treatment, and bringing about an earlier return to work. Although there was initial enthusiasm for this concept, it has been tempered by the lack of documented long-term benefit. For patients with acute low back pain, studies have shown that the back school approach is very effective in returning patients to work. There are many different back schools, each with its own curriculum and goals. The place of these programs in the treatment of spinal disorders remains to be clearly identified.

MEDICATIONS

Analgesics

Salicylate preparations are the most common nonnarcotic analgesics. Commercial preparations are often combined with small amounts of other drugs, such as caffeine. The mechanism of action of salicylates has not been well defined but probably involves prostaglandin modulation. The major side effects of salicylates include gastrointestinal upset, auditory impairment, and a prolonged prothrombin time.

Acetaminophen is becoming an increasingly popular nonnarcotic analgesic. It appears to be somewhat safer than salicylates, but long-term use can result in significant renal disease.

Narcotic analgesics must be used with caution. Habituation and addiction can occur with even very short durations of administration. In general, therefore, they should not be used for chronic disorders. Morphine, codeine, and meperidine are commonly prescribed narcotics. Several morphine derivatives and congeners have been developed and are also commonly used. All narcotics depress the respiratory center; this effect is dose-related. In addition, all narcotics increase sphincter tone and thus should be used judiciously in patients with a history of biliary colic, renal stones, and prostatic hypertrophy. The most common side effect is constipation, so most patients receiving narcotics benefit from an accompanying laxative.

Nonsteroidal Anti-Inflammatory Agents

More than 20 nonsteroidal anti-inflammatory drugs (NSAIDs) are currently available. They can be grouped according to their chemical class (Table 6-1). These drugs have an analgesic and anti-inflammatory effect. The analgesic action is probably due to cyclooxygenase inhibition with

TABLE 6–1. **Nonsteroidal Anti-Inflammatory Agents**

Group	Chemical Name	Trade Name
Salicylates	Aspirin	Bayer
	Enteric-coated	Ecotrin, Easprin
	Time-release	Zorprin
Substituted salicylates	Diflunisal	Dolobid
	Aspirin with antacid	Ascriptin
Proprionic acid derivatives	Ibuprofen	Motrin, Rufen, Advil, Nuprin
	Naproxen	Naprosyn
	Sodium naproxen	Anaprox
	Fenoprofen calcium	Nalfon
	Ketoprofen	Orudis
	Flurbiprofen	Ansaid
	Oxaprozin	Daypro
Pyrrole acetic acid derivatives	Sulindac	Clinoril
	Indomethacin	Indocin
	Tolmetin sodium	Tolectin
	Diclofenac	Voltaren
	Ketorolac tromethamine	Toradol
Oxicam	Piroxicam	Feldene
Fenamate	Meclofenamate sodium	Meclomen
Pyrazalones	Phenylbutazone	Butazolidin
Pyranocarboxylic acid	Etodolac	Lodine
Naphthylakanones	Nabumetone	Relafen

resultant decreased prostaglandin production. The anti-inflammatory effect is probably due to inhibition of a leukocyte activation.

Because of the many NSAIDs currently available, there is sometimes confusion about what drug to prescribe. In general, the response to an NSAID is idiosyncratic: there is no way of knowing which drug will be most beneficial for a particular patient. Therefore, the clinician should prescribe an NSAID for a short duration, assess the patient's response, and then decide whether to continue with that drug or to change to an NSAID of another chemical class.

Various side effects and toxic reactions can occur with the NSAIDs. The most common are gastrointestinal upset, headache, dizziness, and rashes. Older patients are particularly prone to gastrointestinal bleeding, and this may occur without patient recognition. For this reason, H_2 blockers are sometimes prescribed with the NSAID. In addition, follow-up examinations should include a complete blood count. Al-though rare, bone marrow suppression and renal toxicity have been reported, and blood testing should be done at serial intervals in patients receiving long-term NSAID treatment.

Muscle Relaxants

Various medications are used to provide muscle relaxation. Some of these, such as diazepam, have major depressive central nervous system effects. Others, such as cyclobenzaprine, have a more selective effect on skeletal muscles. The rationale for their use is that many patients with spinal disorders have a secondary muscular spasm that in itself causes pain. A good example is hyperextension injury of the cervical spine. Plain x-rays often show loss of cervical lordosis due to muscle spasm, and these patients may benefit from muscle relaxants. There is no indication that one particular agent is more effective than another.

KEY POINTS

1. Bed rest is of limited use and may be detrimental for periods of longer than 48 to 72 hours.
2. Fitness training is of value in the treatment and prevention of some spinal problems, but exercise is not a panacea.
3. Many of the nonoperative modalities currently used have little if any scientific validity and have no use when prescribed alone.
4. The judicious use of analgesics and nonsteroidal anti-inflammatory agents may help reduce symptoms during the time of recovery from spinal injury.
5. The success of nonoperative treatment depends in large part on the patient's participation in his or her care. In almost all instances, treatment can be transferred entirely to the patient's responsibility as a home program.

BIBLIOGRAPHY

BOOKS

Bourdillon JF, Day EA, Bookhout MR. Spinal manipulation (5th ed). Oxford, Butterworth-Heinemann, 1992

Mayer TG, Mooney V, Gatchel RJ. Contemporary conservative care for painful spinal disorders. Philadelphia, Lea & Febiger, 1991

White A, Anderson R (eds). Conservative care of low back pain. Baltimore, Williams & Wilkins, 1991

JOURNALS

Deyo RA, Walsh N, Martin D, Schoenfeld L, Ramamurthy S. A controlled trial of transcutaneous electronic nerve stimulation (TENS) and exercise for chronic low-back pain. N. Engl. J. Med. 322: 1627–1634, 1990.

Faas A, Chavannes AW, van Eijk JTM, Gubbels JW. A randomized, placebo-controlled trial of exercise therapy in patients with acute low-back pain. Spine 1993; 18: (11) 1388–1395.

Gilbert JR, Taylor DW, Hildebrand A, Evans C. Clinical trial of common treatments for low-back pain in family practice. Br. Med. J. 291: 791–794, 1985.

Hansen FR, Bendix T, Skov P, Jensen CV, Kristensen JH, Krohn L, Schioeler H. Intensive, dynamic back-muscle exercises, conventional physiotherapy, or placebo-control treatment of low-back pain: A randomized, observer-blind trial. Spine 1993; 18:98–108.

Quebec Task Force on Spinal Disorders. Scientific approach to the assessment and management of activity-related spinal disorders: A monograph for clinicians. Report of the Quebec Task Force on spinal disorders. Spine 1987; 7(suppl):S1–S59.

Spratt KF, Weinstein JN, Lehmann TR, Woody J, Sayre H. Efficacy of flexion and extension treatments incorporating braces for low-back pain patients with retrodisplacement, spondylolisthesis, or normal sagittal translation. Spine 1993; 18:1839–1849.

Textbook of Spinal Disorders, by Stephen I. Esses.
J. B. Lippincott Company, Philadelphia © 1995.

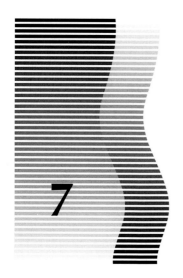

Basic Principles of Surgery

7

SURGICAL GOALS
  Decompression
  Stabilization
  Correction of
    Deformity
SURGICAL
  APPROACHES
  Posterior
  Anterior
  Other
DECOMPRESSION
  Nerve Root
  Dural Sac

STABILIZATION
  Rationale for Fusion
  Physiology of Spinal
    Fusion
  Bone Graft
  Types of Spinal
    Fusion
  Spinal Implants
SPECIAL
  CONSIDERATIONS
  Surgical
    Complications
  Spinal Cord
    Monitoring

Although there have been sporadic attempts to treat spinal problems with surgery since the time of the Egyptian dynasties, spinal surgery is a new field. Only in the last 50 years has surgical treatment of spinal disorders become an accepted therapeutic modality. Because the surgical experience has been rather short, the proper place of many surgical spine procedures remains to be determined. One must be cautious when assessing operative fads until careful long-term follow-up is available. To this end, many centers are now realizing the importance of well-documented prospective outcome studies. These have been sadly lacking in the past and make critical evaluation of many surgical spinal procedures difficult.

Surgery should not be used as a last resort in treatment; it is just one of many treatment options for various spinal conditions. In some instances, it can be the preferred choice; in other situations, alternative therapies may be superior.

Specific surgical procedures and their indications will be discussed in conjunction with the spinal disorders they are used for. In this chapter, however, basic principles will be reviewed along with special considerations that pertain to the field of spinal surgery.

SURGICAL GOALS

There are three fundamental goals of spinal surgery: decompression of neural elements, stabilization of unstable spinal levels, and, occasionally, correction of deformity. Many surgical cases have more than one of these goals. For each surgical procedure, the surgeon and patient must be clear as to the specific objectives. Preoperative planning by the surgeon and open discussions with the patient are vital.

Decompression

Decompression involves the removal of any material that places undue pressure on neural tissue. The latter may include the spinal cord, spinal nerves, conus medullaris, or cauda equina. Offending elements are usually disc, bone, or tumor. Rarely, other elements, including blood and pus, can cause undue pressure that results in neurologic dysfunction.

Preoperative planning requires precise localization of the compressive lesion. This requires a meticulous physical examination and confirmation using one or more imaging techniques. In addition, every attempt is made to identify the nature of the compression to plan operative strategy.

Successful decompressive surgery requires the removal of the compressive lesion. Although this principle is obvious, it has not always been adhered to, primarily because of technical considerations. For example, consider a metastatic tumor deposit in the vertebral body at T7 causing spinal cord compression by extension posteriorly into the spinal canal. Decompression of the spinal cord would necessitate removal of the tumor mass extending into the canal. In the past, however, because many surgeons were not familiar with anterior spinal approaches, this type of case was often treated by laminectomy (Fig. 7-1). It is not surprising, therefore, that the results of surgery were so poor. In general, anterior compression in the cervical and thoracic spine requires anterior decompression. In the lumbar spine, below the level of the conus medullaris, it is possible to retract the dural sac with less danger, and thus some anterior lesions can be removed through a posterior approach.

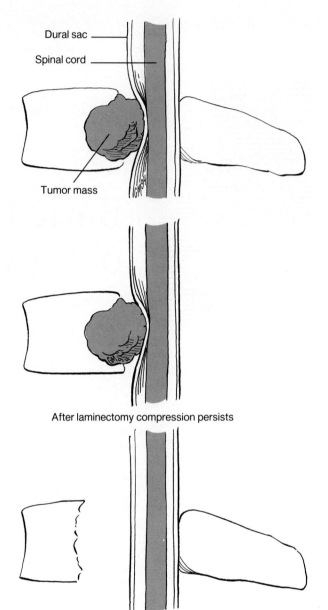

After laminectomy compression persists

Removal of tumor by anterior approach eliminates compression

FIGURE 7–1. Anterior compression of the spinal cord.

Stabilization

As discussed in Chapter 5, in some instances certain levels of the spine are considered unstable—that is, the kinematics have been altered such that motion is accompanied by pain, neurologic injury, or deformity. In other situations, motion of specific spinal levels is accompanied by pain due to pathologic changes in the intervertebral disc or facet joints. In both of these scenarios, the goal of surgical treatment is to stabilize the affected levels of the spine and eliminate motion. Although it may be possible to temporarily immobilize segments of the spine using rigid implants, they cannot withstand loading indefinitely: all materials ultimately fail with continued stress. Thus, with regard to spinal surgery, permanent stabilization is synonymous with fusion. A spinal fusion exists when there is bone solidly bridging one vertebra to another. Fusions are classified depending on where this bridging bony mass is positioned.

Correction of Deformity

Spinal deformity can occur in any of the three anatomic planes. Occasionally a surgeon may wish to correct the deformity. Indications include pain, neurologic dysfunction, pulmonary compromise, progression, or cosmesis. In the past, the deformity was usually corrected by traction or serial casting before surgery. With the development of modern spinal instrumentation, many deformities can now be corrected intraoperatively. Almost always, this is accompanied by the risk of neurologic injury; thus, such surgery should be undertaken judiciously only by the experienced spinal surgeon. The implants used to correct the deformity will eventually fail unless a fusion procedure is done concomitantly. It is often said that after surgery, there is a race between implant failure and the development of an adequate fusion mass.

SURGICAL APPROACHES

Posterior

The most common surgical approach to the spine is directly posterior—that is, posterior to or behind the spinal cord (Fig. 7-2). The spinous processes, laminae, and facet joints of the cervical, thoracic, and lumbar spine can be exposed. In most instances, the patient is positioned prone (Fig. 7-3). This requires very secure control of the airway. Excessive pressure on the eyes, nipples, and genitalia must be prevented; also, undue traction on the brachial plexus or pressure on the ulnar nerve must be avoided. When working on the thoracolumbar region, any abdominal pressure is avoided, because this will result in increased operative blood loss. This occurs because with abdominal pressure, the vena cava is compressed and venous return is diverted to Batson's plexus, increasing the pressure in the spinal venous complex and epidural veins. Various frames that allow abdominal decompression and x-ray access for the prone patient have been developed. These provide many advantages when compared with the use of chest rolls or bolsters.

A midline incision is carried down to the deep fascia, and subperiosteal dissection is done to retract the paravertebral muscles. These muscles have segmental innervation from the posterior primary rami. MacNab has shown that there is some denervation of the paravertebral muscles after posterior exposure, but this rarely leads to clinical sequelae. This approach is extensile—that is, it can be extended in either direction. In addition, it is relatively free of complications.

Occasionally, the approach is performed with the patient on his or her side in a lateral position. This is most frequently used for unilateral exposure in the lumbar spine.

The midline incision is the most commonly used for the posterior approach (Fig. 7-4). However, there are modifications in which a paramedian incision is used and the muscle fibers of the sacrospinalis muscle are split. The advantages of this approach include preservation of the midline structures, which may be providing some stability, as in cases of spondylolysis, and the ability to expose lateral structures more easily.

Anterior

The standard anterior approach to the cervical spine involves dissecting longitudinally between the fibers of the platysma muscle and developing a plane anterior to the sternomastoid muscle. The skin incision may be longitudinal or transverse. This muscle is then retracted laterally, along with the carotid sheath (Fig. 7-5). Occasionally, the omohyoid muscle may have to be divided to optimize the exposure. The trachea and esophagus are retracted medially. With these structures mobilized, the prevertebral fascia is identified and can be split longitudinally. This approach can be used to expose from C2 distally to T1 or T2. Some landmarks may be useful in

(text continues on page 153)

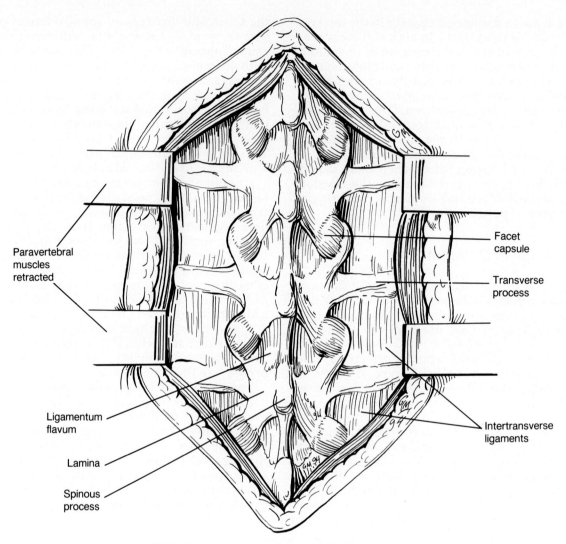

Paravertebral muscles retracted

Facet capsule

Transverse process

Ligamentum flavum

Lamina

Spinous process

Intertransverse ligaments

FIGURE 7–2. Posterior exposure of the lumbar spine.

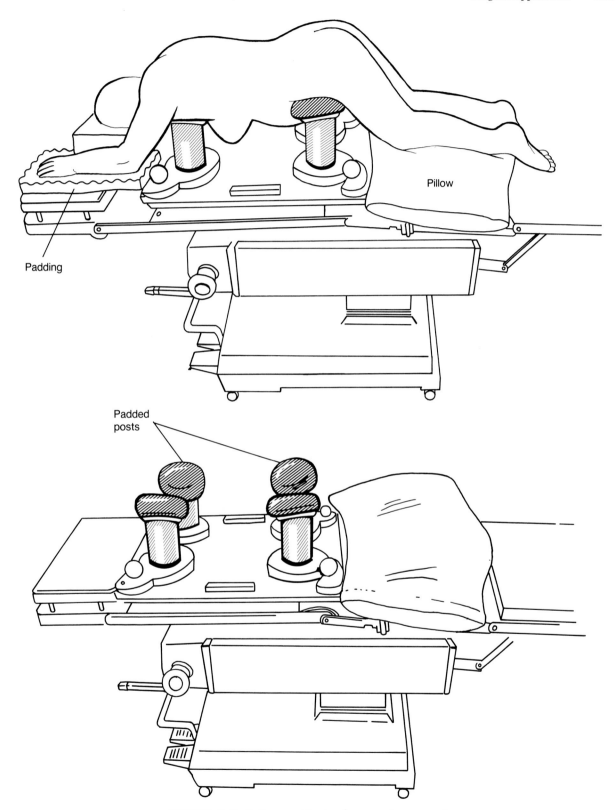

Padding

Pillow

Padded
posts

FIGURE 7–3. Patient positioning for posterior approach.

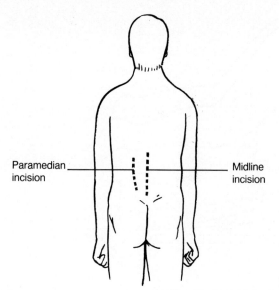

FIGURE 7–4. Posterior spinal incisions.

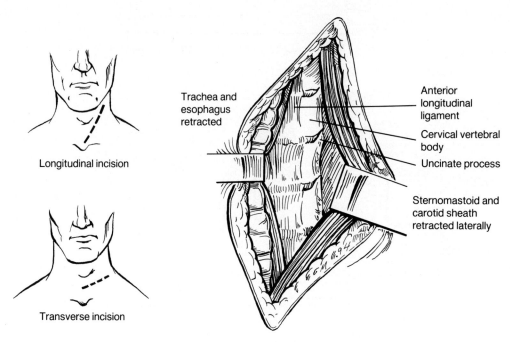

FIGURE 7–5. Anterior approach to the cervical spine.

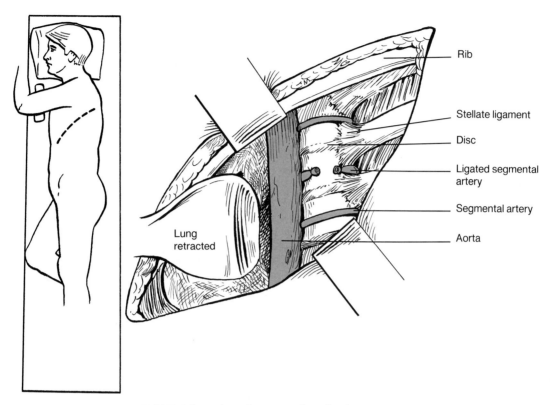

Rib

Stellate ligament

Disc

Ligated segmental
artery

Segmental artery

Aorta

Lung
retracted

FIGURE 7–6. Anterior approach to the thoracic spine.

planning the incision. The hyoid bone is located anterior to the third cervical vertebra. The thyroid cartilage is anterior to the fourth and fifth vertebrae, and the cricoid cartilage is anterior to the sixth vertebra.

The most common anterior approach to the thoracic spine involves a thoracotomy (Fig. 7-6). This is usually done on the left side because mobilization of the aorta is easier than that of the vena cava. In addition, it is easier to repair the aorta than the thin-walled vena cava if injury to one of these vessels occurs. Once the skin and subcutaneous tissues have been incised through a curvilinear incision, the chest may be opened either by transecting the intercostal muscles or by excising a rib. The latter allows more working area. The pleura is then incised and the lung gently retracted. The segmental vessels over each vertebral body to be exposed are identified and ligated. The aorta can then be gently mobilized and retracted.

To expose the thoracolumbar junction, the diaphragm must be taken down. Before incising the diaphragmatic fibers, the peritoneum and its contents must be mobilized off the inferior surface of the diaphragm and the retroperitoneal space opened.

There are three major anterior approaches to the lumbar spine (Figs. 7-7 and 7-8): the anterolateral approach, made through a flank incision with the patient on his or her side; the anterior retroperitoneal approach, with the patient supine through a longitudinal paramedian incision; and an anterior transperitoneal approach, through a midline incision.

The anterolateral flank approach provides excellent exposure from L1 to L4 and does not involve any manipulation of the vena cava. It is extensile proximally and can be confluent with anterior exposure of the thoracic spine. Its disadvantages are that it involves muscle-splitting, and thus there is increased postoperative pain.

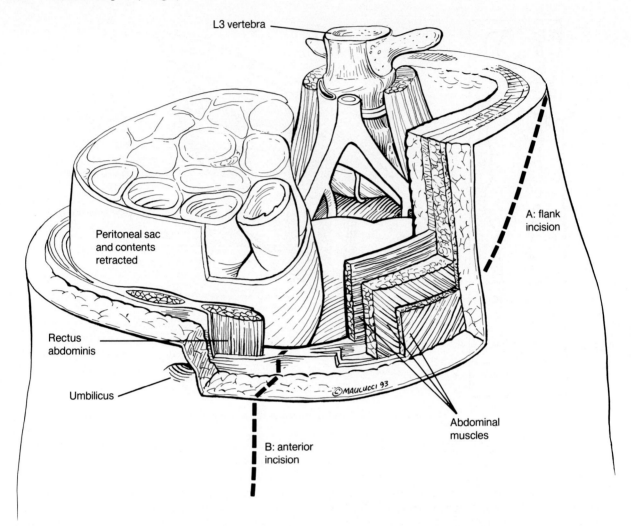

L3 vertebra

Peritoneal sac
and contents
retracted

A: flank
incision

Rectus
abdominis

Umbilicus

©MAULUCCI 93

Abdominal
muscles

B: anterior
incision

FIGURE 7–7. Anterior retroperitoneal approaches to the lumbar spine.

This approach does not provide generous access to the lumbosacral junction and may be associated with damage to the sympathetic chain.

The anterior retroperitoneal approach does not involve transection of muscle fibers. The rectus abdominis is mobilized medially and the retroperitoneal space opened. The peritoneum is not entered, its contents being retracted to one side. This approach allows excellent exposure of the lower lumbar spine. Exposure more proximally, however, requires mobilization of the great vessels and the bifurcation.

Anterior exposure of the lumbar spine through a transperitoneal approach is rarely necessary. It involves opening the peritoneal cavity and thus may be associated with intraoperative contamination and postoperative volvulus, ileus, or adhesions.

Other

Although used only occasionally, there are other surgical approaches that reach specific areas of the spine. There are two ways in which the anterior aspect of the atlas can be exposed (Fig. 7-9). A direct anterior approach through the mouth involves dissection through the posterior pharyngeal wall. Occasionally, splitting of the hard palate is necessary to increase the exposure.

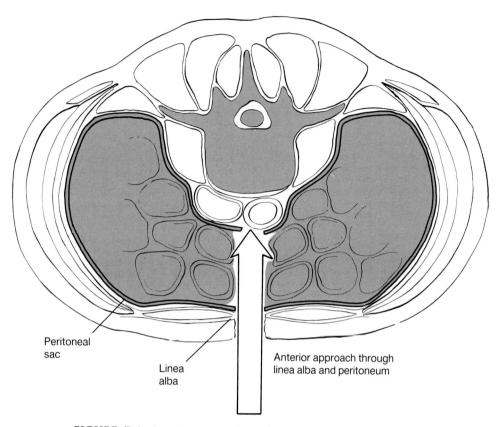

FIGURE 7–8. Anterior transperitoneal approach to the lumbar spine.

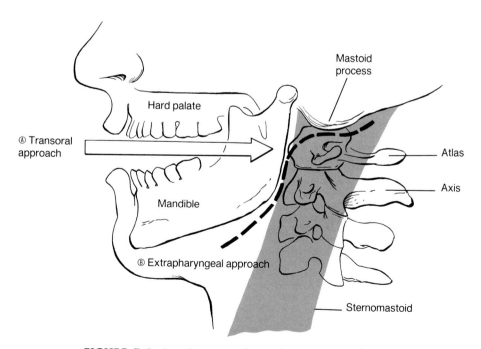

FIGURE 7–9. Anterior approaches to the upper cervical spine.

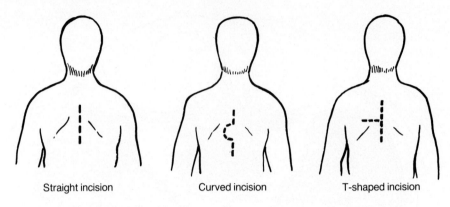

Straight incision   Curved incision   T-shaped incision

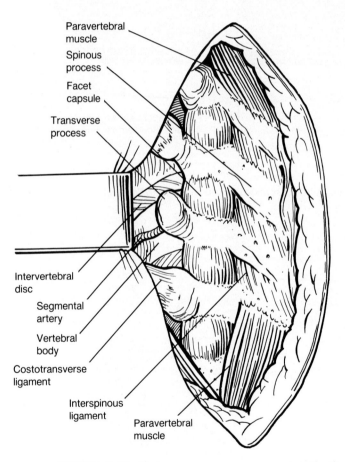

Paravertebral
muscle

Spinous
process

Facet
capsule

Transverse
process

Intervertebral
disc

Segmental
artery

Vertebral
body

Costotransverse
ligament

Interspinous
ligament

Paravertebral
muscle

FIGURE 7–10. Costotransversectomy approach to the thoracic spine.

An alternative is to detach the sternomastoid muscle from its origin off the mastoid process and to dissect posterior to the carotid sheath.

The anterior cervicothoracic junction may be exposed by splitting the sternum. The trachea and esophagus are retracted medially, and the common carotid artery is retracted laterally. To gain optimal exposure distally, the left innominate vein can be ligated.

The cervicothoracic junction and upper thoracic spine can also be exposed through a transaxillary approach. With the patient in the lateral decubitus position, an incision is made at about the level of the third rib. The rib is then excised to gain more working room. The pleura is incised and the lung retracted. Segmental vessels are ligated or cauterized. The pericardium and great vessels can then be easily retracted. This approach allows excellent exposure of the upper thoracic vertebrae. The main disadvantage of this approach is the depth of the wound, which necessitates long instruments and good illumination.

The lateral aspects of the vertebral bodies can be accessed through a costotransversectomy approach (Fig. 7-10). This is a posterolateral approach in which the heads of the ribs at one or more levels are excised. In some instances, the transverse process can also be divided and removed. The approach remains extrapleural with retraction of the pleura and the lung anteriorly. The skin incision can be straight, curved, or "T"-shaped.

DECOMPRESSION

Nerve Root

Cervical nerve root compression is a cause of arm pain, paresthesia, and weakness. A thorough history and physical examination should allow determination of the specific nerve root or roots involved. Using one or more imaging techniques, confirmation of the symptomatic root can be made. The key to successful surgical nerve root decompression is accurate identification of the site and source of compression. The cervical root can be compressed by disc or bone (Fig. 7-11). Disc herniation can occur medially or laterally and may be contained or extruded through the posterior longitudinal ligament. Identification of

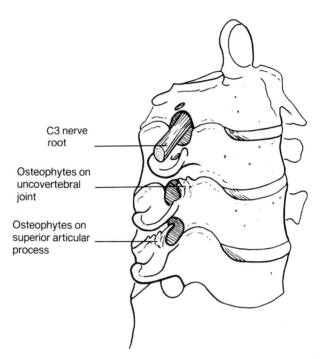

FIGURE 7–11. Osteophyte causing compression of the cervical nerve root.

the exact site of disc compression will allow selection of the appropriate surgical approach. The bony boundaries of the cervical neural foramen are the pars lateralis above and below, the uncovertebral joint anteromedially, and the facet joint posterolaterally. In most instances, bony stenosis of the foramen is due to osteophyte formation of the uncovertebral joint and collapse of the height of the foramen from disc degeneration. Under these circumstances, an anterior surgical approach is appropriate. The uncovertebral osteophytes can be removed and the height of the foramen can be restored by distracting the disc space and inserting a bone graft (Fig. 7-12). In those rare instances in which there are osteophytes from the facet joint causing nerve root compression, a posterior approach is appropriate. Through this exposure, the inferior part of the superior articular process and the superior part of the inferior articular process can be removed. This posterior approach may also be useful for some cases of disc herniation. To remove the offending disc protrusion, however, the nerve root must be retracted, and this may result in some tension on the nerve root and dura.

In the figure labels: C3 nerve root; Osteophytes on uncovertebral joint; Osteophytes on superior articular process

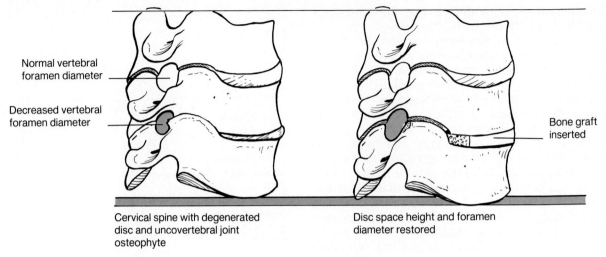

Normal vertebral foramen diameter

Decreased vertebral foramen diameter

Bone graft inserted

Cervical spine with degenerated disc and uncovertebral joint osteophyte

Disc space height and foramen diameter restored

FIGURE 7–12. Anterior cervical discectomy and fusion for bony foraminal stenosis.

Thoracic nerve root compression is rare (see Fig. 1-37) but should be included in the differential diagnosis of chest wall pain. Typically, the patient complains of lancinating pain radiating around the chest unilaterally. Physical examination may demonstrate a sensory change in a single dermatome. In most instances, the nerve root compression is a result of a disc herniation. Because the spinal cord does not tolerate significant retraction, which a posterior approach would require, the usual surgical approach is an anterior transthoracic discectomy. A costotransversectomy may be used, but visualization of the posterior annulus and posterior longitudinal ligament from this approach can be technically difficult.

Sciatica, lumbar nerve root pain, is a well-recognized clinical problem. As in the cervical and thoracic spine, the key ingredient to successful surgical management is precise localization of the compressive lesion. Commonly, the nerve root is compressed by a disc herniation. This may occur with or without concomitant neural foraminal entrapment. Bony stenosis can cause nerve root compression as it enters, traverses, or exits the foramen. (This will be discussed in greater detail in Chapter 11.) The lumbar nerve roots are not as tightly tethered as the cervical roots, and the cauda equina can tolerate considerably more retraction than the spinal cord. For these reasons, most nerve root decompressions in the lumbar spine can be done through a posterior approach.

Dural Sac

A wide variety of conditions can lead to compromise of the spinal canal and dural sac compression. These include disc herniations, spondylosis, fractures, and tumors. When spinal cord compression occurs anteriorly in the cervical spine, the usual surgical approach is an anterior decompression. In some instances, anterior compression occurs over three or more levels; in these cases, anterior decompression is a major undertaking, with significant attendant risk. Surgeons have advocated posterior decompression for these situations, by multiple laminectomy or laminoplasty. The latter technique preserves stability and has been widely used for a condition known as ossification of the posterior longitudinal ligament. Although in this condition the compressive lesion is situated anteriorly, posterior laminoplasty or laminectomy at multiple levels can allow the spinal cord to translate posteriorly and effect an indirect decompression (Figs. 7-13 and 7-14). This occurs as the result of the lordotic posture of the cervical spine and does not occur in the thoracic spine, where there is a kyphosis. In this region, anterior compression must be managed by anterior decompression. Thoracic disc herniations can cause significant spinal cord compression (Fig. 7-15).

Dural sac compression is most common in the lumbar spine. Various decompressive techniques have been described, but the optimal surgical approach depends on the specific nature of the offending compressive lesion, the level or levels

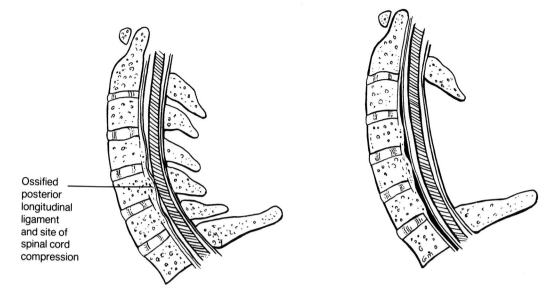

Ossified
posterior
longitudinal
ligament
and site of
spinal cord
compression

FIGURE 7–13. Multiple-level laminectomy of the cervical spine.

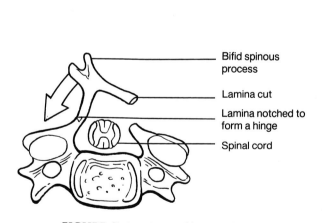

Bifid spinous
process

Lamina cut

Lamina notched to
form a hinge

Spinal cord

FIGURE 7–14. Cervical laminoplasty.

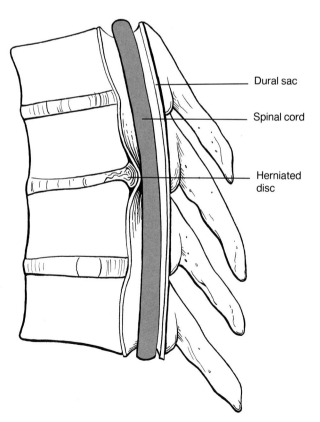

Dural sac

Spinal cord

Herniated
disc

FIGURE 7–15. Thoracic disc herniation causing spinal cord compression.

affected, the patient's medical and surgical history, and the surgeon's training.

STABILIZATION

Rationale for Fusion

A spinal fusion is a bony union of contiguous vertebrae. In other words, there is bony bridging from one vertebra to another. This bony bridging may occur in a variety of places and determines the fusion type. A spinal fusion results in elimination or significant reduction of motion between the involved levels.

A basic principle of orthopedic surgery is that joint pain can be relieved by eliminating motion of that joint. As discussed in Chapter 1, there are three joints between the vertebrae: the intervertebral disc and the two facet joints. In some instances, pathology of one or more of these joints results in pain. Pain relief may be achieved by following the orthopedic principle of eliminating motion by performing a fusion. *Arthrodesis* is the obliteration of a joint and is sometimes used synonymously with the term fusion. This is not strictly correct, as will be discussed later in this chapter in the section on types of spinal fusion.

Apart from eliminating motion to treat pain, spinal fusion has also been undertaken for other purposes. These include maintaining spinal alignment in cases of progressive deformity, stabilizing unstable injuries, and in association with debridement for infectious conditions.

Physiology of Spinal Fusion

The physiologic sequence of events that lead to a successful spinal fusion is similar to that of fracture healing. There are three phases: inflammatory, reparative, and remodeling.

The two major components of a spinal fusion are the tissue bed and the graft material. During the inflammatory phase of healing, the graft bed is of prime importance. Ideally, it consists of healthy, bleeding, decorticated bone. From this bed comes an inflammatory exudate containing viable bone marrow cells, monocytes, and multinuclear phagocytes. Some of the bone marrow cells have the potential for differentiating into various cell lines. Some of the pleuripotent mesenchymal cells become osteogenic and contribute to bone formation in the fusion mass. If autogenous bone is used as graft material, it may have some viable osteoprogenitor cells that can also contribute to the fusion mass. During the reparative phase, bone matrix formation occurs, and some of the grafted material is resorbed and replaced by viable, newly formed host bone. The remodeling phase may occur over 2 to 3 years. The fusion mass adheres to Wolff's law, which states that the architecture of bone responds to the pattern of loading to which it is subjected.

Bone Graft

The nature and quantity of the bone graft material are essential factors in a successful spinal fusion. There are three basic ways in which bone graft can enhance the development of a fusion. The first, called *osteogenesis*, is the potential of some bone grafts to provide viable osteoprogenitor cells that can directly contribute to bone formation. The second is the ability of certain graft materials to induce pleuripotent cells to differentiate along osteogenic lines. This process is called *osteoinduction*, and there are probably various osteoinductive factors. The best known is *bone morphogenic protein* (BMP), which is present in bone matrix. The third, *osteoconduction*, is the process by which the graft can provide a scaffold on which host bone can be made. Hydroxyapatite is the best-known osteoconductive substance.

Various bone graft materials have been used in spinal surgery, and the advantages and disadvantages of each remain controversial. Clearly, however, autogenous cancellous bone provides the optimum osteogenic, osteoconductive, and osteoinductive qualities. Bone graft harvesting is associated with some morbidity. The usual site for harvesting autograft is the iliac crest, and the quantity of bone available is limited. *Allograft* is tissue taken from other members of the same species. Allograft bone can be harvested from femoral heads obtained at the time of total hip replacement or from fresh cadavers. Various processes are used to sterilize allograft to avoid disease transmission; these processes are also used to reduce the immunogenicity of the transplanted tissue. Allograft does not have the potential for providing viable osteoprogenitor cells. The tissue may be osteoinductive, but most of the processing techniques, such as freeze-drying or demineralization, depress this effect. Synthetic graft material is still investigational. It is hoped that we will be able to synthesize bone

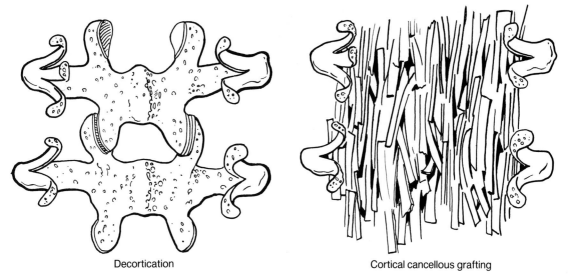

Decortication   Cortical cancellous grafting

FIGURE 7–16. Posterolateral fusion of adjacent transverse processes and posterior elements.

graft substitutes that are both osteoinductive and osteoconductive.

Autograft is the optimal bone graft material. Allograft may be indicated for use in certain cases, such as when there is inadequate autograft.

Types of Spinal Fusion

Spinal fusion implies bony bridging from one vertebra to another. Fusions can be categorized as to the position of this bony bridging. The first fusions were done by placing bone from spinous process to spinous process. This became modified to include the entire posterior arch and arthrodesis of the facet joints. Posterior fusions of this nature are not commonly performed today, largely because although the posterior column of the spine is immobilized, significant motion can still occur in the anterior column at the fused levels.

Posterolateral fusion includes not only the posterior elements but also the transverse processes (Fig. 7-16). Although originally designed for cases of spondylolysis or posterior pseud-arthroses, it is now the most common type of fusion done in North America. The major advantage is biomechanical. The bony fusion is situated not only in the posterior column but also more anteriorly at the level of the transverse processes. This creates a stiffer fusion and results in decreased motion both anteriorly between the

vertebral bodies and posteriorly in the facet joints.

Bone graft can be placed between the vertebral bodies after anterior discectomy (Fig. 7-17) in a procedure called *anterior interbody fusion*. The large surface area provided by the end plates favors the success of this type of fusion. Further-

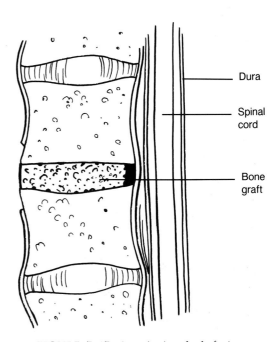

Dura

Spinal cord

Bone graft

FIGURE 7–17. Anterior interbody fusion.

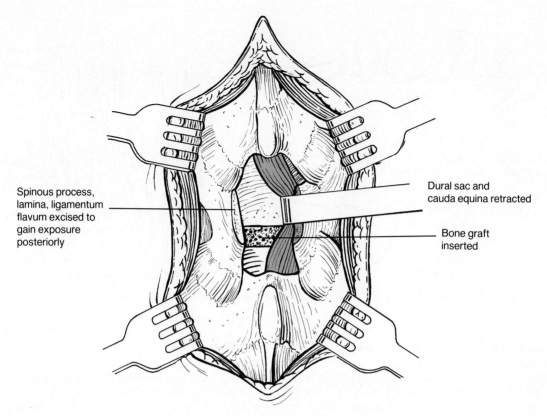

Spinous process,
lamina, ligamentum
flavum excised to
gain exposure
posteriorly

Dural sac and
cauda equina retracted

Bone graft
inserted

FIGURE 7–18. Posterior interbody fusion.

more, an anterior interbody fusion is extremely rigid and eliminates motion in the anterior column. The disadvantages are that this technique requires an anterior exposure to the spine, which does not allow posterior decompression when necessary and may not eliminate all motion in the facet joints.

An interbody fusion may be done in the lumbar spine through a posterior approach (Fig. 7-18), referred to as a *posterior lumbar interbody fusion* (PLIF). This technique has become increasingly popular in recent years. The major disadvantages are the significant retraction of the dural sac and nerve roots required to place the grafts and the possibility of postoperative graft retropulsion, creating neurologic injury.

Some surgeons perform *circumferential fusion,* also known as 360° fusion (Fig. 7-19), in selected cases. This involves both anterior and posterior fusion at the same levels, either in one operation or as staged procedures. The original goal of this technique was to improve fusion rates. Some surgeons advocate this procedure because it results in the greatest stiffness at the fused levels. However, this stiffness results in altered kinematics at adjacent levels that with time may be deleterious.

Spinal Implants

Spinal implants were originally developed to immobilize vertebrae while a bony fusion was healing. These internal fixation devices included plates bolted to the spinous processes and screws placed through the facet joints. Although these implants reduced the pseudarthrosis rate, physicians became aware that meticulous attention to the actual grafting technique was more crucial than the types of implants being used.

In the early 1960s, Dr. Paul Harrington in Houston, Texas, began implanting stainless steel rods connected to the spine by laminar hooks. These implants were originally used to correct scoliosis (Fig. 7-20). In his early work, Harrington did not perform a concomitant fusion. Ulti-

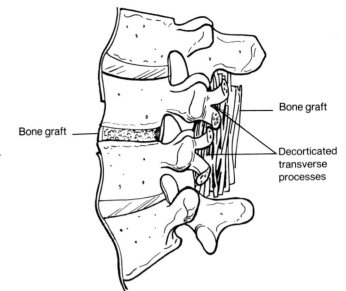

FIGURE 7–19. Circumferential fusion.

Bone graft

Bone graft

Decorticated transverse processes

Bone graft

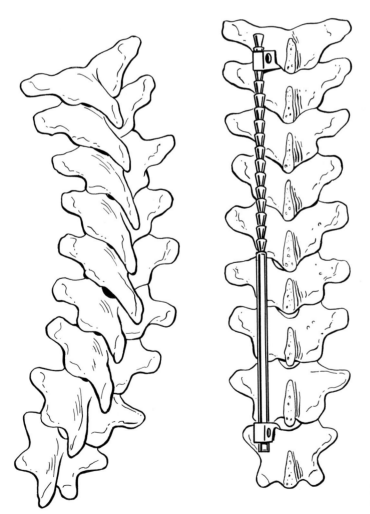

FIGURE 7–20. Harrington rod for correction of scoliosis.

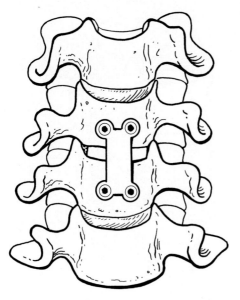

FIGURE 7–21. Anterior cervical plate.

mately, because of repetitive stress-loading on the metallic implants, they failed, and Harrington realized that the rods could be used to correct deformity and hold the spine in a corrected position while a fusion was developing.

Thus, there are two major reasons why implants are used. The first is to temporarily immobilize the spine in the hopes that this will increase the rate of successful fusion. The second is to correct deformity and hold the spine in the corrected position while a fusion is developing.

Spinal implants are constantly being developed and modified, but they all basically consist of two components: one that allows secure purchase to the vertebra, and the other that connects these fixation points. These transfixion devices include rods, plates, and cables. The implants used to secure purchase include hooks, wires, and screws.

Many studies have sought to determine how these implants can be designed to improve pullout strength and resistance to cyclic loading of

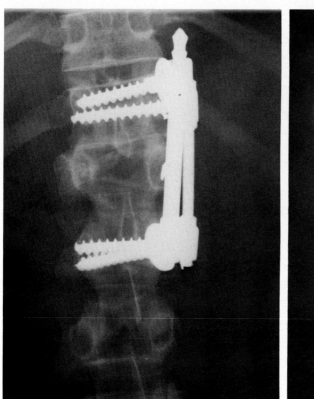
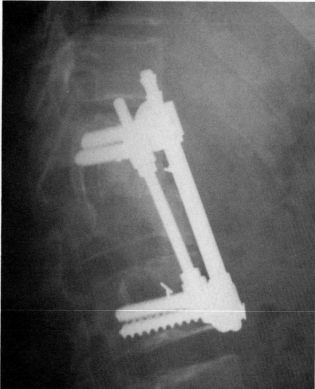

FIGURE 7–22. Anterior Kostuik-Harrington system.

the spine. In fact, the most significant factor is not the implant itself but the quality of the bone.

It is beyond the scope of this textbook to describe all the spinal implants available. Some commonly used fixation devices are shown in Figures 7-21 through 7-25. Others will be described in the sections on the conditions for which they were specifically designed.

SPECIAL CONSIDERATIONS

Surgical Complications

Surgical complications may be divided into those associated with any orthopedic surgical procedure and those unique to spinal surgery. The former include postoperative infection, deep vein thrombosis, and so forth; for further information, the reader is referred to the general orthopedic literature. The complications unique

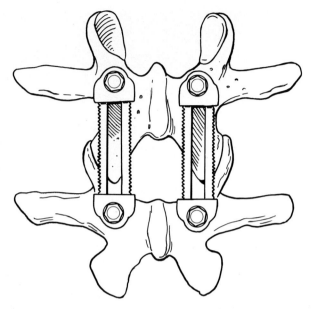

FIGURE 7–23. Posterior plating system.

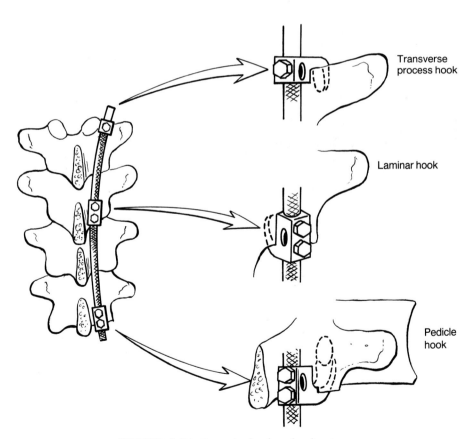

FIGURE 7–24. Posterior hook and rod system.

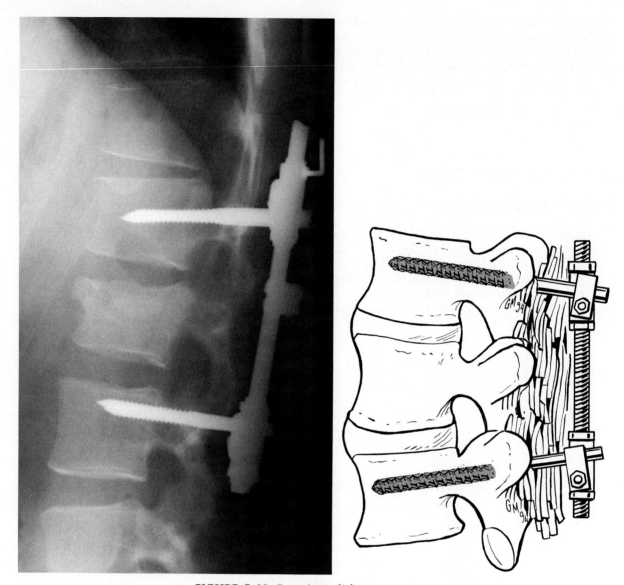

FIGURE 7–25. Posterior pedicle screw system.

to spinal surgery have become increasingly common because of the development of more aggressive operative approaches and the growing number of surgical procedures being done.

Because many spinal procedures require exposure of a large operative field, blood loss can be significant. Techniques to minimize blood loss include attention to surgical positioning with decompression of the abdomen, hypotensive anesthesia, autologous blood transfusions, and the use of hemostatic agents. In posterior surgery of the spine, positioning the patient so that there is no compression of the abdomen en-

sures that venous return occurs through the vena cava. Pressure on the abdomen causes venous blood to preferentially travel through Batson's plexus, with resultant increased epidural blood loss. Hypotensive anesthesia can reduce intraoperative blood loss by up to 50%. The degree to which the blood pressure is lowered must be meticulously monitored and evaluated. If the blood pressure is dropped too much or for too long, there can be renal dysfunction, cardiovascular dysfunction, reactive hemorrhage, and thromboembolic events. Furthermore, some patients undergoing spinal surgery may have compromise of the arterial supply to the spinal cord. With hypotension, vascular profusion to the cord may be diminished sufficiently to cause neural damage. Autologous blood transfusions can be done in one of two ways. The first is by phlebotomizing the patient during the month before surgery and storing the blood, which is transfused as needed during the perioperative period. The second method of autotransfusion is to collect the blood lost during surgery, wash it, and then return it to the patient. This requires the use of a Cell Saver system in the operating room. Hemostatic agents include bone wax, absorbable gelatin, regenerated cellulose, and microfibrillar collagen. The latter three are used topically at the site of bleeding to induce and accelerate the clotting cascade.

One of the major concerns in spinal surgery is the risk of injury to neurologic structures. Several techniques have been developed to monitor spinal cord function, as discussed in the following section. These techniques do not prevent acute catastrophic intraoperative injury to the cord but allow neurologic monitoring during decompressive procedures, instrumentation of the spine, or correction of deformity. The cluneal nerves, which provide sensation to the skin over the gluteal area, are vulnerable when bone graft is harvested from the posterior iliac crest. They are at risk if the bone graft incision extends more than 8 cm lateral to the posterior superior iliac spine.

Another complication of spinal fusion procedures is the failure of bone to incorporate into a solid mass; this is known as a *pseudarthrosis* or *nonunion* (Fig. 7-26). The incidence of pseudarthrosis varies considerably, depending on the technique of fusion used, the number of levels being fused, and the means of evaluating the fusion mass. Cigarette smoking significantly reduces fusion rates. Pseudarthroses may be diagnosed in two ways. First, motion may be detected at the level of the supposed fusion either by flexion-extension radiographs or by surgically exposing the area and visualizing motion at that level. Second, a gap or break in bony continuity may be demonstrated within the fusion mass bridging the vertebrae, using plain radiographs, computed tomographic (CT) scans, tomography, or magnetic resonance imaging (MRI) (Fig. 7-27).

With the increasing popularity of spinal implants, there has been an increase in the incidence of implant failure. Any implant subjected to stress will eventually fail; thus, implants are not a substitute for a solid bony fusion. Many im-

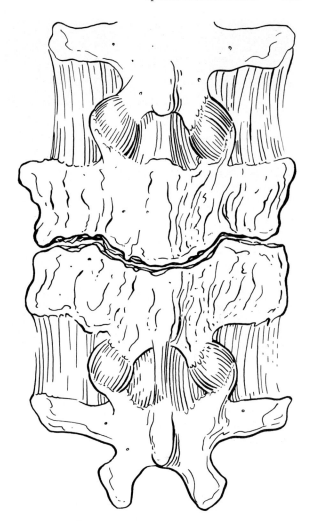

FIGURE 7–26. Pseudarthrosis.

plant failures are due to delayed union or nonunion of the fusion, with resulting persistent stress-loading of the implant. As spinal instrumentation systems become more sophisticated, there has been an increase in the number of implant failures that occur from mechanical disassembly or loosening (Fig. 7-28). Finally, as very rigid spinal systems are being developed, implant breakage can occur once a fusion has successfully healed. This is due to a mismatch in the modulus of elasticity between the implant system and the fusion mass itself. As was discussed in Chapter 5, all materials, including bone, have a certain degree of elasticity. If a fusion mass permits more motion, or is more elastic, than the implant, the latter will ultimately fail due to continued stress-loading (Fig. 7-29).

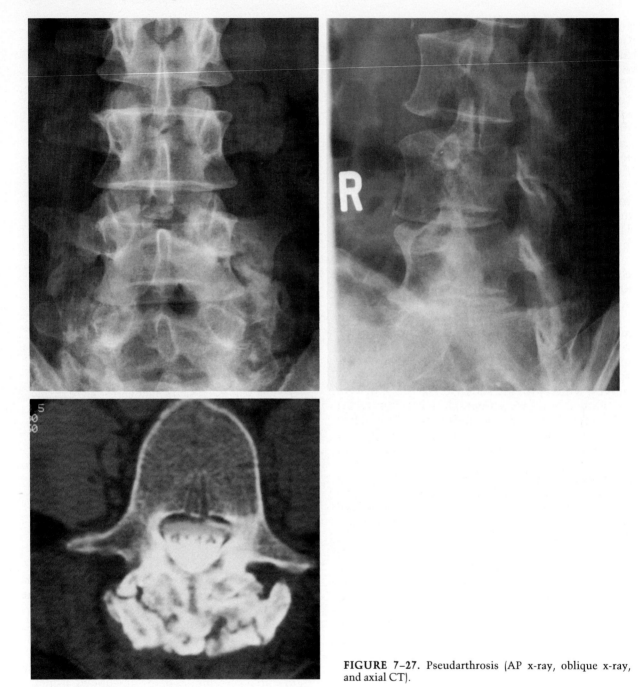

FIGURE 7-27. Pseudarthrosis (AP x-ray, oblique x-ray, and axial CT).

Spinal Cord Monitoring

One of the most catastrophic complications that can occur as the result of spinal surgery is injury to the spinal cord. This may be the result of direct injury to the spinal cord, indirect injury by overly aggressive correction of deformity, or impairment of the blood supply to the cord. Because most spinal surgery is performed under general anesthesia, various techniques have been developed to monitor spinal cord function and allow the surgeon to know when the spinal cord function is being jeopardized. The oldest tech-

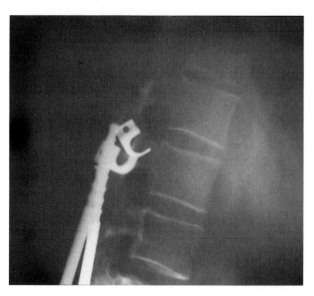

FIGURE 7–28. Mechanical disassembly.

nique, the *wake-up test*, was originally used during scoliosis surgery and continues to be the most common monitoring modality. After the deformity has been corrected, the anesthesia is lightened such that the patient can respond to verbal commands. The patient is asked to move the hands and feet to ensure normal motor response.

Spinal cord function can also be monitored electrically (Fig. 7-30). The principle involved is that an evoked potential can be produced by electrically stimulating a nerve, and this will be propagated along that nerve up the spinal cord and to the cerebral cortex. The various evoked potential monitoring techniques depend on where the stimulus is given and where the evoked potential is monitored. In North America, most spinal cord monitoring is done with the stimulus being delivered to a peripheral nerve. Recording is usually done from the cerebral cortex by using needles inserted subdermally in the scalp. This

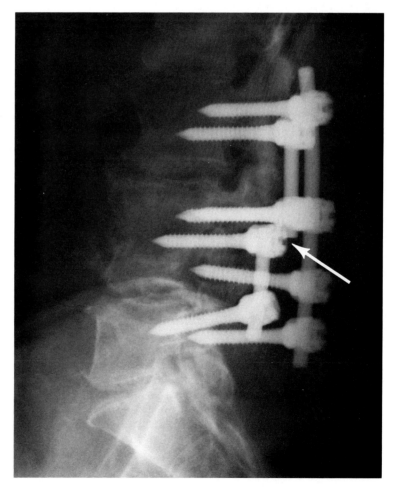

FIGURE 7–29. Implant breakage.

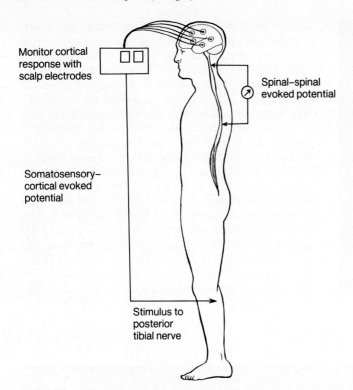

Monitor cortical response with scalp electrodes

Spinal–spinal evoked potential

Somatosensory–cortical evoked potential

Stimulus to posterior tibial nerve

FIGURE 7–30. Spinal cord monitoring during surgery.

method of monitoring is called *somatosensory cortical evoked potentials*. Alternatively, recordings may be made along the spinal cord; this is referred to as *somatosensory spinal evoked potentials*.

In Japan, there has been interest in stimulating the spinal cord rather than the peripheral nerves and recording from the spinal cord directly through needles placed in the epidural space. This technique is referred to as *spinal spinal evoked potentials*. With this method of monitoring, either electrode may be used to stimulate or to record; therefore, both ascending and descending pathways can be evaluated.

Spinal cord monitoring has limitations. The quality of the recording is affected by numerous factors, including stimulus and recording parameters, blood pressure, and anesthetic agents. Most of the ascending stimulus travels through the posterior column and thus does not give information pertaining to the status of the entire spinal cord pathways, the most important being the motor tracts. Much work has been done on

motor evoked potentials, and it is hoped that this research will give us a means to specifically evaluate the motor pathways.

KEY POINTS

1. Various surgical approaches have been developed to allow safe access to any area of the spinal column.
2. Surgical decompression of the spine involves the removal of any material placing pressure on the neural elements.
3. Stabilization of the spine usually requires a fusion, which is the bridging of one vertebra to another by solid bone.
4. Correction of spinal deformity usually involves the implantation of metallic devices. These are meant to temporarily hold the spine in a corrected position while a bony fusion develops.

BIBLIOGRAPHY

BOOKS

Bauer R, Kerschbaumer F, Poisel S. Operative approaches in orthopaedic surgery and traumatology. New York: Thieme, 1987.

Garfin SR, ed. Complications of spine surgery. Baltimore: Williams & Wilkins, 1989.

Homma S, Tamaki T. Fundamentals and clinical applications of spinal cord monitoring. Tokyo: Saikon Publishing Co, 1984.

Hoppenfeld S, DeBoer P. Surgical exposures in orthopaedics: The anatomic approach. Philadelphia: JB Lippincott, 1994.

White AH, Rothman RH, Ray CD. Lumbar spine surgery. St. Louis: CV Mosby, 1987.

JOURNALS

Deyo RA, Cherkin DC, Loeser JD, Bigos SJ, Ciol MA. Morbidity and mortality in association with operations on the lumbar spine. The influence of age, diagnosis, and procedure. J Bone Joint Surg [Am] 1992;74:536–543.

Deyo RA, Ciol MA, Cherkin DC, Loeser JD, Bigos SJ. Lumbar spinal fusion. A cohort study of complications, reoperations, and resource use in the medicare population. Spine 1993;18:1463–1470.

Esses SI, Huler RJ. Indications for lumbar spine fusion in the adult. Clin Orthop 1992;279:87–101.

Esses SI, Sachs BL, Dreyzin V. Complications associated with the technique of pedicle screw fixation: A selected survey of ABS members. Spine 1993;18:2231–2240.

Tabaraud F, Boulesteix JM, Moulies D, Longis B, Lansade A, Terrier G, Vallat JM, Dumas M, Hugon J. Monitoring of the motor pathway during spinal surgery. Spine 1993;18:546–550.

West JL III, Anderson LD. Incidence of deep vein thrombosis in major adult spinal surgery. Spine 1992;17:S254–S257.

Zucherman J, Shu K, Picetti G III, White A, Wynne G, Taylor L. Clinical efficacy of spinal instrumentation in lumbar degenerative disc disease. Spine 1992;17:834–837.

Textbook of Spinal Disorders, by Stephen I. Esses.
J. B. Lippincott Company, Philadelphia © 1995.

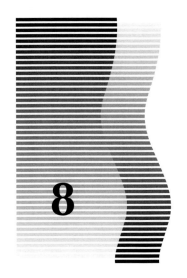

Degenerative Disease of the Spine

8

LUMBAR SPINE
 Clinical Presentation
 Diagnostic Evaluation
  X-ray
  *Computed
   Tomography*
  *Magnetic Resonance
   Imaging*
  Discography
  Facet Blocks
 Treatment
  Nonoperative
  Operative

THORACIC SPINE
 Clinical Presentation
 Diagnostic Evaluation
 Treatment
  Nonoperative
  Operative
CERVICAL SPINE
 Clinical Presentation
 Diagnostic Evaluation
  X-ray
  *Computed
   Tomography*
  *Magnetic Resonance
   Imaging*
  Discography
  Facet Blocks
 Treatment
  Nonoperative
  Operative

The term *degenerative* refers to a situation in which there has been a loss of normal structure and function. For reasons that are not yet clear, a degenerative process occurs in various components of the spinal column over time. This "aging" or "maturational" process occurs at different rates in different people and in different parts of the spine. In general, degenerative disease of the spine is said to be present when radiographic changes are associated with this process, but biochemical and histologic changes occur well before gross radiologic manifestations. The two regions where the degenerative process is most profound are the intervertebral discs and facet joints. Because the changes are not dissimilar to those of osteoarthritis, the degenerative condition is sometimes referred to as osteoarthritis of the spine or *spondylosis*.

Over time, the collagen architecture of the annulus fibrosus becomes distorted. Tears occur in the lamellae due in part to altered collagen cross-linking. There is a decrease in the water and proteoglycan content of the annulus fibrosus. Degenerative changes in the nucleus are primarily characterized by decreased water content. There is a loss of proteoglycan and a relative increase in the amount of collagen. These changes all lead to

173

altered mechanical properties of the disc, making it less resilient to stress.

Changes in the facet joints include a loss of cartilage and formation of osteophytes and cysts. The joints themselves become hypertrophic. These changes can result in very distorted anatomy.

Although the degenerative process primarily affects the intervertebral discs and facet joints, there are changes in other structures, including the vertebral end plates and ligamentum flavum.

As a result of all of these changes, abnormal motion can occur. These changes can also lead to a decrease in the size of the spinal canal or the size of the neural foramina. When this occurs, patients may develop neurologic symptoms with pain or weakness in an extremity. (Degenerative spinal stenosis is discussed in Chapter 11.)

In most people, pain from the degenerative process is not severe enough to warrant medical consultation. This chapter, however, deals with patients who experience significant local pain from degenerative disease of the spine. Situations in which the degenerative process results in nerve root or dural sac compression and dysfunction are discussed in Chapter 11.

LUMBAR SPINE

Clinical Presentation

Most patients with symptomatic degenerative disease of the lumbar spine are over age 40. In many of these patients, symptoms arise as a result of pathology at multiple levels. In younger patients, it is not uncommon that a single isolated level gives rise to symptoms.

Certain factors accelerate the degenerative process in the lumbar spine. These include vibration, such as occurs while seated in a tractor or large truck; repetitive bending and lifting, as is done in manual labor; and smoking. The clinician should ask about these risk factors, particularly in the younger patient with multiple-level degenerative disease.

When symptomatic, the primary complaint associated with degenerative disease of the lumbar spine is pain, almost always associated with activity. The abnormal movement patterns in this condition probably stimulate pain fibers in the annulus fibrosus and facet joint capsule. Prolonged sitting may also exacerbate symptoms.

The sitting position places more load on the lumbar intervertebral discs than other postures, such as standing or lying supine. Pain fibers innervating the intervertebral disc may be stimulated by long seated periods. The seats in most cars are not particularly well designed; thus, riding in a car usually causes worsening of symptoms.

Patients may complain of stiffness, particularly in the morning. In these patients, a small degree of activity helps relieve symptoms.

Physical examination of these patients is not particularly remarkable. There may be some secondary paravertebral muscle spasm. Usually a decreased range of motion is detected. There may be evidence of osteoarthritis affecting other joints.

Diagnostic Evaluation

X-RAY

Typical x-ray findings of degenerative disease in the lumbar spine include intervertebral disc space narrowing, osteophyte and syndesmophyte formation, hypertrophy of the facet joints, and loss of the cartilage space within those joints. As the degenerative process continues, there is reactive bone formation adjacent to the end plates (Fig. 8-1). Rarely, this sclerotic reaction is pronounced and results in *idiopathic vertebral hyperostosis*. It is much more common in females than males and seems to selectively affect the inferior aspect of the L4 vertebral body.

The degenerative phenomenon leads to altered kinematics that can occasionally be detected on dynamic radiographs. When there is more than 4 mm of translation in flexion and extension, this may indicate pathologic motion, referred to as *segmental instability*. There may be evidence of instability on static films as indicated by anterior, posterior, or lateral listhesis.

COMPUTED TOMOGRAPHY

The computed tomography (CT) scan is ideal for imaging the bony anatomy. Degenerative changes in the facet joints can be well appreciated. The hypertrophy of the joints occasionally results in a "ram's horn" appearance (Fig. 8-2). As the disc collapses in height, bulging occurs, with redundancy of the annulus fibrosus. This can be appreciated on good-quality CT scans.

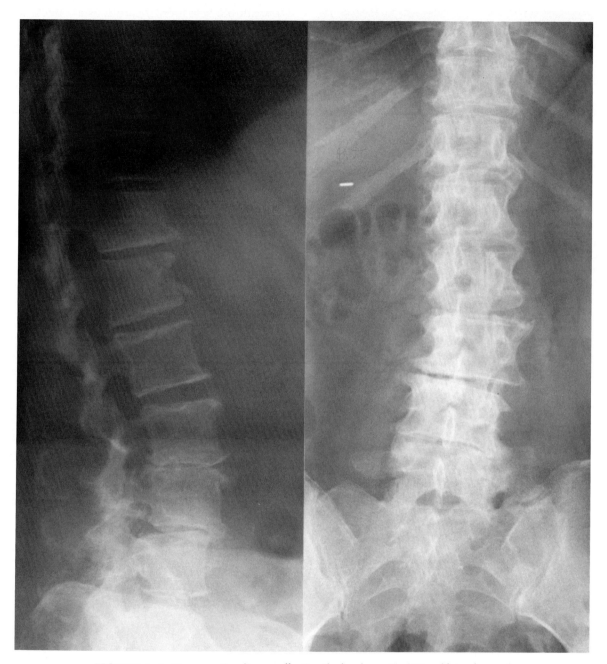

FIGURE 8–1. Degenerative disease affecting the lumbar spine (AP and lateral x-rays).

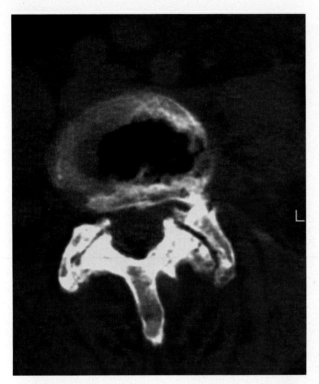

FIGURE 8–2. CT scan showing lumbar facet arthropathy.

MAGNETIC RESONANCE IMAGING

Magnetic resonance imaging (MRI) is the most sensitive imaging modality for detecting degenerative disease affecting the intervertebral disc. The earliest changes include loss of water content, which can be easily identified by loss of signal intensity on T2-weighted images; this is called "black disc disease" (Fig. 8-3). Cartilage usually appears as intermediate signal intensity on T2-weighted images and as high signal intensity on gradient echo images. Degenerative changes in the cartilage of the facet joint can be appreciated on axial MR images. Buckling, redundancy, and hypertrophy of the ligamentum flavum is best appreciated on T1-weighted images (Fig. 8-4). Changes in the end plate and adjacent bone marrow appear as altered signal intensities on T1- and T2-weighted images (Fig. 8-5).

DISCOGRAPHY

All of the aforementioned diagnostic studies are purely morphometric: they give information about the appearance of the spine but not about the pathology, if any, giving rise to symptoms.

For example, the identification of a "black disc" on an MR scan at the L5–S1 level does not necessarily mean this is the source of pain in a patient complaining of low back discomfort. This is why provocative tests such as discography have been developed. Their goal is to reproduce symptoms in an effort to identify the pain source.

Discography involves the injection of contrast agent into the center of an intervertebral disc. At the time of injection, the patient is asked if there is pain. The patient is then asked whether this pain, if present, is concordant or discordant with his or her typical symptoms. Assessment of the dye pattern is then made by x-ray and CT scanning. Under normal conditions, the annular fibers should contain the contrast to the center of

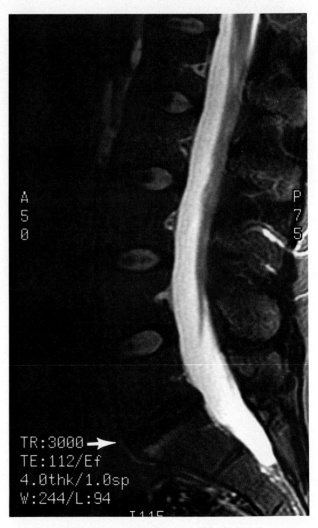

FIGURE 8–3. MRI showing "black disc."

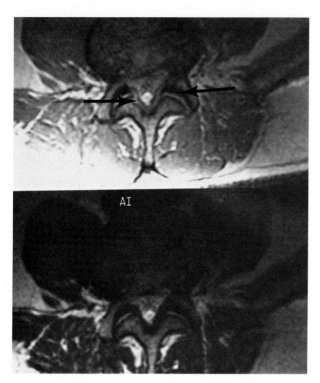

FIGURE 8-4. MRI showing altered joints and hypertrophic ligamentum.

generative disease of the lumbar spine. A few well-controlled studies have called into question the reliability of facet blocks. At present, the results of facet blocks should not be used exclusively either for patient assessment or treatment. It is of interest to note that injection of hypotonic saline into the lumbosacral facet joint capsule can result in pain in the region of the posterior thigh.

Treatment

NONOPERATIVE

All too often, patients diagnosed with symptomatic degenerative disease of the lumbar spine are given the impression that nothing can be done and that they will have to learn to live with it. The degenerative process itself is irreversible,

the disc. When there are degenerative changes with tearing of the annulus, extravasation of the dye into the periphery of the disc can be seen.

Although CT discography may be useful in the identification of a herniated nucleus pulposus (see Chap. 9), its use in the evaluation of symptomatic degenerative disease is controversial. Grossly degenerative intervertebral discs may be asymptomatic. Injection of seemingly normal discs in asymptomatic patients may be painful. For this reason, the results of discography should not be used as the sole modality in patient assessment. Advocates of discography believe that the concordant response of the patient on dye injection is the most important factor in determining further treatment.

FACET BLOCKS

A diagnostic facet block is a test in which local anesthetic is injected into one or more facet joints. The patient is then asked whether this has resulted in any pain relief. The rationale for this test is that degenerative disease of the facet joint can be the primary source of symptoms in a subgroup of patients with low back pain due to de-

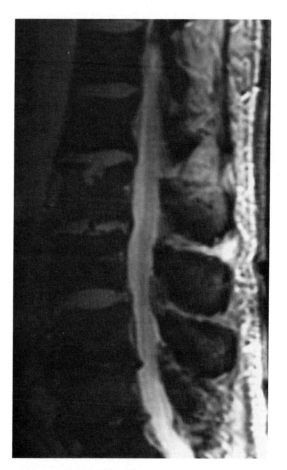

FIGURE 8-5. Sagittal MRI showing degenerative changes in lumbar spine.

but many steps can be taken to provide symptomatic relief and to decrease the rate of further degenerative changes.

Several risk factors are associated with an accelerated degenerative process, including repetitive lifting in a forward-flexed posture, exposure to whole-body vibration, and prolonged driving. The patient should be asked about these activities, and some modification of lifestyle or work should be suggested if possible. Patients who smoke should be encouraged to quit. Obese patients should be enrolled in a supervised weight-loss program.

There is some theoretical advantage to strengthening the paravertebral and abdominal muscles: it may result in decreased loading of the lumbar spine and help stabilize abnormal motion. For this reason, an exercise program should be encouraged. Care should be taken, however, because mobilization of the spine may result in exacerbation of pain. In general, isometric exercises should be encouraged.

The episodic and judicious use of medications may be valuable in these patients. Anti-inflammatory agents may depress the arthritic process of the facet joints; they may also modulate pain (see Chap. 6). Analgesics may be useful in acute exacerbations of back pain due to degenerative disease. However, the anti-inflammatory agents and analgesics are generally not intended for long-term use.

Lumbosacral orthoses may be useful in some patients (see Chap. 5). They are thought to exert two major effects. First, they can theoretically decrease the load on the lumbar spine by increasing intra-abdominal pressure. Second, they can limit motion of the lumbar spine. Although these advantages have not been scientifically validated, empiric data show some pain relief in certain patients. They may be of maximal benefit in patients with segmental instability or spondylolisthesis.

Treatment should be provided in a positive manner, and the clinician should remain supportive. Patients should know they are not doomed to progressive problems. Many patients are worried, consciously or subconsciously, that they will "end up in a wheelchair." The clinician should explain that in most instances as the process continues there is actually a diminution in motion. This is due to stabilization by osteophytes, ankylosis of the facet joints, and fibrosis of ligaments. In some instances, this diminution of motion results in resolution of symptoms.

OPERATIVE

The standard surgical approach for degenerative disease of the lumbar spine has been fusion. The rationale for arthrodesis is based on the orthopedic principle of arthrodesis for painful joints of the extremity. It is thought that if specific levels of the spine affected by the degenerative phenomenon could be identified as being symptomatic, then fusion of those levels would result in pain relief.

Results of surgery have been inconsistent. This may be due to a variety of problems, including our inability in many cases to identify the source of pain accurately. Also, we do not understand how the degenerative process results in pain. There may be biochemical changes that stimulate pain receptors irrespective of motion.

There are numerous factors to consider before proposing operative treatment to a patient, including the confidence with which the pain source can be identified and the patient's age, lifestyle, and occupation. The number of levels being considered for treatment must also be assessed because the more levels being fused the greater the magnitude of surgery and the potential for complication or failure.

In most cases, surgery should not be considered for patients with multiple-level disease who have demonstrated a proclivity to an accelerated degenerative process. In general, surgery should not be offered before nonoperative methods have been thoroughly tried. The optimal surgical candidate is young, has strictly single-level disease, and does not plan to carry out heavy manual labor or engage in high-level sports postoperatively.

There is considerable controversy over the technique of lumbar fusion. The most common approach is a posterolateral fusion. Some surgeons have advocated an anterior interbody fusion, arguing that some motion, however small, may continue to exist in the anterior column despite a solid posterolateral fusion and that this persistent motion may stimulate pain fibers in the intervertebral disc and be a source of ongoing symptoms of low back pain. More recently, some clinicians have suggested that the only way to address all pain sources effectively is by discectomy, interbody fusion, facetectomy, and a posterolateral fusion, the so-called 360° or *circumferential fusion* (see Fig. 7–19). To date, there have been no good studies comparing the results of these various surgical approaches.

THORACIC SPINE

Clinical Presentation

Assessing and treating patients with midback or interscapular pain is exceedingly difficult. Degenerative disease of a thoracic disc and arthropathy of thoracic facets can cause local pain; the difficulty arises from the fact that numerous visceral conditions can cause similar complaints (eg, herpes, disorders of the heart, pulmonary problems, intra-abdominal disease). Thus, while taking the history, it is crucial to do a full functional inquiry and to obtain complete details about the patient's symptoms.

Symptomatic degenerative disease of the thoracic spine can occur in all age groups. Often there is a prior history of trauma. An intervertebral disc can be significantly damaged during a compression fracture, particularly when there is significant end plate involvement. The bone of the vertebral body will heal, but the intervertebral disc can remain symptomatic.

Physical examination may show local pain with palpation. In the situation discussed here, the neurologic examination is normal. Patients may have some reproduction of their pain with forward-flexion or hyperextension. When most symptoms are due to the intervertebral disc, the pain is increased by flexion; when the facet joint is more involved, hyperextension causes an increase in symptoms.

Diagnostic Evaluation

Plain radiographs are not particularly useful in the diagnostic evaluation of these patients. There may be evidence of decreased intervertebral disc space height at the involved level. Hypertrophic changes of the facet joints may also be identified, but they may be more easily seen on axial CT scanning. Occasionally a degenerative disc calcifies and becomes apparent on x-ray (Fig. 8-6).

With the advent of MRI, the status of thoracic intervertebral discs can be assessed noninvasively. Degenerative changes are most easily recognized on T2-weighted images. Decreased signal intensity reflects desiccation. There may also be altered signal intensity on both T1- and T2-weighted images in the adjacent end plates (Fig. 8-7).

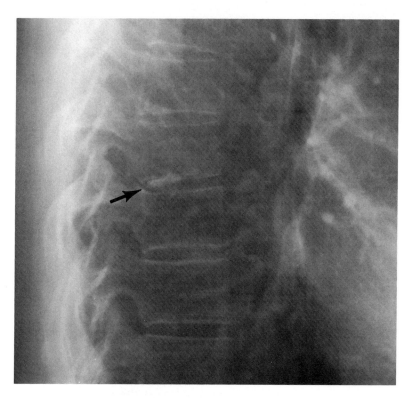

FIGURE 8–6. Thoracic calcified disc.

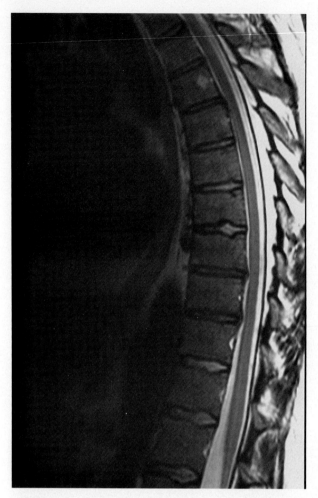

FIGURE 8–7. MRI showing degenerative changes in thoracic spine.

Because the degenerative process accompanies aging, it is expected in a significant number of people of middle age or older. Therefore, the clinician must ensure that a degenerative disc identified on MRI is indeed the source of the patient's back pain. This is why CT discography and facet blocks continue to be used as diagnostic tests. Because discograms are almost always done on levels already demonstrated to be abnormal on MRI, their primary use is to determine whether the patient's typical pain is reproduced. Whether this is scientifically valid has yet to be shown conclusively. Most clinicians recommend doing discography not only at the index level but also at the discs above and below; in this way, some internal control may be achieved. Recent work has questioned the usefulness of facet joint block. If a thoracic facet block with local anesthetic results in temporary symptomatic relief, it should probably be repeated at least two additional times to ensure that the results are legitimate.

Treatment

NONOPERATIVE

Nonoperative treatment of degenerative disease of the thoracic spine is similar to that of the lumbar spine: lifestyle modification, exercise, and drug therapy. Lifestyle modification includes identifying and eliminating activities that contribute to symptoms. This may mean a change in recreational and work activities. Exercise is encouraged, both to strengthen muscles and to improve endurance. Strengthening is concentrated on the paravertebral muscle groups. Aerobic exercise to improve endurance reduces muscular fatigue, improves posture, and may alter pain perception. Most of the nonsteroidal anti-inflammatory agents are not intended for long-term use, but they can be effective in controlling acute exacerbations of symptoms. This is also true of the analgesics and the muscle relaxants.

OPERATIVE

Surgery for symptomatic degenerative disease of the thoracic spine without neurologic involvement is rarely necessary. It is indicated in well-selected patients with single-level disease in whom it is absolutely clear that the degenerative level is responsible for symptoms.

Two surgical approaches have been proposed: an anterior discectomy and fusion, and a posterolateral fusion. There is no good information to compare these approaches. The anterior procedure requires a thoracotomy, however, which is a major undertaking.

CERVICAL SPINE

Clinical Presentation

The cervical spine is particularly susceptible to the degenerative process, in part because of its large range of motion and the five-joint complex making up each spinal motion unit. These five joints are the intervertebral disc, the two zygoapophyseal joints, and the two uncovertebral joints. The degenerative process may begin in any of these joints but with time will cause secondary changes in the others. For example, the intervertebral disc may be primarily affected. As the disc narrows, the normal kinematics of that segment is altered, and the other four joints are subjected to abnormal forces. This can lead to degenerative arthritis of those joints.

Neck pain as a result of spondylosis is common. The pain may radiate into the shoulder blade or chest or up to the skull. There may be associated headaches or blurred vision. Patients may have an arm complaint, not as the result of nerve root compression but rather due to a referred pain phenomenon. Dysphagia can result from large anterior osteophytes. Osteophytes extending laterally from the uncovertebral joints can cause vertebral artery compression, which may be manifest as dizziness, blurred vision, and tinnitus.

Physical examination may show a spasm of the paravertebral, trapezius, or sternomastoid mus-

cles; this may be secondary to pain. In association with the degenerative process, this can result in a decreased range of motion. Movement of the cervical spine may precipitate or exacerbate symptoms.

A thorough neurologic examination must always be done to rule out a deficit. A shoulder examination should also be done to ensure that the symptoms are indeed originating from the neck.

Diagnostic Evaluation

X-RAY

Plain radiographs of the cervical spine may show narrowing of the intervertebral disc space height, anterior osteophytes, arthrosis of the facet joints, and osteophytes from the uncovertebral joints (Fig. 8-8). The most commonly

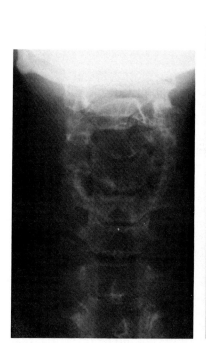
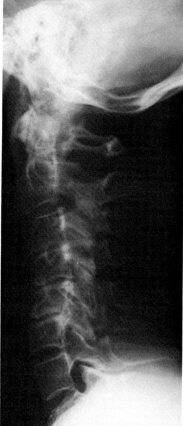
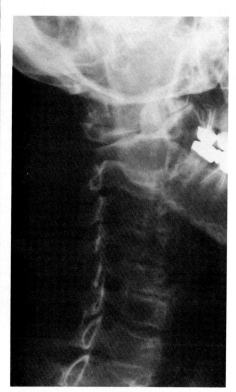

FIGURE 8–8. Plain x-rays of cervical spine showing degenerative disease (AP, lateral, and oblique x-ray).

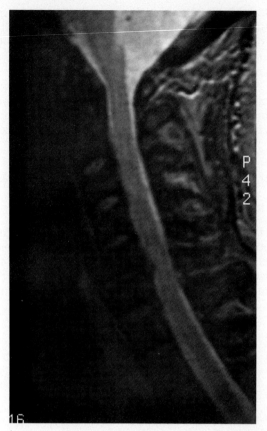

FIGURE 8–9. MRI showing extensive degenerative changes; patient is asymptomatic.

affected level is C5–C6, followed by the C6–C7 level.

COMPUTED TOMOGRAPHY

Computed tomography (CT) provides good demonstration of the bony changes associated with degenerative spondylosis. Osteophytes can be evaluated both on axial and sagittal cuts. However, CT does not allow optimal evaluation of disc pathology. It can be used to show disc herniations, but these may not always be present, even with advanced degenerative changes.

MAGNETIC RESONANCE IMAGING

Magnetic resonance imaging (MRI) is a powerful tool in the assessment of patients with symptomatic cervical spondylosis. Decreased signal intensity on T2-weighted images results from disc desiccation. T1-weighted images can show osteophytes and joint arthrosis. Because MRI is a sensitive imaging modality, pathology may be demonstrable in more than 40% of asymptomatic people over age 40 (Fig. 8-9). MRI remains a morphometric test, and the clinician must correlate MRI findings with symptoms.

DISCOGRAPHY

As in the lumbar and thoracic spine, cervical discography (Fig. 8-10) remains controversial. Although the discogram may add to the clinician's knowledge, it should not be used by itself to predicate treatment.

FACET BLOCKS

Facet blocks in the cervical spine are subject to the same criticisms as facet blocks used elsewhere. There is little scientific documentation to validate their use. Repeating the test and comparing results at different levels probably gives much more useful information than carrying out facet blocks at one or more levels at one point in time.

Treatment

NONOPERATIVE

Nonoperative treatment of cervical degenerative disease provides good to excellent results in over 75% of patients. A multidisciplinary approach includes immobilization, physical therapy, and medication. Immobilization can be achieved using the collar or braces described in Chapter 5. They are most beneficial during acute exacerbations of pain by reducing motion at the symptomatic levels. Physical therapy can be useful in decreasing the secondary muscle spasm that can contribute to symptoms; this is where heat, electrical stimulation, and exercise have their maximum benefit. Medications include analgesics, nonsteroidal anti-inflammatories, and muscle relaxants. Patients must be informed of possible complications and side effects of these medications.

This treatment should be given in a positive, caring manner. Patients should be reassured that nonoperative treatment can provide good long-term results.

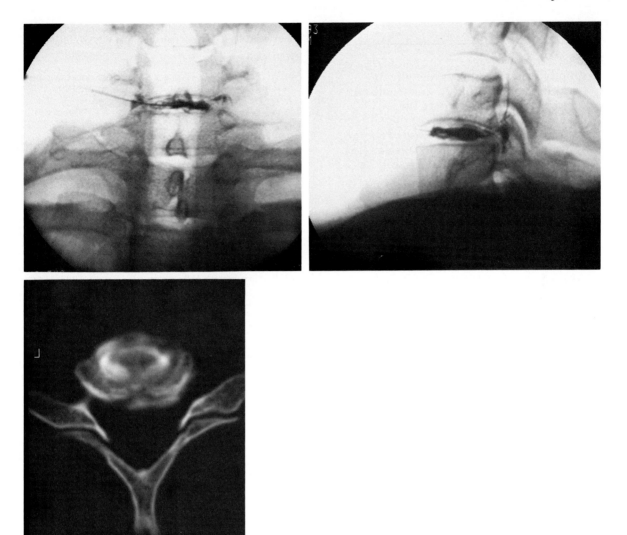

FIGURE 8–10. Cervical CT discography (AP, lateral discogram, and axial CT).

OPERATIVE

Although surgical treatment is occasionally warranted for this condition, the overall results of operative treatment are not good. This is due in large part to inappropriate patient selection and the inability in many instances to localize symptomatic levels accurately. The ideal candidate for surgery is young, has one affected level, and has failed nonoperative treatment; the association between degenerative disease and symptoms must be clearly established. Relative contraindications include multiple-level disease, degenerative changes at levels adjacent to the suspected symptomatic level, and increasing age.

The surgical procedure proposed for these patients is fusion. In almost all instances, the preferred approach is an anterior interbody fusion. Using the anterior approach, a complete discectomy can be done, and with careful sculpting of the graft, normal intervertebral disc space height and normal lordosis can be restored.

Until diagnostic testing improves to the point where we can show irrefutably that a specific cervical spinal motion unit is giving rise to symptoms, surgery for neck pain without neurologic involvement should be discouraged.

KEY POINTS

1. Degenerative disease of the spine, or spondylosis, is a process that affects many components of the spinal column.
2. Many factors can accelerate the degenerative process of the spine.
3. Although degenerative disease of the spine is frequently identified on imaging studies, it usually does not cause symptoms.
4. Almost all patients with symptomatic degenerative disease without neurologic symptoms or signs can be managed nonoperatively.

BIBLIOGRAPHY

BOOKS

Cooper PR, ed. Degenerative disease of the cervical spine. Neurosurgical Topics. Baltimore: American Association of Neurological Surgeons, 1992.

Frymoyer JW, Gordon SL. New perspectives on low back pain. Park Ridge, Illinois: American Academy of Orthopaedic Surgeons, 1989.

Wilkinson M, ed. Cervical spondylosis: Its early diagnosis and treatment. 2nd ed. Philadelphia: WB Saunders, 1971.

JOURNALS

Aprill C, Bogduk N. The prevalence of cervical zygapophyseal joint pain: A first approximation. Spine 1992;17:744–747.

Bough B, Thakore J, Davies M, Dowling F. Degeneration of lumbar facet joints. J Bone Joint Surg [Br] 1990;72:275–276.

Connor PM, Darden BV. Cervical discography complications and clinical efficacy. Spine 1993;18:2035–2038.

Fujita K, Nakagawa T, Hirabayashi K, Nagai Y. Neutral proteinases in human intervertebral disc. Role in degeneration and probable origin. Spine 1993;18:1766–1773.

Gibson MJ, Buckley J, Mawhinney R, Mulholland RC, Worthington BS. Magnetic resonance imaging and discography in the diagnosis of disc degeneration. J Bone Joint Surg [Br] 1986;68:369–373.

Modic MT, Steinberg PM, Ross JS, Masaryk IJ, Carter JR. Degenerative disk disease: Assessment of changes in vertebral body marrow with MR imaging. Radiology 1988;166:193–199.

Natarajan RN, Ke JH, Andersson GBJ. A model to study the disc degeneration process. Spine 1994;19:259–265.

Nelson DA. Intraspinal therapy using methylprednisolone acetate: twenty-three years of clinical controversy. Spine 1993;18:278–286.

Okada A, Harata S, Takeda Y, Nakamura T, Takagaki K, Endo M. Age-related changes in proteoglycans of human ligamentum flavum. Spine 1993;18:2261–2266.

Vanharanta H, Floyd T, Ohnmeiss DD, Hochschuler SH, Cruyer RD. The relationship of facet tropism to degenerative disc disease. Spine 1993;18:1000–1005.

Textbook of Spinal Disorders, by Stephen I. Esses.
J. B. Lippincott Company, Philadelphia © 1995.

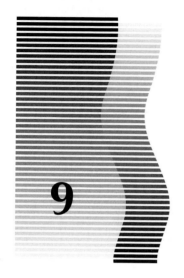

9

Herniated Disc Disease

LUMBAR HERNIATED
  DISC DISEASE
  Clinical Presentation
  Physical Examination
  Diagnostic Evaluation
    Electromyography
    Somatosensory
      Evoked Potentials
    X-ray
    Myelography/
      Computed
      Tomography
    CT Discography
    Magnetic Resonance
      Imaging
  Nonoperative
    Treatment
  Operative Treatment
    Indications
    Chemonucleolysis
    Discectomy
  Central Disc
    Herniation

THORACIC
  HERNIATED DISC
  DISEASE
  Clinical Presentation
  Diagnostic Evaluation
  Treatment
CERVICAL
  HERNIATED DISC
  DISEASE
  Clinical Presentation
  Diagnostic Evaluation
  Nonoperative
    Treatment
  Operative Treatment

The anatomy of the intervertebral disc has already been discussed in Chapter 1. The organization of collagen in the annulus fibrosus makes it strong in tension. Although there are many different molecular types of collagen present in the disc, most of it is type I or II. Type I collagen is primarily located in the outer lamellae of the annulus fibrosus. Type II collagen is predominantly located in the inner fibers of the annulus and in the nucleus pulposus. It has been suggested that the arrangement of collagen varies circumferentially in such a way that the posterolateral regions are the weakest and most prone to injury. This would explain why most disc herniations occur in those areas. The outer fibers of the annulus fibrosus blend with the anterior and posterior longitudinal ligaments. The anterior longitudinal ligament is much stronger than the posterior longitudinal ligament. This also helps explain why anterior disc herniations are so uncommon and why most occur posterolaterally (that is, lateral to the posterior longitudinal ligament) rather than directly posteriorly.

Normally, the collagen fibers of the annulus fibrosus are continuous and thus contain the nuclear material. If the annular fibers become disrupted, displacement of the nuclear material can occur. This situation is termed *herniated nucleus pulposus* (HNP). Four degrees of hernia-

185

tion can occur (Fig. 9-1). In *intraspongi nuclear herniation*, nuclear material migrates from the central region of the disc and into the annular fibers but does not cause any change in the configuration of the outermost annular fibers. *Protrusion* occurs when the nuclear material causes a bulging of the outermost annular fibers; this is also referred to as a *prolapsed* intervertebral disc. An *extruded* intervertebral disc rupture occurs when the nuclear material escapes through all the annular fibers but still remains connected to nuclear material within the disc. A *sequestered* intervertebral disc refers to nuclear material that has extruded through the fibers of the annulus fibrosus and lies in the spinal canal as a free fragment.

Other terms referring to herniated disc disease are found in the literature and medical records. Their use should be discouraged because this adds to the confusion in terminology and does not refer to specific pathologic states. Terms such as bulging disc, ruptured disc, and slipped disc should be avoided.

LUMBAR HERNIATED DISC DISEASE

Clinical Presentation

Large epidemiologic studies have suggested that the following are risk factors for herniated disc disease in the lumbar spine: smoking, prolonged daily driving of motor vehicles, and frequent repetitive lifting of heavy objects and twisting. It is more common in males than females and has a maximal incidence in the third and fourth decades of life. First-degree relatives of patients with disc herniations have an increased prevalence of disc herniation.

Clinical presentation of a herniated nucleus pulposus can be the onset of back pain, leg pain, or both. Back pain may be caused by stimulation of the pain fibers in the outer layers of the annulus fibrosus. Alternatively, distortion of the posterior longitudinal ligament, which is richly innervated by pain fibers, may result in back pain. Leg pain can result from compression of a nerve root by an HNP. Figure 9-2 shows how herniation of the L4–L5 disc can compress the fifth lumbar nerve root and how herniation of the lumbosacral disc causes compression of the first sacral nerve root. *Sciatica* is pain along the course of the sciatic nerve. It is a symptom, rather than a pathologic entity, that can be caused by an

HNP. The clinician must rule out a compressive lesion of the sciatic nerve peripherally before ascribing the pain to a herniated disc (Fig. 9-3).

Many patients present initially with back pain and then develop sciatica, with diminution of the back pain as their leg symptoms increase. *Radicular* pain is pain in the distribution of a specific nerve root. The most common levels for lumbar HNP are L4–L5 and L5–S1. For this reason, radicular symptoms almost always refer to symptoms below the level of the knee, in the L5 or S1 dermatome.

Leg symptoms are usually most predominant proximally and diminish distally. Leg symptoms can vary from numbness to dysesthesia to true pain.

In over half the patients with sciatica from an HNP, a specific nerve root can be identified simply by history. It is important to question the patient about weakness. Motor involvement of the tibialis anterior may make it difficult for patients to go downstairs, whereas involvement of the gastrocnemius–soleus muscle group may make going upstairs difficult.

Any maneuver that increases intraspinal pressure, such as straining at stool, coughing, or sneezing, may exacerbate symptoms.

Physical Examination

Physical examination of the patient begins with an evaluation of posture. Often there is a functional scoliosis, an involuntary attempt by the patient to reduce nerve root irritation. In most instances the disc herniation is lateral to the nerve root and the scoliosis has its concavity away from the side of the lesion. If the disc herniation is medial to the nerve root, the patient may bend to the painful side.

Range of motion of the lumbar spine may be limited due to paravertebral muscle spasm or guarding. Forward flexion may increase the symptoms of sciatica.

Palpation may show tenderness in the sciatic notch due to irritation of the nerve.

The signs of nerve root tension were discussed in Chapter 3. Well-leg raising often indicates a sequestered HNP; indeed, the most specific sign for lumbar disc herniation is a contralaterally positive straight leg raising examination. A femoral stretch test usually indicates a disc herniation at the L3–L4 level or above.

A meticulous neurologic examination is necessary to detect motor weakness, sensory changes, and deep tendon reflex asymmetry.

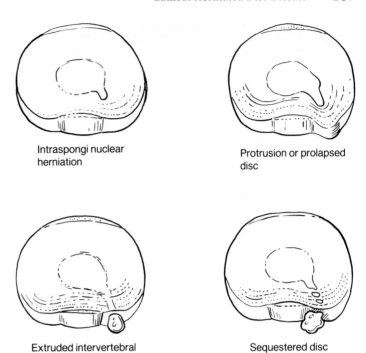

Intraspongi nuclear
herniation

Protrusion or prolapsed
disc

Extruded intervertebral
disc rupture

Sequestered disc

FIGURE 9–1. Four degrees of disc herniation.

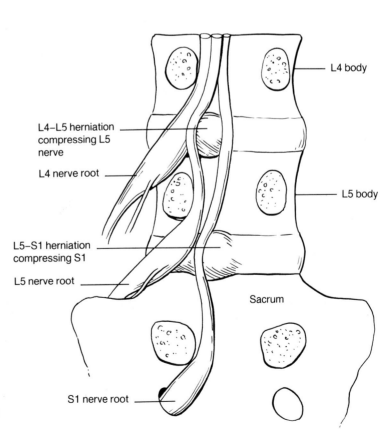

L4 body

L4–L5 herniation
compressing L5
nerve

L4 nerve root

L5 body

L5–S1 herniation
compressing S1

L5 nerve root

Sacrum

S1 nerve root

FIGURE 9–2. Disc herniation causing nerve
root compression.

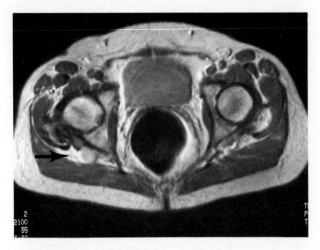

FIGURE 9–3. Cyst following total hip replacement.

Diagnostic Evaluation

ELECTROMYOGRAPHY

Electromyography (EMG) is an objective way in which the motor fibers of a nerve root can be assessed. Electric activity in a muscle is examined at rest and with voluntary muscle contraction. Normally, there is no spontaneous activity when the muscle is at rest. After demyelination, however, which usually occurs 2 to 3 weeks after the onset of nerve compression, there is spontaneous electric activity in the muscle at rest. This may be detected as fibrillation potentials or fasciculations. After denervation, voluntary muscle contraction may elicit abnormal motor unit potentials. They may be of higher amplitude, increased duration, or increased number of phases. The EMG may be useful in objectively documenting motor dysfunction and ascertaining the degree and duration of denervation.

SOMATOSENSORY EVOKED POTENTIALS

Somatosensory evoked potentials, discussed in Chapter 7, have been used to measure the sensory integrity of specific nerve roots. Dermatomal stimulation is done in the autonomous areas and recording is done at the level of the cortex.

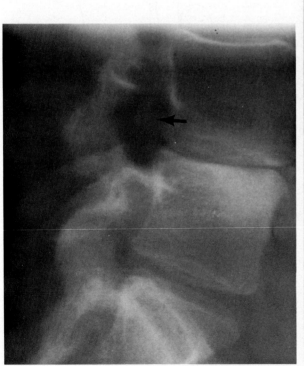
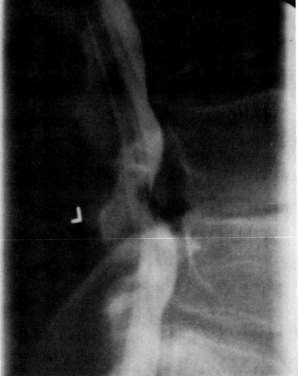

FIGURE 9–4. Ossified fragment in canal.

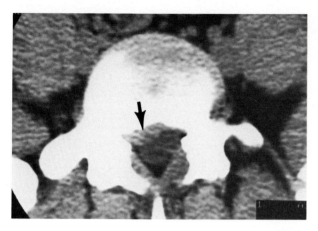

FIGURE 9–5. Plain CT showing herniated nucleus pulposus (HNP).

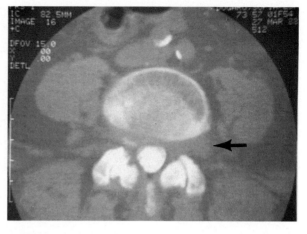

FIGURE 9–6. CT myelography showing lateral disc herniation.

X-RAY

Plain radiographs are not particularly useful in the investigation of patients with HNP. However, in young patients the herniation may be associated with an avulsion of the end plate. In these instances, a small ossified fragment may be identified in the spinal canal at the level of the intervertebral disc (Fig. 9-4). An estimated 30% of symptomatic HNPs are associated with some element of spinal stenosis. Thus, examination of the oblique x-rays can be useful.

MYELOGRAPHY/COMPUTED TOMOGRAPHY

Myelography in combination with computed tomography (CT) scanning is more useful than either alone (Figs. 9-5 through 9-7). Although the nonionic water-soluble contrast agents are not associated with the side effects attendant on the use of oil-based dyes, myelography is still an invasive procedure and has risks (see Chap. 4). Myelography is no longer the primary imaging modality used for the assessment of suspected HNP, but there are specific indications for myelography and CT scanning. These include the presence of significant spinal deformity, which makes it difficult to interpret MR images; the presence of metallic implants, precluding MR scanning; and significant claustrophobia of the patient, which makes MR scanning too uncomfortable.

CT DISCOGRAPHY

CT discography involves the injection of contrast into the center of the intervertebral disc, followed a few hours later by CT scanning. Nuclear disc material has been shown to have an affinity for water-soluble contrast media. Thus, CT discography is useful in distinguishing between recurrent disc herniation and epidural scar tissue. CT discography is particularly useful in the diagnosis of foraminal disc herniation (Fig. 9-8). CT discography is more accurate, sensitive, and specific than myelography, CT scanning, or both for lumbar HNP. Nevertheless, because it is an invasive procedure, it is not recommended as the primary diagnostic technique. Discography is contraindicated in cauda equina syndrome.

MAGNETIC RESONANCE IMAGING

Magnetic resonance imaging (MRI) is the optimal imaging modality for patients with suspected lumbar disc herniation (Fig. 9-9). One major advantage is that far lateral disc herniations,

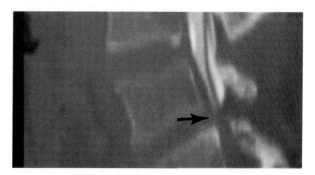

FIGURE 9–7. Sagittal CT myelogram showing a complete block.

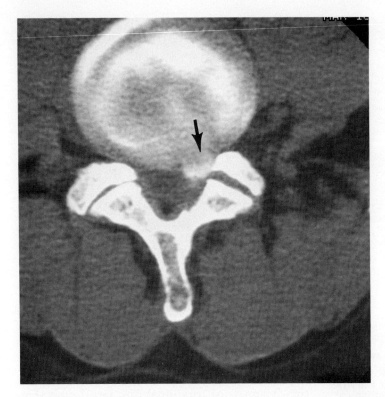

FIGURE 9–8. CT discogram showing foraminal disc herniation.

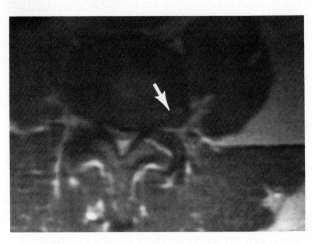

FIGURE 9–10. MRI showing lateral disc herniation.

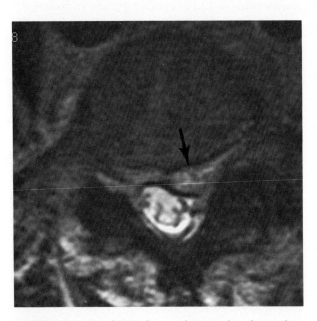

FIGURE 9–9. Axial MRI showing herniated nucleus pulposus (HNP).

which would be overlooked on myelography, can be easily identified (Fig. 9-10). In addition, it is possible to differentiate sequestered disc herniations from disc protrusions and extrusions. Extruded fragments are best seen on T2-weighted images and are characterized by a very high signal intensity with a surrounding area of decreased signal intensity. The use of gadolinium has made it possible to distinguish between recurrent disc herniations and postoperative scarring (Fig. 9-11). The sensitivity and specificity of MRI in the diagnosis of herniated disc disease of the lumbar spine compares well with myelography and CT and CT discography. MRI is noninvasive and does not require exposure to ionizing radiation.

Nonoperative Treatment

Any rational discussion of treatment assumes that the natural history of the condition without treatment has been documented. In general, patients with lumbar HNP tend to get better. The longer one waits, the more likely the patient is to have spontaneous resolution of symptoms. Studies have shown that fewer than 10% of patients who do not have treatment still cannot work 3 months after the onset of symptoms. Unfortunately, we cannot identify these patients at the onset of their symptoms. We do not know the natural history of lumbar herniated disc disease as a function of the precise pathology present. Given our socioeconomic climate, it is unfortunate but true that a number of nonorganic factors influence a patient's recovery.

Because more than 90% of patients will recover without treatment, it is difficult to show the beneficial effect of a given treatment modality. Many types of interventions that have been touted as useful have not been shown to have any significant benefit when subjected to scrupulous scientific investigation. Because patients suffering from HNP have pain and are disabled, they are susceptible to becoming victims of ineffective but costly advice and treatment.

As discussed in Chapter 6, very few modalities have been shown to alter the natural history of lumbar disc disease. Rest may be of benefit but is not recommended for more than 72 hours. Gentle back exercises, especially a McKenzie extension routine, may hasten recovery (see Fig. 6-2). In the past, pelvic traction was advocated for the treatment of acute sciatica, but this is ineffective in altering the disc herniation in any way, nor does it affect the time to recovery.

Operative Treatment

INDICATIONS

Most patients with a lumbar HNP do not require operative treatment, but it is reasonable to offer intervention to patients who have profound or progressive weakness, those with pain persisting for more than 3 months, and those who develop a cauda equina syndrome. Under any of these circumstances, an imaging study must confirm the presence of neural compression at the level suspected by clinical examination.

At present we cannot identify early on the patients who will not get better within 3 months, but we may be able to in the future. There is speculation that these patients have very large extrusions or sequestered fragments.

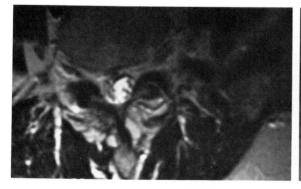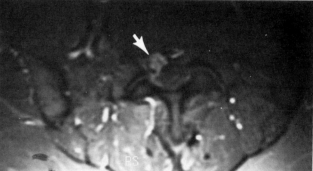

FIGURE 9–11. MRI with and without gadolinium.

TABLE 9–1. **Indications for Chymopapain**

Pain less than 6 months
Leg pain greater than back pain
Positive nerve root tension signs
Nerve root dysfunction
Imaging defect correlating with clinical findings

TABLE 9–2. **Relative Contraindications
to Chymopapain**

Patient older than age 50
Previous surgery at affected level
Increased ESR in females
Bony stenosis

CHEMONUCLEOLYSIS

Various substances have been used in an attempt to dissolve or shrink the disc and thus remove neurologic compression. These have included chymopapain, collagenase, aproteinin, chondroitinase, and cathepsins. *Chymopapain*, derived from the papaya, is approved for use in most countries. After injection into the disc, nuclear material is dissolved. Many double-blind prospective trials have shown that chymopapain has a significant therapeutic effect. Its indications and relative contraindications are given in Tables 9-1 and 9-2. Absolute contraindications include a sensitivity to chymopapain, severe neurologic lesions, multiple-level disc herniations, and a sequestered disc fragment. There is a significant allergic response, which can range from a benign rash to fatal anaphylaxis; the incidence of the latter has been reported between 0.18% and 1%. There have been rare reports of central nervous system (CNS) hemorrhage and acute transverse myelitis. Paravertebral back spasm occurs in 20% to 30% of patients, and some reduction in disc height is detected in almost all patients. Because of these complications, chymopapain fell into disfavor. Recently, however, skin testing has been developed to allow for preinjection detection of sensitivity.

The technique of injection is shown in Figure 9-12. The patient is awake and in the lateral decubitus position. The needle is introduced about one handbreadth lateral to the midline and angled obliquely to enter the affected disc. Accurate needle placement is confirmed using an image intensifier.

It is not possible to predict the degree to which a disc will be dissolved by a chymopapain injection. Occasionally, significant disc degradation occurs, with resultant intervertebral disc space collapse. This can lead to symptomatic foraminal stenosis.

The most common cause for unsuccessful chymopapain injection is the presence of a sequestered disc fragment. With newer imaging techniques, it should be possible to identify these patients more accurately before treatment is instituted.

With increasing interest in minimally invasive surgical techniques, methods have been developed for percutaneous discectomy. Some of these are simply mechanical, with cannulas placed through the skin into the intervertebral disc and special instruments for removing the nuclear material. Devices to perform *automated percutaneous discectomy* consist of a probe with a rotating blade and port on the end for suction and removal of the sliced nuclear material (Fig. 9-13). Recently, lasers have been used for percu-

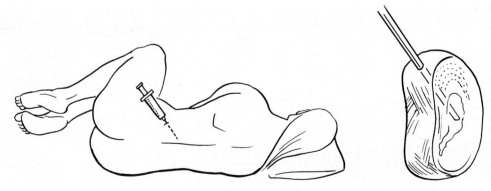

FIGURE 9–12. Injection technique for chymopapain.

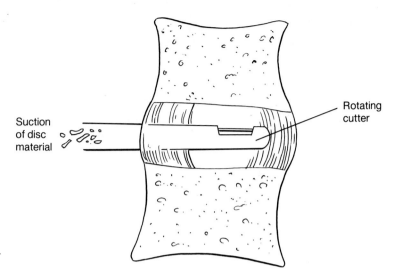

Suction of disc material

Rotating cutter

FIGURE 9–13. Automated percutaneous discectomy.

taneous discectomy. A cannula positioned in the intervertebral disc allows the introduction of a laser beam to destroy disc material.

All the percutaneous techniques are thought not only to remove nuclear material but also to decrease intradiscal pressure. These techniques are of value only in contained disc herniations. At present it is impossible to safely remove a sequestered disc fragment percutaneously.

DISCECTOMY

Discectomy is the excision of all or part of an intervertebral disc by an open surgical procedure. In the past, discectomy was almost always accompanied by *hemilaminectomy* (removal of half of a lamina), *laminectomy* (removal of all of a lamina), or *laminotomy* (removal of part of a lamina). These were done purely for technical reasons. With the surgical instruments then available, it was thought safer to remove some of the bone from the posterior neural arch to better expose the dura and nerve root (Fig. 9-14). With improvements in surgical instrumentation and better intraoperative lighting, we can now perform a discectomy without removing any bone.

The standard technique consists of a midline incision made over the affected disc level. The paravertebral muscles are retracted and the lamina of the vertebrae above and below the index disc is identified. The ligamentum flavum is incised and carefully removed. It should now be possible to identify the dura and nerve root (Fig. 9-15). In most instances, the nerve root is displaced laterally because of the underlying disc herniation. The root is gently retracted medially

and protected. If the disc herniation is sequestered, the fragment is removed. If there is a protrusion or extrusion, the annular fibers must be incised with a small knife. A special instrument, the pituitary rongeur, is then introduced through the annular fibers, and the nuclear material can be removed (Fig. 9-16). There is no need to remove the intervertebral disc in its entirety; it is usually necessary only to remove the material causing neural compression.

Microdiscectomy is the use of a microscope in performing disc excision. By providing magnification and illumination, the microscope allows for a smaller incision and limited dissection. In

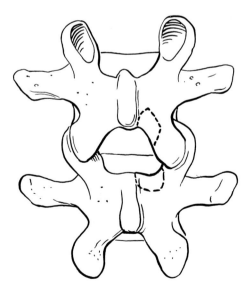

FIGURE 9–14. Lumbar laminotomy.

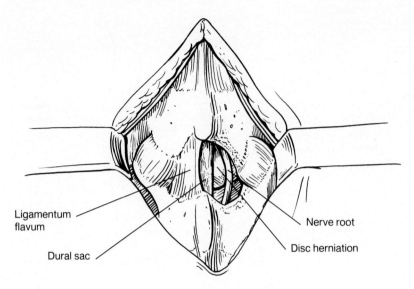

Ligamentum flavum

Dural sac

Nerve root

Disc herniation

FIGURE 9-15. Surgical exposure of nerve root.

general, the reported results for microdiscectomy are similar to those of discectomy.

About a third of patients with symptomatic disc herniations have an element of lateral recess stenosis. It is important to identify these patients so that at the time of surgery a concomitant foraminotomy can be undertaken (Fig. 9-17).

It is difficult to review the reported results of surgery for herniated disc disease because most studies are retrospective, involve a single-author review, and often use different rating systems.

Although there may be no difference between surgical and nonsurgical treatment in regard to pain relief and return to work in the long term, surgical patients do better early on with respect to resolution of symptoms and return to work. There is some evidence that surgical results are not as good if there has been sciatica for longer than 12 weeks. In cauda equina syndrome, surgical results are optimal if operative intervention is instituted within the first 6 hours. In general, the worst results from discectomy occur in patients who have worker's compensation and when there is minimal clinical evidence of sciatica. Factors associated with the development of significant low back pain after discectomy include worker's compensation, cigarette smoking, and age over 40 years.

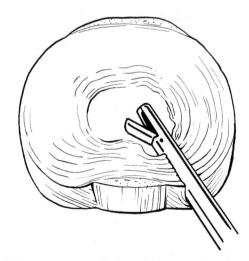

FIGURE 9-16. Removal of nuclear material with a pituitary rongeur.

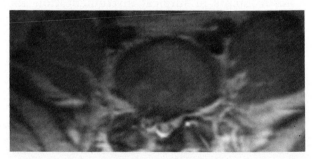

FIGURE 9-17. Lumbar herniated nucleus pulposus (HNP) with spinal stenosis.

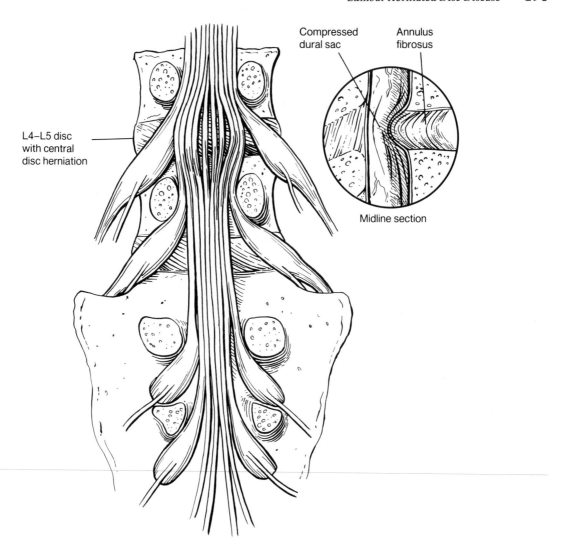

Compressed
dural sac

Annulus
fibrosus

L4–L5 disc
with central
disc herniation

Midline section

FIGURE 9–18. L4–L5 central disc herniation resulting in cauda equina syndrome.

Central Disc Herniation

A small central disc herniation can put tension on and deform the posterior longitudinal ligament. The posterior longitudinal ligament is richly innervated with pain fibers, and occasionally a small central disc herniation can be associated with marked low back pain. If a central disc herniation becomes larger, neurologic compression results. Because of the anatomy of the cauda equina, the sacral roots on both sides are affected. Cauda equina syndrome is characterized by bilateral leg pain, perianal anesthe-

sia, urinary retention, and loss of rectal tone. Although rare, it can result from a large central disc herniation (Fig. 9-18).

Cauda equina syndrome is an absolute indication for urgent surgical intervention. The operative approach is similar to that described above, but because the dural sac itself may have to be retracted, a laminectomy is considered prudent. This will prevent iatrogenic neural injury by compression from retraction. The prognosis in cauda equina syndrome from a central disc herniation is worse for return of bowel and bladder function than for motor and sensory function.

THORACIC HERNIATED DISC DISEASE

Clinical Presentation

Intervertebral disc herniation occurs much less frequently in the thoracic spine than in the lumbar or cervical spine. The major reason for this is that there is much less motion in the thoracic spine and, therefore, the annular fibers are less prone to fail. The most common levels for thoracic disc herniations are T9 to T12, levels with more motion than the rest of the thoracic spine.

Patients may present with three major symptoms. The first is back pain, which is usually not well localized and may be described as aching. The second symptom is due to thoracic nerve root irritation, which may result in a band of tenderness around the chest (Fig. 9-19). Physical examination may detect a dermatomal dysesthesia or loss of sensation to pinprick or light touch. Third, the patient may have symptoms of spinal cord compression such as weakness in the lower limbs, bowel or bladder dysfunction, or ataxia. This is not uncommon because the spinal canal is small in the thoracic area, and even a small disc herniation may result in spinal cord compression.

Even major neurologic deficits may not be associated with pain. Therefore, the clinician must do a careful neurologic examination to ascertain the affected level. In many instances, the diagnosis is made late or completely overlooked. Disc herniation should be included in the differential diagnosis of chest or breast pain, myelopathy, and lower extremity weakness.

Diagnostic Evaluation

In the past, many patients suffering from herniated thoracic disc disease were not accurately identified due to limited and insensitive diagnostic tests. Plain radiographs are not generally helpful, although occasionally calcification of an old herniated disc can be seen. Although myelography was used in the past, it is not as sensitive for thoracic herniations as for lumbar disc herniations. This is because the thoracic kyphosis makes it difficult to obtain equal distribution of the contrast dye throughout the thoracic spine. With the patient supine, the dye collects in the midthoracic region; with the patient prone, dye tends to drain away from the thoracic area. Myelography with CT scanning has improved our ability to identify herniated thoracic discs, particularly if a large volume of contrast material is used and the radiologist is meticulous (Fig. 9-20). CT discography has not been widely advocated in the thoracic spine, primarily because of the risk of pneumothorax.

MRI allows us to identify herniated discs noninvasively and much more accurately. Sagittal and axial images permit precise localization and an assessment of the degree of spinal cord compression, if any. It is extremely useful for identifying lateral herniations causing nerve root compression (Fig. 9-21).

Treatment

The natural history of thoracic disc herniations has not been well documented, but many herniations resolve with time. However, if there is spinal cord compression and associated neurologic deficit, neither the clinician nor the patient has the luxury of observation. The duration and degree of spinal cord compression correlate with irreversible spinal cord damage. For this reason, any significant neurologic deficit is an indication for urgent surgery.

The spinal cord is extremely sensitive to pressure, and any retraction on the spinal cord can result in permanent injury. For this reason, lami-

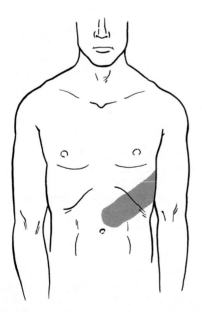

FIGURE 9–19. Thoracic herniated disc causing band of chest tenderness.

nectomy is usually not recommended for thoracic herniations. Costotransversectomy has been advocated by some surgeons, but it may not provide optimal visualization, particularly if the herniation is central. Furthermore, if the herniation is central, some manipulation of the spinal cord may be necessary. An anterior transthoracic approach allows excellent visualization and does not require any retraction on the spinal cord. Most surgeons recommend complete excision of the disc, but there is debate as to whether a concomitant fusion is necessary. If a fusion is not done, some kyphotic deformity may occur and can lead to symptoms.

CERVICAL HERNIATED DISC DISEASE

Clinical Presentation

Due to the large motions that occur in the cervical spine, the intervertebral discs are subject to significant stress. The annular fibers, particularly in the posterior and posterolateral regions, can fail, with resultant nuclear herniation. Herniated material can cause spinal cord or nerve root compression.

Because most cervical disc herniations occur only after significant degenerative change, many patients present with a long history of neck pain. With herniation of the nuclear material, the pa-

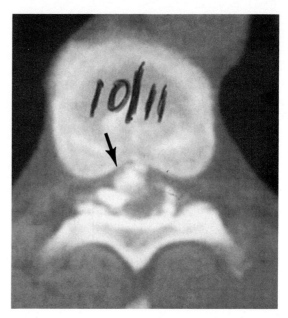

FIGURE 9–20. CT myelogram showing thoracic disc herniation.

tient's symptoms then change from neck pain to neck pain with additional arm symptoms. The upper extremity symptoms may include paresthesias, dysesthesias, pain, and weakness. Holding the arm elevated in a position of comfort is a classic finding of cervical disc herniation. It is important to note by history and physical examination the specific nerve root level affected. At

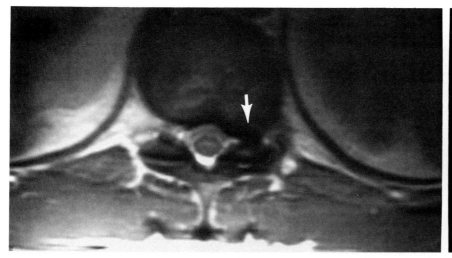
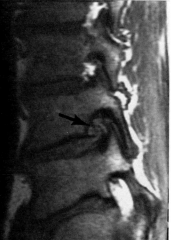

FIGURE 9–21. Axial and sagittal MRI showing thoracic disc herniation into foramen.

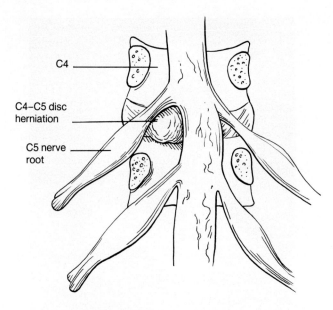

FIGURE 9–22. Compression of the fifth cervical nerve root by a C4–C5 disc herniation.

the C4–C5 disc level, for example, the fifth cervical root can be compressed by a disc herniation (Fig. 9-22). Occasionally a patient may not have any symptoms referable to the neck and may present with painless weakness in the upper extremity or with myelopathy.

Diagnostic Evaluation

As with disc herniations elsewhere, plain radiographs are not particularly useful. There may be some changes indicative of a degenerative process at the affected level (eg, disc space narrowing, spur formation, or subluxation).

Myelography in combination with CT scanning is more effective and sensitive than either test alone (Fig. 9-23). The CT scan should be done with very thin slices, and sagittal reformations should be generated.

Some investigators have advocated the use of CT discography in the investigation of the herniated disc (Fig. 9-24). However, injection of the contrast dye at a level in which there is significant cord compression can cause or exacerbate neurologic symptoms.

MR scanning is the primary investigative tool for herniated cervical disc disease (Fig. 9-25). Very thin axial sections should be taken. Software is continually being developed with resul-

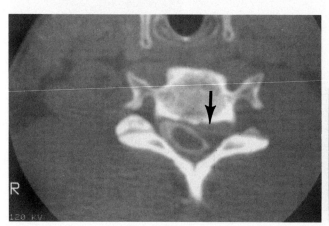
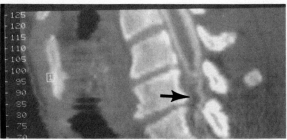

FIGURE 9–23. Axial and sagittal CT myelogram showing cervical disc herniation.

tant improvement in the generated images. Unfortunately, cervical MRI requires the subject's head and face to be placed in a small enclosed space, and the examination, particularly the T2-weighted images, may take 30 to 40 minutes to complete. Many patients who do not consider themselves claustrophobic have found this to be uncomfortable and anxiety-producing. Some patients may require sedation before MR examination of the cervical spine.

In patients with upper extremity symptoms without objective findings of neurologic deficit, EMG examination may be of great value because it can be used to localize the symptomatic nerve root. Nerve conduction studies should also be done in these patients to detect concomitant peripheral nerve entrapment syndromes. However, EMG findings may be normal even in patients with very marked compressive cervical radiculopathy because the cervical sensory route may be selectively compromised. In addition, the EMG may be normal due to overlapping motor innervation of a single muscle.

Nonoperative Treatment

Many nonoperative modalities have been suggested for the treatment of herniated cervical disc disease, but as outlined in Chapter 6, most have not been subjected to scientific scrutiny. Immobilization, either by the use of an orthosis or by bed rest, has been widely used. Although it

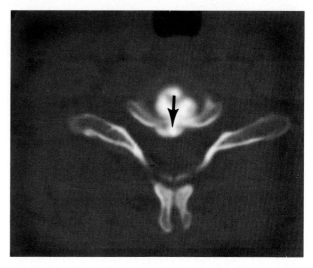

FIGURE 9–24. CT discogram showing cervical herniated disc.

probably does not alter the natural history of the herniated cervical disc, it may cause some decrease in pain by limiting cervical motion and thus the irritation of a compressed root. Although traction has been advocated, its maximum benefit is for foraminal stenosis (see Chap. 11). There is no evidence that traction, either in-

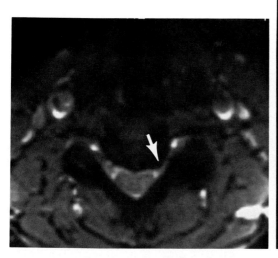
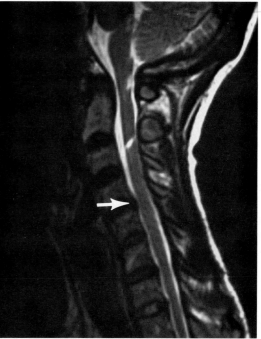

FIGURE 9–25. MRI showing C4–C5 disc herniation.

termittent or continuous, affects herniated nuclear material in any way. In general, physical modalities are used to control symptoms rather than alter the natural history of this condition.

Operative Treatment

Surgical intervention is indicated when a cervical disc herniation causes spinal cord dysfunction, profound weakness in the upper extremity, or prolonged arm pain. Two surgical approaches have been advocated—posterior and anterior. The posterior approach is best reserved for lateral herniations in patients who have primarily radicular symptoms. The posterior approach usually consists of a hemilaminectomy with removal of part of the facet joint on one side. It allows good visualization of the nerve root (Fig. 9-26). The anterior approach is ideal when the herniation is central and when there are significant symptoms of neck pain in association with radicular or spinal cord symptoms. The anterior approach allows for complete disc excision and decompression of the spinal cord. The risk of neurologic injury at the time of elective anterior cervical disc excision is less than 1%. There is some controversy as to whether disc excision should always be accompanied by an anterior interbody fusion. Most surgeons agree that performing a fusion at the time of disc excision prevents the development of a kyphotic deformity and decreases the incidence of postoperative neck pain. However, it is associated with the potential of significant complications. Each patient considered for surgery should be individually assessed to determine the optimal operative approach.

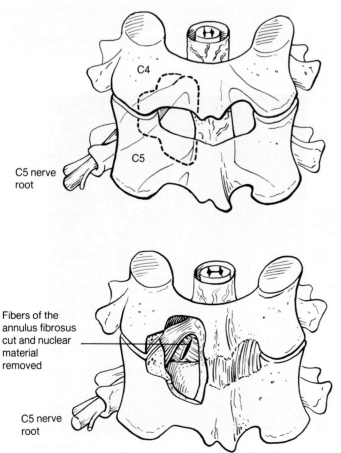

FIGURE 9–26. Posterior surgical approach for herniated cervical disc.

KEY POINTS

1. Herniations of the intervertebral disc can be categorized as intraspongi, prolapsed, extruded, or sequestered. Most herniations are asymptomatic.
2. Most symptomatic herniations can be managed nonoperatively. If a disc herniation causes significant neurologic deficit or unremitting, profound pain, surgery may be indicated.
3. MRI is the best imaging modality for demonstrating herniated disc disease.

BIBLIOGRAPHY

BOOKS

Warkins RG, Collis JS Jr, eds. Lumbar discetomy and laminectomy. Rockville, Maryland: Aspen Publications, 1987.

JOURNALS

Bohlman HH, Emery SE, Goodfellow DB, Jones PK. Robinson anterior cervical discectomy and arthrodesis for cervical radiculopathy. Long-term follow-up of one hundred and twenty-two patients. J Bone Joint Surg [Am] 1993;75:1298–1307.

Brown CW, Deffer PA Jr, Akmakjian J, Donaldson DH, Brugman JL. The natural history of thoracic disc herniation. Spine 1992;17(6 suppl): S97–S102.

Gunzburg K, Fraser RD, Moore R, Vernon-Roberts B. An experimental study comparing percutaneous discectomy with chemonucleolysis. Spine 1993;18:218–226.

Maigne JY, Deligne L. Computed tomographic follow-up study of 21 cases of nonoperatively treated cervical intervertebvral soft disc herniation. Spine 1994;19:189–191.

Mochida J, Arima T. Percutaneous nucleotomy in lumbar disc herniation. A prospective study. Spine 1993;18:2063–2068.

Ohshima H, Hirano N, Osada R, Matusi H, Tsuji H. Morphologic variation of lumbar posterior longitudinal ligament and the modality of disc herniation. Spine 1993;18:2408–2411.

Quigley MR, Maroon JC. Laser discectomy: a review. Spine 1994;19:53–56.

Revel M, Payan C, Vallee C, et al. Automated percutaneous lumbar discectomy versus chemonucleolysis in treatment of sciatica: A randomized multicenter trial. Spine 1993;18:1–7.

Tsuji H, Hirano N, Ohshima H, Ishihara H, Terahata N, Motoe T. Structural variation of the anterior and posterior anulus fibrosus in the development of human lumbar intervertebral disc: A risk factor for intervertebral disc rupture. Spine 1993;18:204–210.

Tullberg T, Isacson J, Weidenhielm L. Does microscopic removal of lumbar disc herniation lead to better results than the standard procedure? Results of a one-year randomized study. Spine 1993;18:24–27.

Weber H, Holme I, Amlie E. The natural course of acute sciatica with nerve root symptoms in a double-blind placebo-controlled trial evaluating the effect of piroxicam. Spine 1993;18:1433–1438.

Textbook of Spinal Disorders, by Stephen I. Esses.
J. B. Lippincott Company, Philadelphia © 1995.

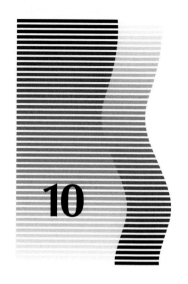

10

Spondylolisthesis

CERVICAL SPINE
LUMBAR SPINE
  Classification
  Clinical Presentation
  Diagnostic Evaluation
  Treatment

Spondylolisthesis is a forward translation of one vertebral body with respect to another. The term is derived from two Greek words, *spondylo* (vertebra) and *olisthesis* (to slide on an incline). Spondylolisthesis can occur anywhere in the spinal column but is most common in the lower lumbar spine. *Spondylolysis* is a break in the vertebra, almost always in the region of the pars interarticularis. A spondylolysis may or may not be associated with a spondylolisthesis. Furthermore, these two entities are not necessarily associated with any clinical symptoms. Thus, the demonstration of a spondylolysis or listhesis does not necessarily implicate it as symptomatic even in patients with back pain. The degree of spondylolisthesis is not associated in any way with the incidence of symptoms.

CERVICAL SPINE

Although rare, spondylolisthesis has been described in the cervical spine. The most commonly affected levels are C2, C4, and C6. The cause is almost always a defect in the pedicles or pars lateralis. When these defects are congenital, they are usually associated with other anomalies. As discussed in Chapter 15, spondylolisthesis at C2 can result from a traumatic fracturing of the

TABLE 10–1. **Classification of Spondylolisthesis**

I. Dysplastic (congenital)
II. Isthmic
  A. Lytic
  B. Elongated pars
  C. Acute pars fracture
III. Degenerative
IV. Posttraumatic
V. Pathologic
VI. Iatrogenic

pedicles. It is important to distinguish between a hangman's fracture and a longstanding anomaly. The presence of other congenital aberrations suggests the latter.

LUMBAR SPINE

Classification

Various classification schemes have been proposed for spondylolisthesis. The most common classification is based on cause (Table 10-1). *Type I* spondylolisthesis is a congenital abnormality that allows a forward slip to occur (Fig. 10-1). It usually occurs at the lumbosacral junction and is due to a deficiency of the upper sacrum or dysplasia of the posterior arch of L5. Because the pars interarticularis remains intact, the posterior arch translates forward with the vertebral body. This causes a kinking of the dural sac. When the slip exceeds 35%, cauda equina symptoms usually result. There is a strong hereditary ele-

ment to this type of spondylolisthesis, and it may be associated with other congenital spinal anomalies.

The basic lesion in *isthmic* or *type II* spondylolisthesis is in the pars interarticularis. *Type IIA* or *lytic* listhesis involves a defect in the pars area (Fig. 10-2). Many causes have been proposed, but it is generally thought to be caused by recurrent microfractures, probably occurring when the articular processes impact the pars in extension. Type IIA spondylolisthesis is twice as common in males than females. It usually occurs by age 6, although some cases develop later. The overall incidence in North American Caucasians is 6%, but the incidence varies greatly among different races and approaches 50% in North American Eskimos. Developmental anomalies such as lumbarization, sacralization, and spina bifida occulta are associated with lytic spondylolisthesis.

The difference between type IIA and IIB isthmic listhesis is that the pars interarticularis is intact in the latter. It probably does result from recurrent microfractures, but rather than a defect the pars heals in an elongated contour (Fig. 10-3). The pars has been compared to pulled toffee in this condition.

Type IIC spondylolisthesis results from an acute fracture of the pars interarticularis. It results from very significant trauma and is rare. It is sometimes difficult to distinguish a type IIA from a type IIC lesion, particularly in patients with back pain following injury. In longstanding lesions, cortication of the defects can be seen on computed tomographic (CT) scanning.

Degenerative or *type III* spondylolisthesis results from intersegmental stability. The major pathology is probably degenerative arthritis of the facet joints (Fig. 10-4). Multiple stress frac-

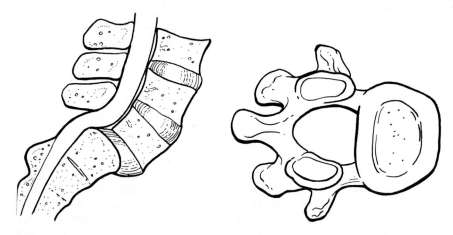

FIGURE 10–1. Congenital spondylolisthesis (type I).

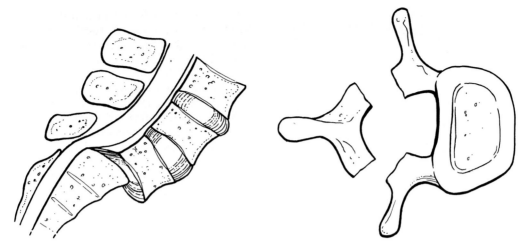

FIGURE 10–2. Lytic spondylolisthesis (type IIA).

tures of the inferior articular process of the vertebra allows anterior translation and leads to a change in the orientation of the articular processes. This process is more pronounced on one side than the other, which gives rise to the rotational component of this deformity. It is far more common at the L4–L5 level than at the L5–S1 level. It is much more common in females than in males and is rare in patients under age 40. When there is an L4–L5 degenerative spondylolisthesis, the L4 root is commonly trapped between the L4 inferior facet and the L5 body. Occasionally, degenerative changes in the facet joints cause the vertebra to translate posteriorly rather than anteriorly; this is called a *retrolisthesis* (Fig. 10-5).

Posttraumatic or *type IV* spondylolisthesis is secondary to a severe injury that fractures some part of the vertebra other than the pars interarticularis.

Pathologic or *type V* spondylolisthesis is usually due to a metabolic bone disease such as osteogenesis imperfecta or osteomalacia. These processes allow attenuation and elongation of the pedicles with resultant forward translation of the vertebra. Occasionally a neoplastic deposit may result in a pathologic spondylolisthesis.

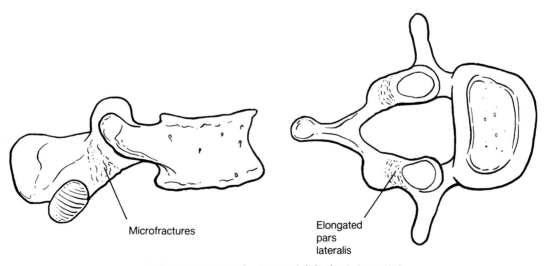

Microfractures

Elongated
pars
lateralis

FIGURE 10–3. Isthmic spondylolisthesis (type IIB).

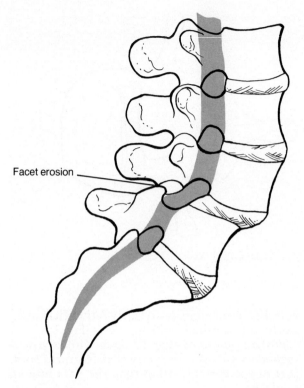

Facet erosion

FIGURE 10–4. Degenerative spondylolisthesis (type III).

Postsurgical or *type VI* spondylolisthesis is iatrogenic. It usually occurs as a result of overly aggressive decompression of the dural sac with removal of all the posterior elements. It can also occur after surgery by fracturing of the pars.

Clinical Presentation

Clinical presentation is determined largely by the type of spondylolisthesis. Dysplastic and isthmic forms usually present during late childhood or early adolescence, possibly due to the increased participation in strenuous sports that occurs at that time. The usual complaint is low back pain. Occasionally there is leg pain in the L5 or S1 distribution, but signs of nerve root compression are rare. In addition to pain, there commonly is an abnormal gait, primarily due to hamstring tightness (see Fig. 3-17). Patients cannot flex their hips with the knees extended and tend to walk with a waddle. They take only short strides. Because the pelvis is thrust forward, there is a postural deformity. Patients develop a transverse abdominal crease with flattening of the buttocks.

Three major pain patterns are associated with degenerative spondylolisthesis: back pain as a result of the degenerative arthritis and segmental instability; claudicant pain due to the spinal stenosis caused by the slip; and leg pain due to a compression neuropathy resulting from foraminal stenosis. The latter is the most common.

On physical examination, a palpable step may be felt over the spinous process at the level above the slipped vertebra (Fig. 10-6). In types I and II spondylolisthesis, the posterior arch of the vertebra translated forward remains in its usual position; this is why the step is felt at the level above. Due to hamstring tightness, straight leg raising may cause pain, but there are usually no true nerve root tension signs. The pelvic rotation causes the transverse abdominal crease mentioned above.

A thorough neurologic evaluation should be part of the physical examination. The clinician should specifically check for any sacral anesthesia due to cauda equina compression. Weakness in the tibialis anterior is common.

Diagnostic Evaluation

Because the translation in spondylolisthesis occurs in the sagittal plane, it is best appreciated on lateral x-rays. Due to the oblique orientation of the lower lumbosacral intervertebral disc spaces, the degree of slip is accentuated when the patient is standing. For this reason, measurements made with respect to the degree of spondylolisthesis should be done on standing lateral films (Fig. 10-7).

The degree of spondylolisthesis can be measured in two ways. The Myerding technique involves dividing the superior aspect of the vertebra below the slip into four equal divisions. Assessment is then made of where the posterior vertebral body of the spondylolisthetic vertebra lies with respect to these four quadrants. If the vertebra lies entirely anterior to the vertebra below, it is a grade V spondylolisthesis or *spondyloptosis* (Fig. 10-8). In a more refined technique for measuring the degree of translation, the percentage slip is calculated. A ratio is constructed of the distance from the posterior vertebral body below the slip to a line drawn parallel to the posterior body of the spondylolisthetic vertebra. This is then divided by the anteroposterior size of the slipped vertebral body.

In addition to translation, there is often significant rotation of the vertebra in the sagittal plane. This leads to a kyphotic deformity at the

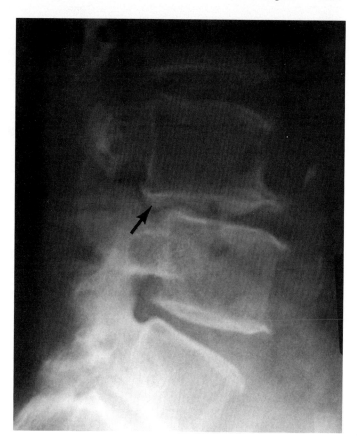

FIGURE 10–5. Retrolisthesis of the lumbar spine.

level of the slip. The slip angle or degree of sagittal rotation can be measured in different ways but is essentially a determination of this kyphosis. In longstanding lumbosacral spondylolisthesis, the superior contour of the sacrum becomes dome-shaped (Fig. 10-9). In these instances, the slip angle is measured by constructing a perpendicular line from the posterior aspect of the sacrum and measuring its intersection with a line parallel to the inferior aspect of L5.

The amount of shear force acting on the spondylolisthesis is largely determined by the degree of vertical orientation of the sacrum. Sacral inclination is the angle measured by a line parallel to the posterior aspect of the sacrum and a vertical line drawn on a standing x-ray.

As the degree of spondylolisthesis and the slip angle become greater, the body of the spondylolisthetic vertebra becomes increasingly parallel to the cassette of an anteroposterior x-ray. This gives rise to the "Napoleon's hat" appearance in significant slips (Fig. 10-10).

Oblique x-rays are the optimal views for assessing the integrity of the pars interarticularis (Fig. 10-11). A defect in the neck of the Scotty

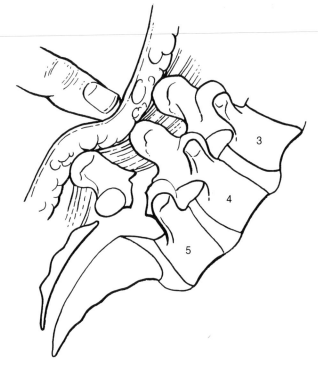

FIGURE 10–6. Palpation of spinous processes with types I and II spondylolisthesis.

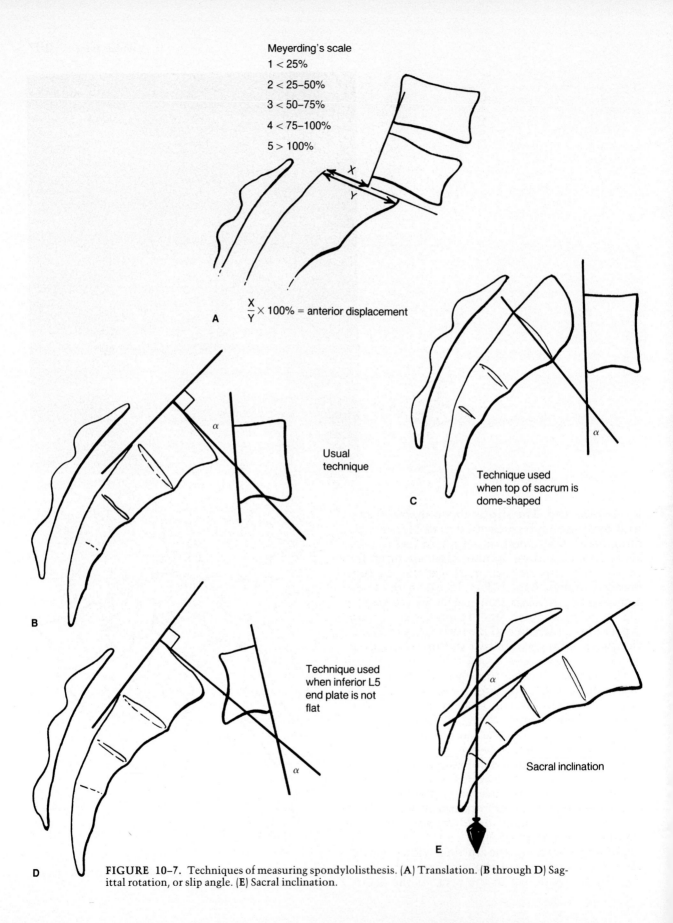

Meyerding's scale
1 < 25%
2 < 25–50%
3 < 50–75%
4 < 75–100%
5 > 100%

$$\frac{X}{Y} \times 100\% = \text{anterior displacement}$$

A

Usual
technique

Technique used
when top of sacrum is
dome-shaped

C

Technique used
when inferior L5
end plate is not
flat

Sacral inclination

E

B

D

FIGURE 10–7. Techniques of measuring spondylolisthesis. (**A**) Translation. (**B** through **D**) Sagittal rotation, or slip angle. (**E**) Sacral inclination.

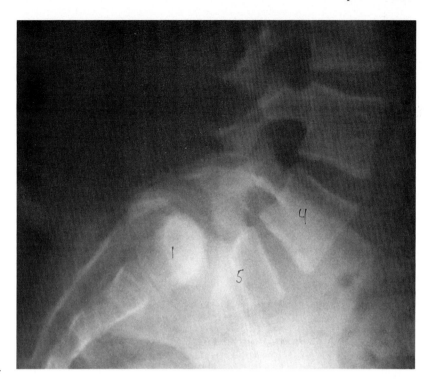

FIGURE 10–8. Spondyloptosis.

dog will be identified in type IIA spondylolistheses (Fig. 10-12). In degenerative spondylolistheses, the oblique views are an excellent way of assessing the degree of resultant foraminal stenosis.

It is important to assess the degree of mobility at the area of the slip. Thus, flexion-extension films should be obtained in most instances.

The CT scan is an excellent way of imaging the pars interarticularis (Fig. 10-13). The size of the defects of type IIA lesions can be measured. The presence of cortication of the defects can be assessed when there is uncertainty as to whether the spondylolisthesis is type IIA or IIC. Often, fibrocartilaginous tissue can be appreciated at the defects; this tissue often causes nerve root compression and leads to radicular symptoms. Sagittal reformations are useful in evaluating foraminal stenosis.

When it is unclear whether a pars defect is acute or chronic, technetium 99 bone scanning may be helpful. A marked increase in radioisotope uptake indicates an acute fracture.

In the past, myelography was done in many instances of spondylolisthesis (Fig. 10-14), but it has been supplanted by MR scanning. When the

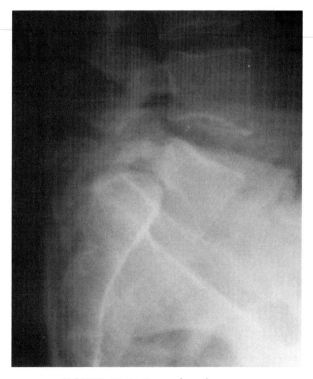

FIGURE 10–9. Dome-shaped sacrum.

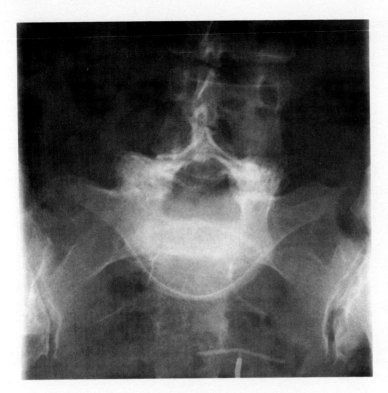

FIGURE 10–10. Napoleon's hat.

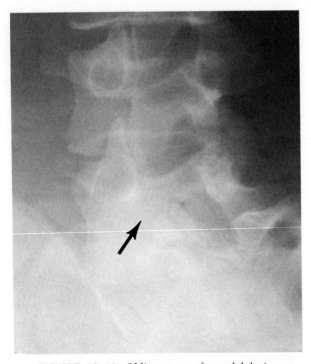

FIGURE 10–11. Oblique x-ray of spondylolysis.

posterior arch of the spondylolisthesis is intact, such as in degenerative cases, the dural sac will become increasingly compressed with advancing slip. It is, in effect, spinal stenosis. When the posterior arch is left behind, such as in isthmic spondylolisthesis, spinal stenosis does not occur. Rather, the dural sac becomes draped over the posterior aspect of the vertebra below the spondylolisthesis. This is readily appreciated on MR scanning.

Apart from imaging studies, other diagnostic techniques may be occasionally useful. Electromyograms may help detect subtle radiculopathy in a patient with a normal neurologic examination. Nerve root blocks may be helpful in identifying the specific nerve root responsible for leg symptoms in selected patients. With a grade 0 or I lytic spondylolisthesis, it may be difficult to ascertain whether the spondylolysis is responsible for a patient's low back pain. Infiltrating the defects with local anesthetic can help determine whether they are responsible for clinical symptoms. Leg pain may be a referred-type symptom that will not be altered by the aforementioned studies but that will resolve with fusion.

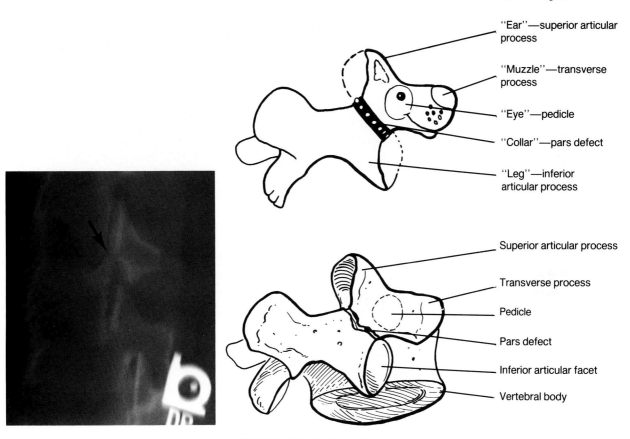

"Ear"—superior articular process

"Muzzle"—transverse process

"Eye"—pedicle

"Collar"—pars defect

"Leg"—inferior articular process

Superior articular process

Transverse process

Pedicle

Pars defect

Inferior articular facet

Vertebral body

FIGURE 10–12. Scotty dog.

Treatment

Most cases of spondylolisthesis can be managed nonoperatively. In asymptomatic patients in whom spondylolisthesis is detected as an incidental finding, no restriction on activities is necessary. Children and adolescents presenting with pain and a grade I or II spondylolisthesis should modify their activities; bracing has also been found useful for these patients. For a type IIC traumatic pars defect, a plaster cast incorporating at least one hip is generally recommended. There have been reports of successful treatment using thoracolumbosacral orthoses. Unilateral defects are much more likely to heal than bilateral defects.

Surgery should be considered for patients who have continued pain despite adequate nonoperative treatment. Various surgical approaches have been advocated. Each patient should be assessed

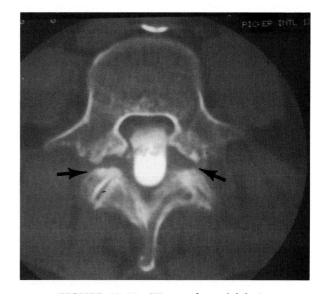

FIGURE 10–13. CT scan of spondylolysis.

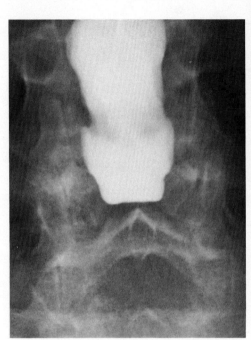
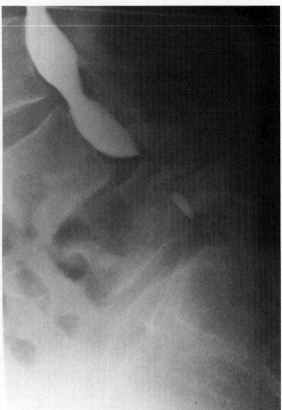

FIGURE 10–14. Myelogram of degenerative spondylolisthesis.

to ascertain the optimal operative approach. In young patients with a grade 0 or I slip and in whom pars interarticularis defects have been identified, direct repair of the pars has been advocated. Various techniques have been used to achieve bony union, including grafting alone, screw repair, figure-of-eight wiring, and specially designed hook-screw implants. The underlying assumption is that the pars defects themselves and the resulting instability give rise to symptoms, but this is not always the case. When there is a significant slip, the intervertebral disc at the level of the slip is thought to contribute to pain. Furthermore, in longstanding slips, the disc at the level above the spondylolisthesis may be abnormal and may be a pain generator.

In young patients with a grade I or II slip who have pain unresponsive to nonoperative treatment, a single-level posterolateral fusion is the procedure of choice. In adults, it is important to investigate the intervertebral disc at the adjacent cranial level. If it is abnormal, a two-level posterolateral fusion to include it should be considered.

Surgery should be considered in young patients in whom there is pain and documented progression of the slip. Surgery should also be considered for young patients presenting with a neurologic deficit. In general, a single-level posterolateral fusion is adequate for most painful spondylolistheses in patients under age 60. The appropriate surgical approach for slips greater than grade II is controversial. Some surgeons think it is necessary to reduce these slips and restore anatomic alignment to ensure a good long-term outcome, but it is unclear as to whether this is necessary. A single-level posterolateral fusion in the presence of a severe slip has an extremely high associated nonunion rate. For this reason, it is recommended that at least two levels be considered for a fusion. Some authors supplement this with an anterior interbody or posterior lumbar interbody arthrodesis.

Adult patients with degenerative spondylolisthesis may also be treated nonoperatively. This is usually most successful when the major complaint is low back pain. When the symptoms are primarily claudication or radiculopathy, surgery should be considered. Although there have been proponents of decompressive surgery alone, most clinicians now think that if the decompression is extensive, it will tend to further destabilize the area and may lead to progression of the slip postoperatively. In these instances, decompression is done in conjunction with a fusion.

KEY POINTS

1. Spondylolysis of the lumbar spine is most common at L5. It is present in about 6% of the population and is usually asymptomatic.
2. Isthmic spondylolisthesis usually occurs by age 6 and very rarely progresses after adolescence.
3. Degenerative spondylolisthesis usually occurs after age 40 and is most common at L4. It can produce symptoms of spinal stenosis.

BIBLIOGRAPHY

BOOKS

Andersson GBJ, McNeill TW, eds. Lumbar spine stenosis. St. Louis: CV Mosby, 1992.

Weinstein JN, Wiesel SW, International Society for Study of the Lumbar Spine, eds. The lumbar spine. Philadelphia: WB Saunders, 1990.

JOURNALS

Boos N, Marchesi D, Zuber K, Aebi M. Treatment of severe spondylolisthesis by reduction and pedicular fixation: A 4–6 year follow-up study. Spine 1993;18:1655–1661.

Boxall D, Bradford DS, Winter RB, Moe JH. Management of severe spondylolisthesis in children and adolescents. J Bone Joint Surg [Am] 1979;61:479–495.

Bradford DS, Boachie-Adjei O. Severe spondylolisthesis, anterior and posterior reduction and stabilization for, long-term follow-up. J Bone Joint Surg [Am] 1990;72:1060–1066.

Burkus JK, Lonstein JE, Winter RB, Denis F. Long-term evaluation of adolescents treated operatively for spondylolisthesis. A comparison of insitu arthrodesis only with in situ arthrodesis and reduction followed by immobilization in a cast. J Bone Joint Surg [Am] 1992;74: 693–704.

Cope R. Acute traumatic spondylolysis. Report of a case and review of the literature. Clin Orthop 1988;230:162–165.

Fredrickson BE, Baker D, McHolick WJ, Yuan MA, Lubicky JP. The natural history of spondylolysis and spondylolisthesis. J Bone Joint Surg [Am] 1984;66:679–707.

Frymoyer JW. Degenerative spondylolisthesis: Diagnosis and treatment. J Am Acad Orthop Surg 1994;2:9–16.

Grobler LJ, Roberson PA, Novotny JE, Pope MH. Etiology of spondylolisthesis: Assessment of the role played by lumbar facet joint morphology. Spine 1993;18:80–91.

Pedersen AK, Hagen R. Spondylolysis and spondylolisthesis. Treatment by internal fixation and bone grafting of the defect. J. Bone Joint Surg [Am] 1988;70:15–24.

Poussa M, Schlenzka D, Seitsalo S, Ylikoski M, Hurri H, Osterman K. Surgical treatment of severe isthmic spondylolisthesis in adolescents: Reduction or fusion in situ. Spine 1993;18:894–901.

Textbook of Spinal Disorders, by Stephen I. Esses.
J. B. Lippincott Company, Philadelphia © 1995.

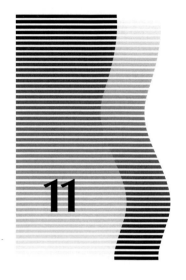

11

Spinal Stenosis

CERVICAL SPINE
  Etiology
  Clinical Presentation
  Diagnostic Evaluation
  Treatment

THORACOLUMBAR
  SPINE
  Classification
  Clinical Presentation
  Diagnostic Evaluation
  Treatment

Stenosis refers to any narrowing of a tubelike structure. Spinal stenosis is a narrowing of the spinal canal. As the space in the spinal canal decreases, the dural sac and nerve roots become compressed (Fig. 11-1). Spinal stenosis can result from many different conditions and can occur anywhere in the spinal column.

There are several ways in which spinal stenosis can result in symptoms. Local pain and discomfort may be due to alterations in kinetics and kinematics as the result of pathologic anatomy. In addition, there may be impingement of the sinuvertebral nerve and posterior primary ramus. Direct mechanical compression of the dural sac and nerve roots can result in pain and weakness in the extremities. It is thought that neural dysfunction may also occur as the result of nutritional or vascular compromise.

Apart from classifying spinal stenosis by cause, it is also possible to categorize stenosis according to anatomic involvement (Fig. 11-2). The narrowing may be only central, causing compression of the dural sac, or it may be lateral, affecting exiting nerve roots.

It is important to distinguish between the incidental finding of stenosis on x-ray or other imaging studies and spinal stenosis that is symptomatic. No direct correlation can be made between the degree of stenosis and the severity of symptoms.

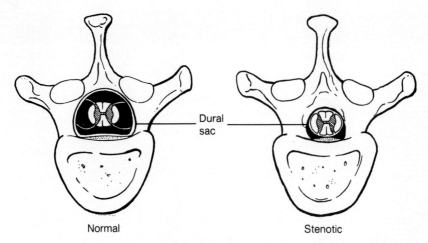

Dural sac

Normal   Stenotic

FIGURE 11–1. Spinal stenosis.

CERVICAL SPINE

Etiology

Stenosis of the cervical spine, although not uncommon, is usually asymptomatic. The usual causes of cervical stenosis are given in Table 11-1. Congenital causes are usually idiopathic but may be associated with other conditions such as achondroplasia or *Klippel-Feil syndrome*. It has been suggested that young people with congenital stenosis are at higher risk for traumatic neuropraxia of the cervical spinal cord when participating in contact sports.

The most common acquired cause of cervical stenosis is degenerative disease or spondylosis (Fig. 11-3). As the intervertebral discs collapse, there may be bulging of annular material into the spinal canal. Buckling of the ligamentum flavum may contribute to spinal cord compression. The neural foramina decrease in height, and compression of nerve roots occurs. Superimposed on these changes, there may be osteophytes centrally or laterally.

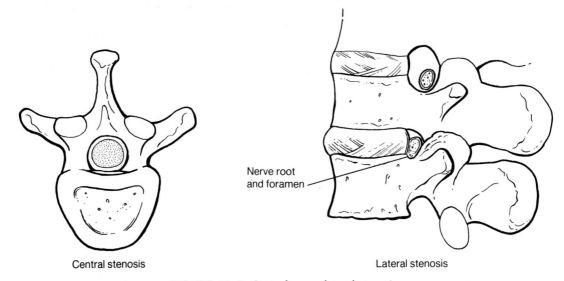

Nerve root and foramen

Central stenosis   Lateral stenosis

FIGURE 11–2. Central versus lateral stenosis.

TABLE 11–1. **Classification of Cervical Spinal Stenosis**

Congenital
  Idiopathic
  Achondroplastic

Acquired
  Spondylosis
  Ossification of the posterior longitudinal ligament
  Paget's disease
  Fluorosis

Paget's disease is a metabolic disorder in which there is an accelerated rate of bone turnover. The size of a vertebra can increase, and central or lateral spinal stenosis can occur. Excessive intake of fluoride will cause an increased amount of bone production and will cause a spinal stenosis not dissimilar to that of Paget's disease.

Ossification of the posterior longitudinal ligament (OPLL) was originally described in the Japanese literature (Fig. 11-4). Initially this condi-

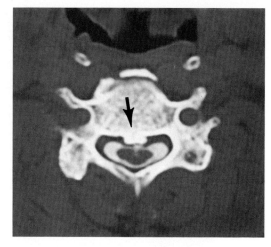

FIGURE 11–4. Ossification of the posterior longitudinal ligament (OPLL).

tion was thought to occur only in Asians, but it has since been identified in Caucasians, although the incidence is much lower. The cause of OPLL has not been identified. There is an association with diabetes mellitus, and dietary factors are thought to contribute to the pathogenesis. OPLL may occur segmentally or continuously (Fig. 11-5). The morphology of the calcification may be classified as square, mushroom, or hill.

Clinical Presentation

Patients with cervical spinal stenosis can present in a variety of ways. There may be symptoms and signs of myelopathy. The spinal cord tracts that are most affected determine the neurologic deficits that are found on clinical examination. In other instances, patients may have symptoms and signs due to compression of a nerve root or roots. Physical examination may elicit weakness in one or both arms. Some patients may exhibit findings compatible with both nerve root and spinal cord compression. It is important to ask about bowel and bladder involvement. Cervical radiculopathy or myelopathy may not be associated with neck pain; perhaps this is why the diagnosis is often overlooked.

Diagnostic Evaluation

X-rays have been used to assess the size of the spinal canal. Many authors have measured the

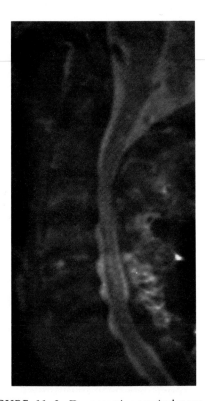

FIGURE 11–3. Degenerative cervical stenosis.

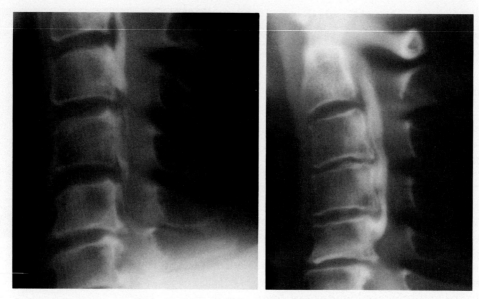

FIGURE 11–5. Segmented versus continuous OPLL.

distance between the posterior aspect of the vertebral body and the base of the spinous process. The range of normal values has varied considerably due to differences in radiographic technique and magnification. This is why a ratio method has been developed that compares the anteroposterior size of the vertebral body to that of the spinal canal (Fig. 11-6). Stenosis is thought to be present when this ratio is less than 0.8.

Computed tomographic (CT) scanning is useful in assessing central and lateral stenosis and is ideal in detecting the extent of OPLL. Similarly, magnetic resonance imaging (MRI)—both in the sagittal and axial planes—can be used to assess the degree of neural compression. The size of the central canal and the neural foramina may be affected by posture, so dynamic imaging can be useful. CT and MRI can be done with the patient's neck flexed, in neutral position, and hyperextended.

Myelography is no longer routinely needed in the assessment of these patients. Electromyograms are useful if there is some uncertainty as to the exact nerve root or roots involved. In addition, they can be useful in excluding peripheral neuropathies.

Treatment

In treatment decision-making, the clinician must carefully consider the type and extent of neurologic deficit. If there is profound myelopathy or radiculopathy, surgical intervention should be considered. Surgical options include laminectomy, laminoplasty, and anterior decompression. The optimal surgical approach depends on the predominant site of stenosis, the amount of lordosis present, and whether the patient has significant neck pain. In general, the anterior approach is best for patients with only one- or two-level disease and patients with significant loss of the normal cervical lordosis. Posterior approaches are best reserved for patients with three or more levels involved and those in whom the cervical lordosis has been maintained. Posterior laminectomy and laminoplasty can be effective

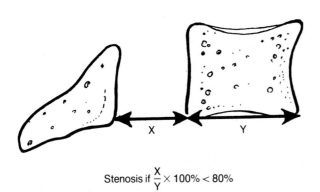

Stenosis if $\frac{X}{Y} \times 100\% < 80\%$

FIGURE 11–6. Measurement of cervical canal size.

even when most of the compression is anterior, provided that there is enough cervical lordosis at the affected levels to allow translation of the cord backward (see Fig. 7-13). Multiple-level laminectomies, particularly in younger patients, may lead to a kyphotic deformity. If this kyphosis becomes significant and is associated with chronic neck pain, then an anterior fusion with strut grafting may be necessary. By maintaining posterior stability, laminoplasty presents this from happening (Fig. 11-7).

Neurologic recovery is best in patients with symptoms of short duration and in whom the deficit is not dense. Prolonged and profound neurologic deficits may not fully recover after surgical decompression.

Nonoperative treatment is basically the same as treatment of degenerative disease without neurologic involvement (see Chap. 8): lifestyle modification, physical modalities, and the judicious use of medications. If a patient has radicular symptoms, then infiltration of that nerve root with steroids may be useful, but no good scientific study has been done to evaluate this nonoperative technique. In addition, there is little scientifically valid information on the use of epidural steroids for cervical myelopathy or radiculopathy.

THORACOLUMBAR SPINE

Classification

The various causes of spinal stenosis in the thoracolumbar spine are listed in Table 11-2.

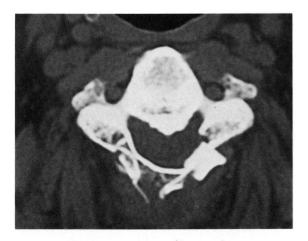

FIGURE 11–7. CT of laminoplasty.

TABLE 11–2. Classification of Thoracolumbar Spinal Stenosis

Congenital
  Idiopathic
  Achondroplastic

Acquired
  Degenerative
  Combined
  Spondylolisthetic
  Iatrogenic
  Posttraumatic
  Miscellaneous

Most congenital stenosis is idiopathic. There are enlarged inferior articular facets and a decreased anteroposterior diameter of the spinal canal. Congenital stenosis may also be associated with other conditions such as achondroplastic dwarfism. Degenerative disease of the spine can result in an acquired stenosis. There is sclerosis and hypertrophy of the laminae and facets. With disc space collapse, there is bulging of the annulus into the canal and buckling of the ligamentum flavum. The most common type of acquired stenosis is due to a combination of acquired and congenital causes (Fig. 11-8). The former are usually degenerative, with a herniation of a disc, and the latter are idiopathic. Iatrogenic stenosis can result from accelerated degenerative changes at either end of a fusion or from a spondylolisthesis following wide laminectomy. Spinal stenosis has been reported as a late complication of fractures, particularly burst-type injuries associated with retropulsion of bone into the canal. Any space-occupying lesion within the spinal canal can cause stenosis. For example, degenerative cysts from the facet joint can produce nerve root compression (Fig. 11-9). Miscellaneous causes include Paget's disease and fluorosis (Fig. 11-10).

Spinal stenosis can also be classified according to the site of compression. There may be central stenosis, in which the dural sac itself is compressed, or there may be stenosis anywhere along the path of the exiting nerve root. The nerve root may be compressed in the *lateral recess*, in the foramen, or on exiting the foramen. The lateral recess is bordered laterally by the pedicle, anteriorly by the posterolateral surface of the vertebral

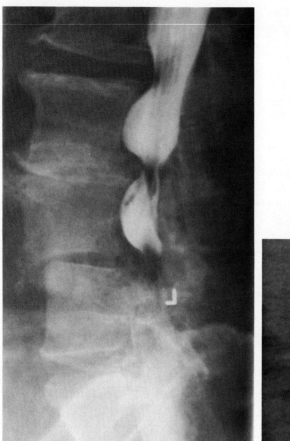

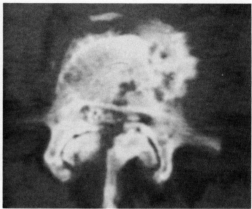

FIGURE 11–8. Combined acquired and congenital stenosis.

body, and posteriorly by the superior articular facet (Fig. 11-11). Lateral recess stenosis is usually caused by hypertrophy of the superior articular facet (Fig. 11-12). The boundaries of the *nerve root foramen* are the vertebral body and intervertebral disc anteriorly, the inferior border of the pedicle superiorly, the pars interarticularis and facet joint posteriorly, and the superior border of the inferior pedicle inferiorly (Fig. 11-13). Foraminal stenosis may result from facet subluxation or osteophyte formation from the facet, or as the result of disc collapse with resultant inferior translation of the superior pedicle (Fig. 11-14). Extraforaminal stenosis is usually due to a lateral disc herniation impinging on the nerve root after it has left the foramen. Degenerative synovial cysts originating from the facet joint can cause nerve root compression and may mimic spinal stenosis (see Fig. 11-9).

Clinical Presentation

Symptoms associated with spinal stenosis are determined by the location of the compression on neural elements. Typically, cauda equina compression from central stenosis results in neurogenic claudication. This is characteristically bilateral leg pain that begins after walking a short distance. Patients often describe a rubbery feeling and weakness in the legs. The pain is usually not well localized and often is more of a dysesthesia than true pain. To alleviate symptoms, the patient usually must stop walking and assume a specific posture, often bending forward, sitting, or squatting. Forward flexion of the lumbar spine usually results in increased space for the cauda equina (Fig. 11-15). This is why many patients can increase their walking distance by leaning forward on a cane or shopping cart.

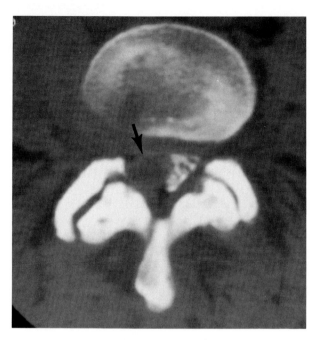

FIGURE 11–9. Synovial cyst.

When the neural compression is primarily of a nerve root, symptoms are those of sciatica. This pain may be much better localized. It may be claudicant and can be associated with weakness in specific well-localized muscle groups.

It is not uncommon to have back pain in addition to the above neurologic symptoms. Paradoxically, leg symptoms worsen with walking but back pain usually improves with activity.

The physical examination should be done both before and after exercise. It is not uncommon to detect weakness, decreased sensation, or a depressed reflex only after the patient has walked far enough to bring on symptoms.

Diagnostic Evaluation

Plain radiographs may be used as a screening test to identify bony stenosis. On the anteroposterior x-ray, the interpedicular distance should be evaluated (Fig. 11-16). On the lateral x-rays, *(text continues on page 224)*

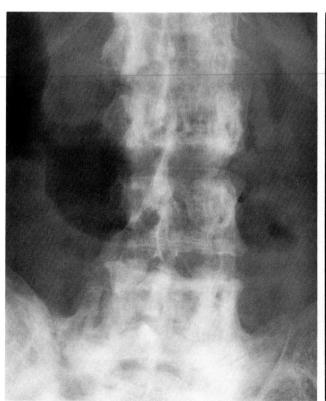

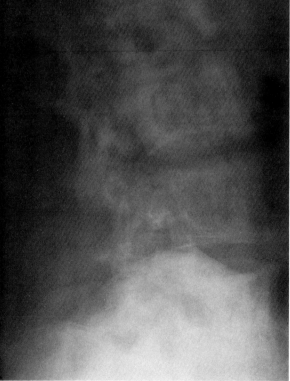

FIGURE 11–10. Paget's disease.

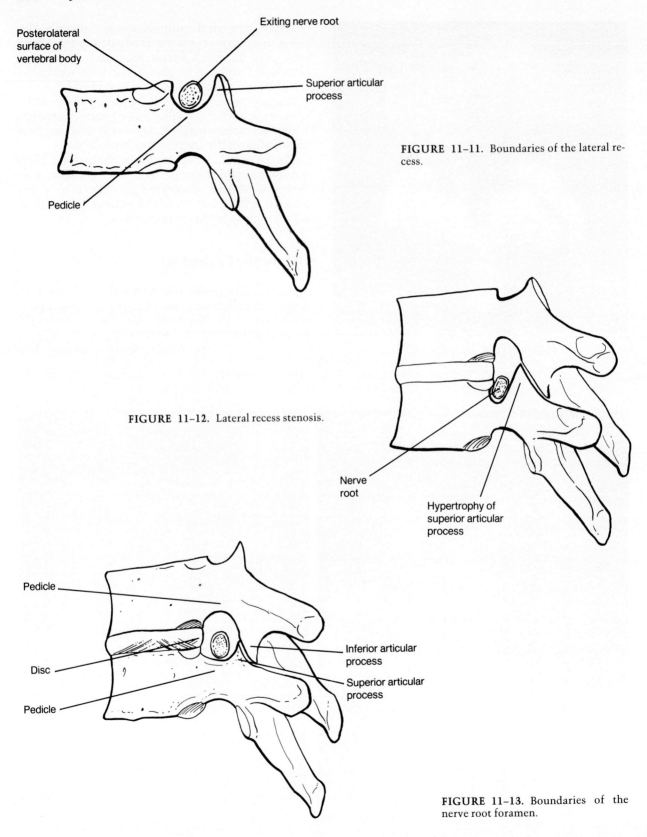

Posterolateral
surface of
vertebral body

Exiting nerve root

Superior articular
process

Pedicle

FIGURE 11–11. Boundaries of the lateral recess.

FIGURE 11–12. Lateral recess stenosis.

Nerve
root

Hypertrophy of
superior articular
process

Pedicle

Disc

Pedicle

Inferior articular
process

Superior articular
process

FIGURE 11–13. Boundaries of the nerve root foramen.

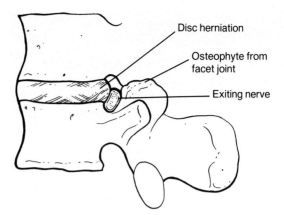

FIGURE 11–14. Foraminal stenosis.

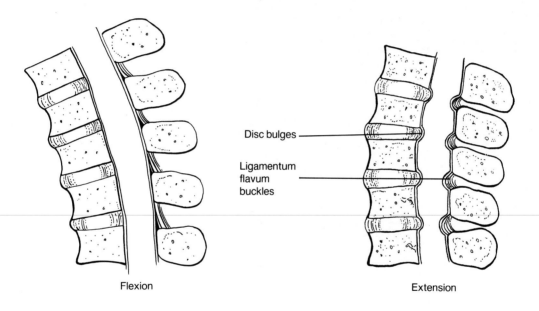

Flexion

Extension

FIGURE 11–15. Forward flexion of lumbar spine increasing canal size.

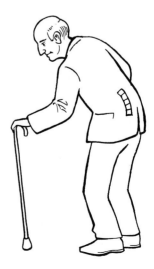

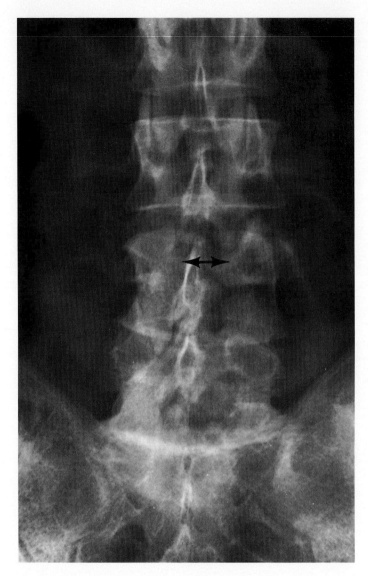

FIGURE 11–16. Anteroposterior (AP) x-ray of stenosis.

the length of the pedicle can be measured as well as the anteroposterior diameter of the spinal canal (Fig. 11-17). A measurement of less than 12 mm is considered abnormal. The presence and degree of a degenerative spondylolisthesis should be evaluated. On oblique x-rays, the neural foramina can be assessed.

In the past, myelography was used routinely in the assessment of stenosis (Fig. 11-18). This is an invasive procedure with attendant risks. It may be technically difficult to instill dye in the subarachnoid space when there is very marked compression. One major advantage of myelography

over other imaging techniques is the fact that it can be dynamic—that is, the spinal canal can be examined with the patient flexed and extended. As discussed above, forward flexion may result in a significant increase in the anteroposterior diameter of the canal.

CT scanning, with and without myelography, has been invaluable in identifying and assessing spinal stenosis. The CT scan without dye in the subarachnoid space can give useful information about the bony boundaries of the canal centrally and the neural foramina more laterally. Because soft tissue, such as the intervertebral disc and lig-

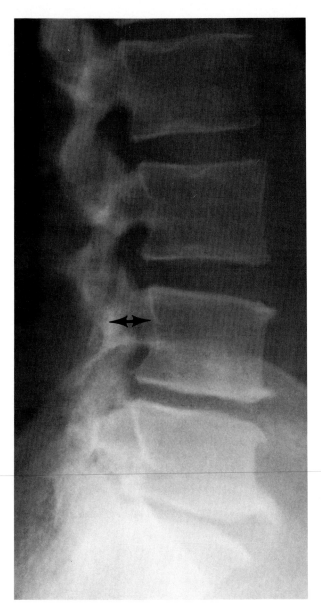

FIGURE 11–17. Lateral x-ray of stenosis.

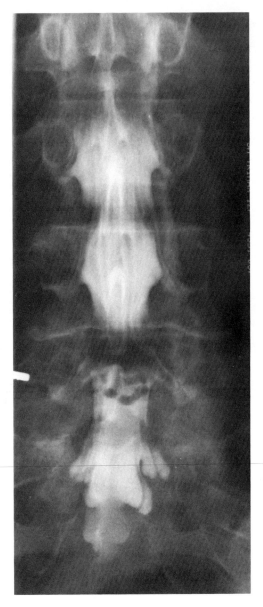

FIGURE 11–18. Myelogram.

amentum flavum, contributes significantly to most cases of stenosis, the postmyelographic CT is useful (Fig. 11-19). A cross-sectional area of less than 100 mm^2 is abnormal. An anteroposterior diameter of the lateral recess of less than 3 mm is similarly abnormal. Sagittal reconstructions are useful in assessing foraminal stenosis (Fig. 11-20).

MR imaging has obviated the need for combined myelography and CT scanning in patients with suspected spinal stenosis; indeed, in most instances, MR provides all the information necessary in diagnosing and treating this condition (Fig. 11-21). T1- and T2-weighted images in both the sagittal and axial planes should be reviewed.

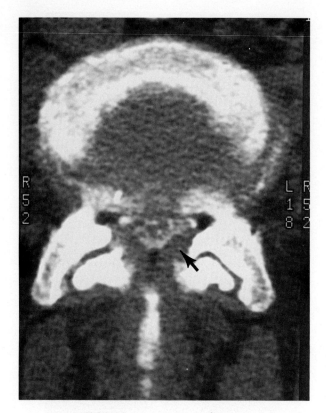

FIGURE 11-19. CT myelogram.

The major problem with all these diagnostic tests is that they may show areas of stenosis that are not symptomatic. The clinician must correlate the diagnostic findings with symptoms. Many older patients with claudication have both spinal stenosis and peripheral vascular disease, so it is a diagnostic challenge to determine to what extent symptoms arise from neurologic versus vascular disease. When confusion exists, electromyograms may be useful.

Treatment

The natural history of lumbar spinal stenosis is one of gradual progression. About 80% of patients, if followed long enough, show significant worsening of symptoms. However, the rate of progression varies. Occasionally, patients may have a sudden exacerbation of their condition that resolves somewhat in 1 to 2 months.

Nonoperative treatment should be tried in all patients. Bed rest of short duration may decrease the mechanical irritation of nerve tissue. Nonsteroidal anti-inflammatory medications and analgesics may provide symptomatic relief. Isometric flexion exercises are occasionally of benefit. Epidural steroid injections have been reported to provide some reduction in symptoms, although their use remains controversial.

For patients with disabling pain resistant to nonoperative measures, surgical decompression may be considered. To ensure successful operative results, the symptomatic compressive areas must be accurately identified. Not all radiographic findings of stenosis represent symptomatic lesions. Nerve root blocks can be done preoperatively if there is doubt concerning symptomatic levels.

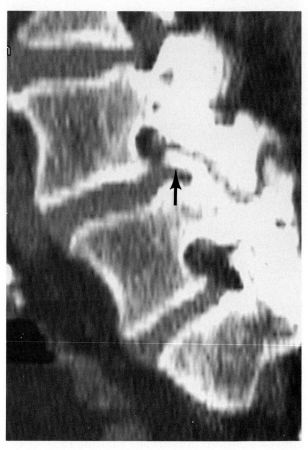

FIGURE 11-20. Sagittal CT myelogram.

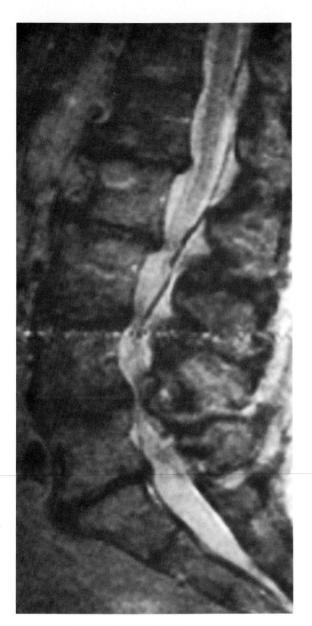

FIGURE 11–21. MRI of stenosis.

The most common surgical approach is laminectomy with or without foraminotomies. Occasionally, the extent of decompression is such that there is potential spinal instability; in these instances, a concomitant fusion is usually recommended, but there is controversy about the exact indications for this.

KEY POINTS

1. Spinal stenosis is a narrowing of the spinal canal. It can be classified according to cause or anatomic location.
2. Symptoms associated with spinal stenosis are usually neurologic. Stenosis of the cervical spine can cause radiculopathy or myelopathy. Lumbar spinal stenosis can produce claudicant leg pain.
3. Surgical decompression may be considered for patients with disabling pain unresponsive to nonoperative modalities and for those with profound neurologic deficits.

BIBLIOGRAPHY

BOOKS

Andersson GBJ, McNeill TW, eds. Lumbar spinal stenosis. St. Louis: CV Mosby, 1992.
Nixon JE, ed. Spinal stenosis. London: Edward Arnold, 1991.
Postacchini F, ed. Lumbar spinal stenosis. Wein, West Germany: Springer-Verlag, 1989.

JOURNALS

Arnoldi AE, Brodsky, Cavchoix J, et al. Lumbar spinal stenosis and nerve root entrapment syndromes: Definition and classification. Clin Orthop 1976;115:4–5.
Bernhardt M, Hynes RA, Blume HW, White AA III. Current concepts review. Cervical spondylotic myelopathy. J Bone Joint Surg [Am] 1993;75:119–128.
Herno A, Airaksien O, Saari T. Long-term results of surgical treatment of lumbar spinal stenosis. Spine 1993;18:1471–1474.
Onel D, Sari H, Donemez C. Lumbar spinal stenosis: Clinical/radiologic therapeutic evaluation in 145 patients: Conservative treatment or surgical intervention? Spine 1993;18:291–298.
Rauschning W. Normal and pathologic anatomy of the lumbar root canals. Spine 1987;12:1008–1019.
Torg JS. Pavlov's ratio: determining cervical spinal stenosis on routine lateral roentgenograms. Contemp Orthop 1989;18:153–160.
Turner JA, Ersek M, Herron L, Deyo R. Surgery for lumbar spinal stenosis: Attempted meta-analysis of the literature. Spine 1992;17:1–8.
Verbiest H. A radicular syndrome from developmental narrowing of the lumbar vertebral canal. J Bone Joint Surg (Br) 1954;36:230–237.
Zdeblick TA, Zou D, Warden KE, McCabe R, Kunz D, Vanderby R. Cervical stability after foraminotomy. A biomechanical in vitro analysis. J Bone Joint Surg [Am] 1992;74:22–27.

Textbook of Spinal Disorders, by Stephen I. Esses.
J. B. Lippincott Company, Philadelphia © 1995.

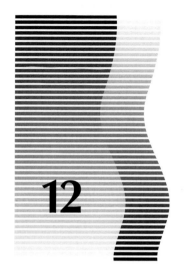

Infections of the Spine

12

VERTEBRAL
  BACTERIAL
  OSTEOMYELITIS
  Etiology
  Clinical Presentation
  Diagnostic Findings
  Treatment
ADULT DISC SPACE
  INFECTION
  Etiology
  Diagnostic Findings
  Treatment
DISCITIS
  Etiology
  Clinical Presentation
  Diagnostic Findings
  Treatment
TUBERCULOSIS OF
  THE SPINE
  Etiology
  Clinical Presentation
  Diagnostic Findings
  Treatment

NONBACTERIAL,
  NONTUBERCULOUS
  OSTEOMYELITIS
  Brucellosis
  Cryptococcosis
  Blastomycosis
  Aspergillosis
  Coccidioidomycosis
EPIDURAL SPACE
  INFECTIONS
  Etiology
  Diagnosis
  Treatment
INTRADURAL
  INFECTIONS
  Meningitis
  Myelitis
POSTOPERATIVE
  INFECTIONS
  Etiology
  Diagnosis
  Treatment

In the past, most cases of spinal infections were due to tuberculosis. Until recently there had been a dramatic decrease in the prevalence of tuberculosis and, thus, spinal infections were uncommon. Today we are seeing a huge increase in both tuberculous and nontuberculous spinal infections. This is due to the aging of our population, the epidemic of AIDS and other conditions rendering patients immunocompromised, and the alarming spread of intravenous drug abuse. In its early stages, spinal infections can present as back pain with few other symptoms or findings. Thus, it is essential to have some index of suspicion and awareness so as not to miss this diagnosis. Most spinal infections can be effectively treated nonoperatively and with no long-term sequelae if diagnosed early. If the infective process goes unchecked, it can lead to permanent neurologic injury and death.

VERTEBRAL BACTERIAL OSTEOMYELITIS

Etiology

About half of all cases of vertebral bacterial osteomyelitis are due to *Staphylococcus aureus*. Hematogenous seeding has been implicated, particularly in older patients. Patients with diabetes mellitus are particularly susceptible to staphylococcal infections. Batson described a venous plexus that drains the pelvis, is valveless, and is close to the lumbar spine. It is by this hematogenous route that urinary tract infections may lead to spinal involvement. These are usually due to *Escherichia coli* and *Proteus. Pseudomonas* is the organism most commonly associated with hematogenous spinal infections from intravenous drug abuse. *Salmonella* is an organism commonly associated with sickle-cell disease.

Clinical Presentation

The most common symptom is back pain, usually worsened by movement. Many patients have a history of fever and sweats. Infections of the lumbar spine can present with abdominal pain or sciatica. Patients may have general malaise and weight loss. Some patients manifest no evidence of infection. A detailed history will often identify the source of the bacterial infection or a preexisting systemic disease rendering the patient susceptible to vertebral osteomyelitis.

Diagnostic Findings

Patients almost always have a fever and increased erythrocyte sedimentation rate (ESR). Occasionally the white cell count is elevated, but this is not a consistent finding. Blood cultures and cultures from other potential sources of infection, such as the urine, may be helpful.

It is hypothesized that the bacteria initially involve the subchondral area of the vertebral body, and thus the earliest radiographic finding is rarefaction of adjacent end plates. As the infection continues, end plate involvement increases to include scalloping and destruction. There is loss of intervening disc space height (Fig. 12-1). A soft tissue shadow, the result of a paravertebral ab-

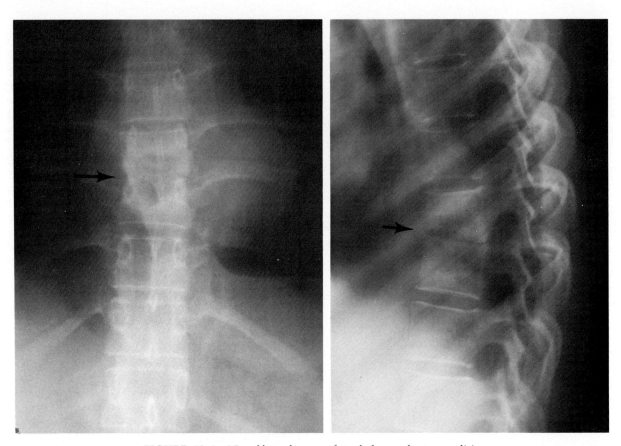

FIGURE 12–1. AP and lateral x-rays of staphylococcal osteomyelitis.

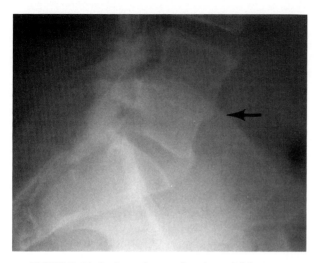

FIGURE 12–2. Lateral x-ray showing solid fusion.

scess, may be identified. If the infective process continues there is reactive new bone formation, and with long-standing infections there may be bony fusion of the adjacent vertebral bodies (Fig. 12-2).

Because the radiographic findings are subtle in the initial stages, technetium 99 bone scanning may be extremely helpful (Fig. 12-3). Although there is almost always increased uptake on the bone scan at the site of infection, it is not a specific test and cannot be used to distinguish infection from tumor, arthritis, or trauma. Gallium scanning may be helpful in this regard.

Computed tomographic (CT) scanning is extremely useful in identifying the extent of bony involvement and soft tissue extension (Fig. 12-4). In addition, CT scanning can be used to identify any involvement of the epidural space with possible dural sac compression.

Before the advent of magnetic resonance imaging (MRI), myelography was occasionally used to define the extent of neural compression. The major risk of this invasive procedure was further spread of the infective process. Currently myelography is probably contraindicated if a spinal infection is suspected.

MR scanning will probably become the imaging modality of choice for infective lesions of the spine; indeed, there is evidence that changes on MRI precede radiographic changes. Typical MRI findings include decreased signal intensity on T1-weighted images in both the vertebral body and intervening intervertebral disc, with an increased signal in these structures on T2-

weighted images (Fig. 12-5). The MRI can be useful in delineating any epidural extension or soft tissue abscess.

The definitive test for vertebral osteomyelitis is a positive tissue culture. Material may be obtained by percutaneous biopsy, occasionally with CT-assisted guidance, or by open surgery. The reported success of needle aspiration varies, due to differences in technique, variations in needle size and type, accuracy in needle placement, and previous antibiotic administration.

Treatment

The cornerstone of treatment is antibiotics, so accurate bacterial identification and sensitivities are crucial. Antibiotics are usually given intravenously for at least 6 weeks, but this is somewhat arbitrary. If the patient has significant pain or deformity, bracing or casting may also be used. The patient should be carefully monitored during antibiotic treatment to ensure a favorable response. This can be demonstrated by a decrease in the ESR and fever, along with shrinkage of any soft tissue extension. Failure to respond in this manner is an indication for surgical treatment. The principles of operative management are thorough debridement of all infected tissues and sta-

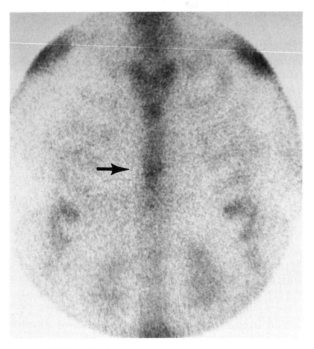

FIGURE 12–3. Technetium-99 bone scanning.

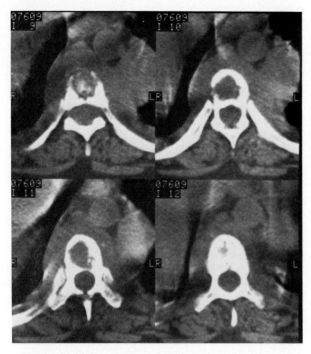

FIGURE 12–4. CT scan of staphyloccal osteomyelitis.

bilization, usually with autogenous tricortical strut grafting. Because these infections affect the anterior column of the spine, surgery is usually done from an anterior approach.

Other indications for surgical treatment include the failure to identify an organism percutaneously. In many instances where an open biopsy is necessary, it is worthwhile proceeding at the same time with formal debridement and stabilization. Onset or progression of neurologic deficit is an indication for surgical management, as is an unacceptable or progressive deformity.

ADULT DISC SPACE INFECTION

Etiology

As discussed in Chapter 2, the intervertebral disc becomes avascular in the adult. Thus, hematogenous feeding of bacteria to a disc is rare. Most adult disc space infections occur by contiguous spread from vertebral osteomyelitis or by direct inoculation of bacteria into the disc at the time of surgery or percutaneous procedures. The latter include discography, percutaneous discectomy, and chemonucleolysis. The most common organism to be implicated in adult disc space in-

fections is *Staphylococcus aureus*. Back pain is the only consistent clinical finding of these disc space infections. Occasionally there may be tenderness to palpation or decreased range of motion due to guarding. One should maintain a high index of suspicion in patients complaining of increasing back pain after spinal procedures. The incidence of discitis following discography is about 1%.

Diagnostic Findings

As with spinal osteomyelitis, the most common diagnostic finding is an increased ESR. This is very nonspecific and not helpful in postoperative patients, because the ESR remains elevated for about 6 months after spinal surgery.

Blood cultures should be done on all patients, although they are not usually positive.

Radiographic changes include a decrease in intervertebral disc space height and reactive sclerosis of the adjacent end plates (Fig. 12-6). Bone scanning may be of value, but increased uptake may also be due to recent surgery or percutaneous manipulation.

MR scanning will probably become an increasingly useful imaging modality, but further experience is needed to accurately differentiate disc infections from MR changes in the intervertebral disc after surgical procedures.

The definitive diagnosis of an adult disc space infection depends on culturing and identifying organisms from disc material. This ma-

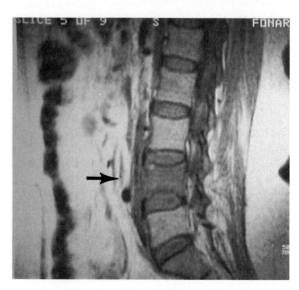

FIGURE 12–5. MRI of early osteomyelitis.

terial is usually obtained by percutaneous aspiration. Fungal infections occasionally occur in the disc space, so appropriate cultures should be obtained.

Treatment

Almost all patients can be successfully treated nonoperatively. Appropriate antimicrobial drugs are necessary and are usually given intravenously for 4 to 6 weeks. Bed rest and bracing are used to control pain. Occasionally disc infections are associated with spinal cord compression. This may be secondary to edema, infective tissue, or reactive granulation tissue. In these instances, surgery may be indicated. The long-term prognosis following the successful treatment of an infected disc space depends on early diagnosis and institution of appropriate antimicrobial drugs. If there is significant disc space collapse and reactive sclerosis, back pain may persist.

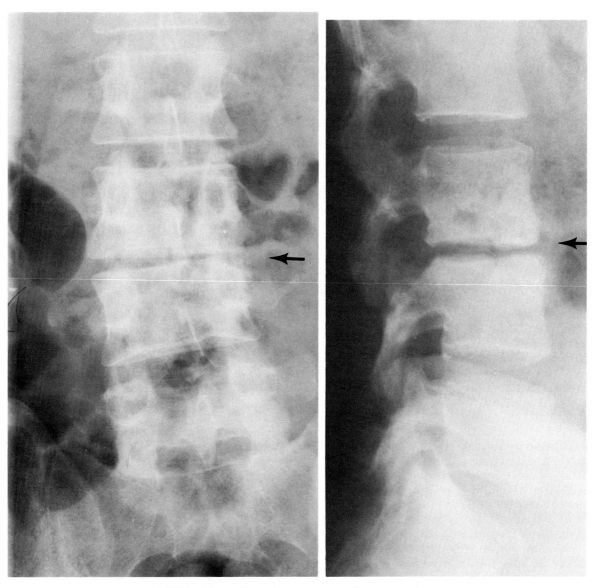

FIGURE 12–6. AP and lateral x-rays of disc space collapse.

DISCITIS

Etiology

Discitis is a distinct childhood entity different from the adult condition discussed above. The latter is always infective, but the childhood condition can be inflammatory or infective. In about half of cases, cultures of disc material are negative. Histology of these specimens occasionally shows a large number of eosinophils, consistent with an inflammatory process. The lumbar spine is the most commonly involved region.

Clinical Presentation

The mean age of patients in most series is about 7 years. The diagnosis is often delayed because of the nonspecific nature of the complaints. The child may be unwilling to stand or walk and may complain of abdominal pain, be irritable, and show signs of general malaise. There may be a previous history of illness or trauma. Fever is not always present. In an attempt to splint the affected area, patients may adopt a peculiar posture such as kyphosis or scoliosis.

Diagnostic Findings

Laboratory studies are not particularly helpful in the diagnosis of discitis. The ESR and the white blood cell count may be elevated. Blood cultures are rarely positive.

The most useful test is a technetium 99 radionuclide scan. This will uniformly show increased uptake in the affected area and is positive well before any plain radiographic changes occur. When plain radiographs are abnormal, they show decreased disc space height. As the process continues, the adjacent vertebral end plates become irregular and eroded.

Experience with MR scanning for this condition is limited, but disc signal changes probably occur before any radiographic abnormalities.

Discitis must be distinguished from *intervertebral disc calcification syndrome*. The latter is almost always cervical, and there is usually a history of preceding trauma or respiratory tract infection. Patients present with pain and torticollis. There may be decreased range of motion of the cervical spine. There is almost always an increase in the white blood cell count, ESR, and temperature. Plain radiographs show disc space calcification without the collapse of the disc space or erosion of the vertebral body associated with infection. Interestingly, this calcification usually disappears with no long-term sequelae.

Treatment

The mainstay of treatment for patients with discitis is resting the affected area. Initially, this necessitates bed rest; as the symptoms decrease, the patient can be ambulated after application of a plaster cast. Because the etiology of this condition is not well understood, there is some controversy as to the need for intravenous antibiotics. It is probably prudent to administer antistaphylococcal drugs if there is a markedly elevated white blood cell count or fever.

TUBERCULOSIS OF THE SPINE

Etiology

The incidence of tuberculosis has been steadily increasing in underdeveloped countries. Until recently, the number of cases in developed countries had been small, but with the spread of *human immunodeficiency virus* (HIV) there has been an increase in the number of immunocompromised patients susceptible to tuberculosis. There are two forms of *Mycobacterium tuberculosis*—human and bovine. The human strain is responsible for most cases and begins as a pulmonary infection. Hematogenous spread can lead to seeding of the tubercles to the cancellous bone of the vertebral body.

Clinical Presentation

Patients with tuberculosis of the spine commonly have back pain. There may be constitutional symptoms, including fever, night sweats, and weight loss. There may be symptoms referable to the lung infection, such as a productive cough and pleuritic pain. The bony destruction associated with the spinal infection is accompanied by deformity, usually a pronounced gibbus. This, in association with spinal cord compression, is known as *Pott's disease*. Soft tissue extension of the tuberculous infection is common and can result in a large psoas abscess (Figs. 12-7 and 12-8). This can give rise to symptoms of pain and swelling in the abdomen or inguinal region.

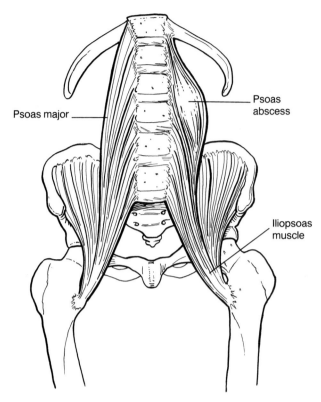

FIGURE 12–7. Left psoas abscess.

Diagnostic Findings

The tuberculin skin test determines whether a patient has been infected with tuberculosis but is not specific for active disease. In addition, some patients with tuberculosis will be rendered anergic, or nonreactive, due to overwhelming immunocompromise. In these patients, the skin test is negative despite active disease. A chest x-ray may demonstrate hilar adenopathy, multinodular infiltrates, and pleural effusions. In about half the cases, there is no pulmonary involvement. Firm diagnosis of active pulmonary disease, therefore, requires the demonstration of acid-fast bacilli on sputum samples.

The spinal infection has a predilection for soft tissue expansion. Anteriorly, the infective process can extend beneath the anterior longitudinal ligament and thus spread to involve multiple vertebrae (Fig. 12-9). This accounts for the radiographic finding of extensive bony destruction, particularly in the anterior half of the vertebral body, and paravertebral soft tissue swelling. The end plates and disc spaces are relatively spared.

The destruction of the vertebral bodies leads to the kyphotic deformity. Bone scans are negative in one third of cases. CT scanning delineates the soft tissue extension and is important for evaluating spinal canal involvement. Dural sac compression can result from direct extension of the infective process or from retropulsion of bony and discal fragments (Fig. 12-10).

The radiographic findings are so typical that when they are seen in a patient with active tuberculosis, further investigations are usually unnecessary (see Fig. 12-10). If there is no active pulmonary tuberculosis, it is usually necessary to do an aspiration biopsy of the involved vertebral region.

Treatment

Both nonoperative and operative treatments have been recommended for spinal tuberculosis. Suggested surgical management has included posterior fusions, drainage procedures, and anterior resections with strut grafting (Fig. 12-11). Despite the numerous surgical approaches recommended, successful treatment can be achieved by chemotherapy alone. The drugs currently used include isoniazid, rifampin, ethambutol, and pyrazinamide. The only disadvantage of medical treatment for spinal tuberculosis is that there can be increasing kyphotic deformity during the first few months of treatment (Fig. 12-12). Surgical treatment is usually reserved for cases in which there is an increasing neurologic deficit or progression of a gibbus deformity, or occasionally in children to prevent further bony destruction and deformity. In these instances, the recommended pro-

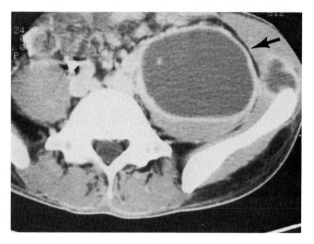

FIGURE 12–8. CT showing psoas abscess.

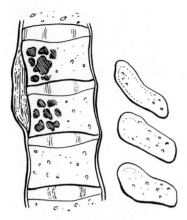

TB may spread inferiorly
to adjacent vertebra along
anterior longitudinal ligament

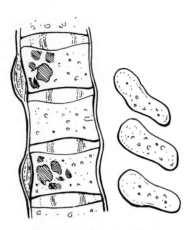

TB may spread to nonadjacent
vertebra along anterior
longitudinal ligament

FIGURE 12–9. Multiple vertebral involvement by tuberculosis.

cedure is anterior decompression and fusion using rib or tricortical iliac crest.

NONBACTERIAL, NONTUBERCULOUS OSTEOMYELITIS

Brucellosis

Undulant fever or brucellosis is caused by gram-negative rods, *Brucella*. This organism is found in animal tissues and can be acquired by humans by direct contact with infected animals or by ingestion of inadequately cooked meat or unpasteurized milk. Systemic symptoms are related to reticuloendothelial involvement by the organism and typically include a fluctuating fever. Osteomyelitis of the spine occurs by hematogenous spread or is due to the presence of the organism in the bone marrow. The lumbar spine is most commonly affected. There may be soft tissue extension, and typically the intervertebral disc is destroyed early in the disease process. This distinguishes it radiographically from entities such as tuberculosis.

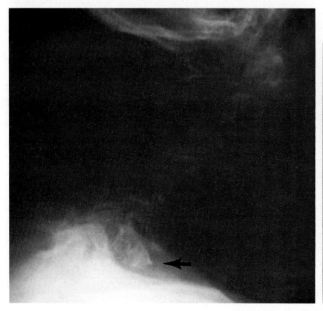

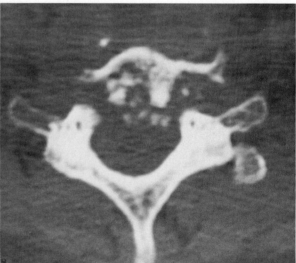

FIGURE 12–10. Spinal involvement in patient with known tuberculosis.

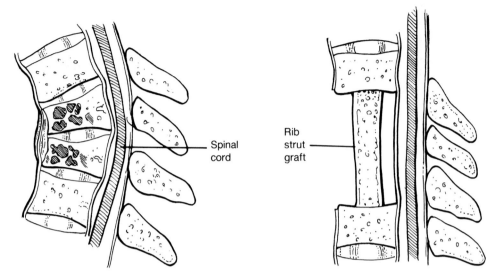

FIGURE 12–11. Anterior resection with strut grafting for tuberculosis.

Diagnostic techniques include a skin test, but this only shows whether the patient has been previously infected with *Brucella*. Blood cultures may be useful, as are *Brucella* titers. The use of these tests may obviate the need for a spinal biopsy. When a biopsy is done, special cultures must be set up.

The usual treatment is tetracycline, although other antimicrobial drugs have been used. Serum titers can be followed to monitor recovery.

Cryptococcosis

Cryptococci are fungi found in bird droppings. Patients become infected by inhaling spores, leading to respiratory colonization. Patients with leukemia, sarcoidosis, and diabetes mellitus are particularly susceptible to this infection. Hematogenous spread from the pulmonary tract leads to seeding of the spine and subsequent osteomyelitis. The cryptococcus has a particular affinity for the central nervous system, and meningitis is not uncommon in this disease. Treatment usually consists of amphotericin B and flucytosine.

Blastomycosis

The blastomycosis fungus is endemic in the southeastern and midwestern United States. There are two portals of infection, the lung and the skin. Spinal osteomyelitis occurs as the result of hematogenous seeding of the organism. Diagnosis almost always requires positive stains on cultures following needle biopsy. Treatment includes amphotericin B, occasionally with added sulfonamides or 2-hydroxystilbamidine.

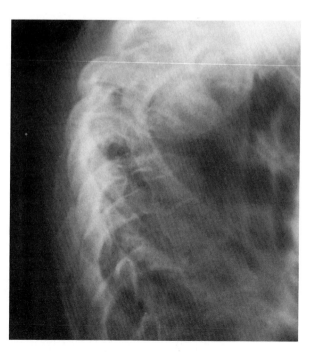

FIGURE 12–12. Old tuberculosis causing marked kyphosis.

Aspergillosis

The fungus *Aspergillus* is common in our environment. It can grow on grain and produces many spores that are released into the air. Fortunately, they are usually of low pathogenicity. Aspergillosis occurs when patients are immunocompromised or when a massive number of spores are inhaled (Fig. 12-13). Hematogenous spread from primary pulmonary disease can lead to spinal osteomyelitis. The organism seeds in the metaphyseal or end plate region of the vertebra, and this is where the first radiographic findings can be detected. A tissue diagnosis requiring biopsy is almost always necessary. Treatment is usually successful with amphotericin B.

Coccidioidomycosis

The chlamydospores of *Coccidioides* are endemic to the southwestern United States, partic-

ularly the San Joaquin Valley; thus, coccidioidomycosis is sometimes called San Joaquin fever. The disease is acquired by inhalation of the spores, causing primary pulmonary infection. Osteomyelitis of the spine occurs as the result of hematogenous spread and radiographically is characterized by punched-out lytic lesions. Occasionally there is soft tissue spread. New serologic tests may cause spinal aspiration to become superfluous. Treatment is with amphotericin B or, in less serious cases, oral ketaconazole.

EPIDURAL SPACE INFECTIONS

Etiology

The epidural space can become infected in one of three ways. There may be direct spread of an infective process from the surrounding bone or intervertebral disc. Occasionally, soft tissue abscesses of surrounding areas can invade the epi-

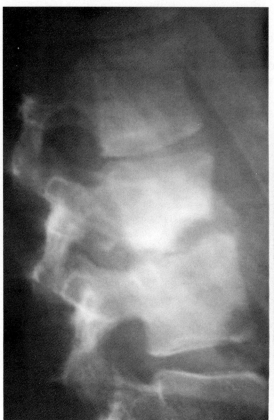
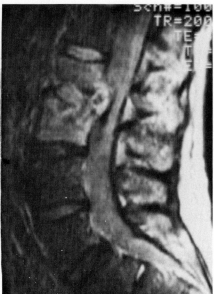

FIGURE 12–13. X-ray and MRI of HIV-positive patient with aspergillosis.

dural space. There may be direct inoculation of organisms into the epidural space. This can occur with the use of epidural catheters, particularly indwelling types. The area may become infected as the result of open surgery. There may be hematogenous spread of organisms to the epidural space. The epidural space extends from the base of the skull to the sacrum, and thus once an infective process begins, it can extend proximally and distally with ease.

Diagnosis

Clinically, epidural infections have four stages. Initially the patient may complain of severe back pain. Following this, there may be radicular pain due to involvement of nerve roots as they exit the spinal canal. As the infection proceeds, the patient may develop weakness and, in the final stage, paralysis.

In the past, diagnostic tests have included myelography and CT scanning. Although they may demonstrate compression of the spinal cord or dural sac, they are inadequate to provide a precise diagnosis. In addition, the introduction of a needle into the subdural space may provide a route by which the epidural infection could extend itself. Consequently, these tests have become supplanted by MRI. Gadolinium-enhanced images may provide additional information.

Treatment

When an epidural abscess is diagnosed or suspected, treatment is surgical. Operative drainage and debridement is the most expedient way of avoiding increasing compromise of neural tissue and preventing permanent neurologic deficit. The specific antibiotics are determined by culture and sensitivity of the offending organism. Usually they are given for 4 to 6 weeks.

INTRADURAL INFECTIONS

Meningitis

Meningitis is an inflammation of the structures within the subarachnoid space: the cerebrospinal fluid (CSF), pia mater, spinal cord, and cranial and spinal roots. The usual clinical presentation includes severe headache, convulsions, or altered consciousness. Neck stiffness is common. Meningitis may be pyogenic, viral, or granulomatous. The most common organisms causing bacterial meningitis are *Haemophilus influenzae*, *Neisseria meningitidis*, and *Diplococcus pneumoniae*. The most common viruses that cause viral or aseptic meningitis are coxsackievirus, echovirus, and herpesvirus. Granulomatous meningitis may be due to tuberculosis, syphilis, fungi, and, rarely, parasites.

The most important diagnostic test when meningitis is suspected is a lumbar puncture. The CSF shows an increase in the number of white cells, protein and sugar concentrations are altered, and the concentration of lactic dehydrogenase may be altered. Gram stain of sedimented CSF may allow identification of bacteria. Cultures should be set up for aerobic, anaerobic, pyogenic, and fungal organisms.

The treatment of meningitis is medical and is determined by the cause and clinical setting.

Myelitis

The term *myelitis* refers to any inflammatory process affecting the spinal cord; thus, there is some overlap between certain types of meningitis and myelitis. For example, certain viral infections mentioned above have a particular predilection for the gray matter of the spinal cord (eg, poliomyelitis). *Treponema pallidum*, which causes syphilis, can affect the white matter of the spinal cord. Apart from these entities, *leukomyelitides* are primary inflammatory conditions of the white matter (eg, multiple sclerosis).

POSTOPERATIVE INFECTIONS

Etiology

Whenever surgery is undertaken, deep or superficial infections can ensue. The overall incidence following spinal surgery without implantation of instrumentation is less than 1%. The infection rate increases when implants are used, but the incidence is difficult to determine and relates not only to the type of implant but also to the duration and site of surgery. Using perioperative prophylactic antibiotics when instrumentation is to be implanted decreases the overall infection rate. The use of laminar air flow and body suits may be considered when undertaking major surgery of prolonged dura-

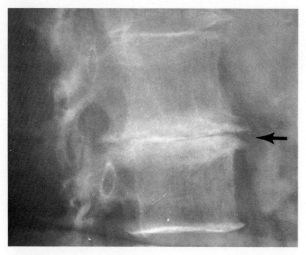

FIGURE 12–14. Anterior graft resorption due to infection.

tion requiring metal implantation. The most common organism associated with postoperative infections is *Staphylococcus aureus*. Patients who undergo major surgery are often nutritionally deprived and protein-depleted, and it is in this population that infection is of particular concern.

Diagnosis

Deep wound infections usually become evident within 1 week postoperatively. Symptoms include increasing pain at the surgical site, fevers, and sweats. Physical examination may show erythema around the incision with drainage. Probing the wound under sterile conditions may reveal a draining tract from the deep operative site. It is sometimes difficult to differentiate a superficial from a deep wound infection. In these instances it is probably prudent to treat the patient as if a deep wound infection were present and consider operative exploration. Sometimes a deep infection does not become evident until some time postoperatively, particularly after anterior surgery. One should suspect a deep infection if there is anterior graft resorption or nonunion (Fig. 12-14).

Treatment

Superficial infections usually respond to meticulous wound care and antibiotics. Deep infec-

tions require operative management. For early deep infections, surgical debridement and lavage is recommended. If the responsible organism is *Staphylococcus aureus*, one may consider leaving the hardware and bone graft in situ and closing the wound over drains or over a suction-irrigation system. For more virulent organisms, it may be necessary to pack the wound and let healing occur by secondary intention. Intravenous antibiotics should be given for about 6 weeks. The particular antibiotics used are determined by culture and sensitivity reports.

KEY POINTS

1. The incidence of spinal infections is increasing, primarily due to the rising number of intravenous drug abusers and immunocompromised patients.
2. The diagnosis of spinal infections is often not made until late in the disease process. A high index of suspicion, blood tests, and imaging studies, including nuclear bone scanning, will lead to an earlier diagnosis.
3. Most infections of the spine can be treated nonoperatively.
4. Operative management of spinal infections may be indicated when there is a progressive neurologic deficit or unacceptable deformity.

BIBLIOGRAPHY

BOOKS

D'Ambrosia R. Orthopaedic infections. Thorofare, NJ: Slack, 1989

Gustillo RB. Orthopaedic infection: Diagnosis and treatment. Philadelphia: WB Saunders, 1989.

JOURNALS

Bircher MD, Tasker T, Crawshaw C, Mulholland RC. Discitis following lumbar surgery. Spine 1988;13:98–102.

Buchelt M, Lack W, Kutschera HP, et al. Comparison of tuberculous and pyogenic spondylitis. An analysis of 122 cases. Clin Orthop 1993;296:192–199.

Charles RW, Mody GM, Govender S. Pyogenic infection of the lumbar spine due to gas-forming organisms. Spine 1989;14:541–543.

Cotty P, Fouquet B, Pleskof L, Audurier A, Cotty F, Groupille P, Valat JP, Alison D, Laffont J. Vertebral osteomyelitis: Value of percutaneous biopsy. J Neurorad 1988;15:13–21.

Dietze DD Jr, Haid RW Jr. Antibiotic-impregnated methylmethacrylate in treatment of infections with spinal instrumentation. Spine 1992;17:981–987.

Fang D, Cheung KMC, Dos Remedios IDM, Lee YK, Leong JCY. Pyogenic vertebral osteomyelitis. Treatment by anterior spinal debridement and fusion. J Spinal Disorders 1994;7:173–180.

Louw JA. Spinal tuberculosis with neurological deficit. Treatment with anterior vasculavised rib grafts, posterior osteotomies and fusion. J Bone Joint Surg [Br] 1990;72:686–693.

Mawk JR, Erickson DL, Chou SN, Seljeskog EL. Aspergillus infections of the lumbar disc spaces: Report of three cases. J Neurosurg 1983;58:270–274.

McGregor A, McNicol D, Collignon P. Aspergillus–induced discitis. A role for intraconazole in therapy. Spine 1992;17:1512–1514.

Medical Research Council Working Party on Tuberculosis of the Spine. A ten-year assessment of a controlled trial comparing debridement and anterior spinal fusion in the management of tuberculosis of the spine in patients on standard chemotherapy in Hong Kong. J Bone Joint Surg [Br] 1982;64:393–398.

Redfern RM, Cottan SN, Phillipson AP. Proteus infection of the spine. Spine 1988;13:439–441.

Thalgott JS, Cotler HB, Sasso RC, LaRocca H, Gardner V. Postoperative infections in spinal implants: Classification and analysis—a multicenter study. Spine 1991;16:981–984.

Upadhyay SS, Saji MJ, Sell P, Sell B, Yau AC. Longitudinal changes in spinal deformity after anterior spinal surgery for tuberculosis of the spine in adults: A comparative analysis between radical and debridement surgery. Spine 1994;19:542–549.

Upadhyay SS, Sell P, Saji MJ, Sell B, Yau ACMC, Leong JCY. 17-year prospective study of surgical management of spinal tuberculosis in children: Hong Kong operation compared with debridement surgery for short- and long-term outcome of deformity. Spine 1993;18:1704–1711.

Textbook of Spinal Disorders, by Stephen I. Esses.
J. B. Lippincott Company, Philadelphia © 1995.

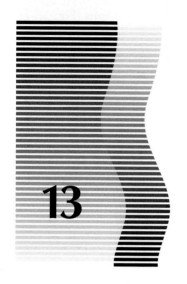

13

Inflammatory Diseases of the Spine

SEROPOSITIVE
  DISEASES
    Rheumatoid Arthritis
      Cervical Spine
    Juvenile Rheumatoid
      Arthritis
      Cervical Spine
    Systemic Lupus
      Erythematosus
      Spinal Cord
SERONEGATIVE
  DISEASES
    Ankylosing
      Spondylitis
      Clinical
      X-ray
      Cervical Spine
      Thoracolumbar Spine

Reiter's Syndrome
  Thoracolumbar Spine
Psoriatic Arthritis
  Thoracolumbar Spine
  Cervical Spine
Other Rheumatologic
  Disorders
Diffuse Idiopathic
  Skeletal
  Hyperostosis
    Thoracolumbar Spine
    Cervical Spine
Fibromyalgia
  Spine
Spinal Arachnoiditis

Various pathologic inflammatory processes affect the spine. Some of these, such as rheumatoid arthritis, involve multiple organ systems with variable derangement of the spinal column; others, such as ankylosing spondylitis, almost always involve the spine.

The classification of rheumatic diseases is continually changing as we gain more information on etiologic mechanisms. For the purposes of this chapter, we have divided the disease processes into seropositive, seronegative, and other rheumatologic disorders. The seropositive diseases discussed are rheumatoid arthritis, juvenile rheumatoid arthritis, and systemic lupus erythematosus. Although spinal involvement does not always occur with these three diseases, the effects on the spine can have significant clinical sequelae. There are numerous seronegative rheumatic diseases; the three that will be discussed here (ankylosing spondylitis, Reiter's syndrome, and psoriatic arthritis) are almost always associated with spinal column involvement, or spondylitis. Until further elucidation of the pathophysiology of conditions such as diffuse idiopathic skeletal hyperostosis and fibromyalgia, it is difficult to classify them. They can be the cause of neck and back pain and thus are included in this chapter.

SEROPOSITIVE DISEASES

Rheumatoid Arthritis

Rheumatoid arthritis (RA) is usually characterized by bilateral, symmetric polyarthritis of small and large joints in the upper and lower extremities. It is more common in women and can present at any time in adult life. Joint disease occurs as a result of synovial inflammation and destruction of articular cartilage. The latter occurs due to the presence of destructive enzymes in the synovial fluid and the formation of *pannus*, a vascular granulation tissue arising from the synovium.

The disease is considered seropositive because in most instances an immunoglobulin of the M class can be detected in a patient's serum. This immunoglobulin is also referred to as *rheumatoid factor*.

RA affects the spine, but for reasons that are not well understood, this involvement is almost always restricted to the cervical spine. Significant manifestation of the rheumatoid process in the thoracolumbar region is rare.

CERVICAL SPINE

Involvement of the cervical spine in patients with RA is common: the incidence is 30% to 80%. In the upper cervical spine, the changes seen on plain x-rays include erosion of the odontoid, atlantoaxial subluxation, and basilar impression (Fig. 13-1). In the lower cervical spine, x-ray changes include subluxation, narrowing of the disc spaces with very little osteophyte formation, and vertebral end plate erosions (Fig. 13-2). These changes occur as the result of zygoapophyseal joint erosion and proliferation of pannus.

When presented with a patient who has RA, it is important to ask specifically about symptoms referable to the neck: headache, neck pain, paresthesias in the upper and lower extremities, weakness in the upper and lower extremities, and paraparesis. In some patients, the presenting clinical manifestation of cervical spine involvement is quadriparesis or death. The physical examination must be meticulous. It is often difficult to identify neurologic deficits in a patient with advanced multiple joint involvement.

Review of plain radiographs should include measuring the distance of the odontoid process to the anterior arch of C1. Basilar impression, an upward migration of the odontoid into the foramen magnum, can be measured in a variety of ways. *Chamberlain's line* is drawn from the hard palate to the posterior aspect of the foramen magnum. The tip of the odontoid process should lie at or below this line. *McGregor's line* is drawn from the hard palate to the lowest part of the occiput. An odontoid extending more than 4.5 mm above this line is considered abnormal. These lines are shown in Figure 13-3. These measurements can occasionally be difficult due to erosion of the odontoid. In this case, upward migration of the odontoid can be determined using the *Red-*

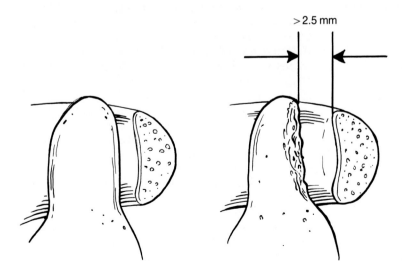

>2.5 mm

FIGURE 13–1. Erosion of the dens with atlantoaxial subluxation in rheumatoid arthritis.

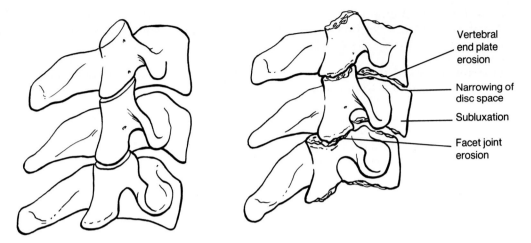

FIGURE 13–2. Changes in the lower cervical spine from rheumatoid arthritis.

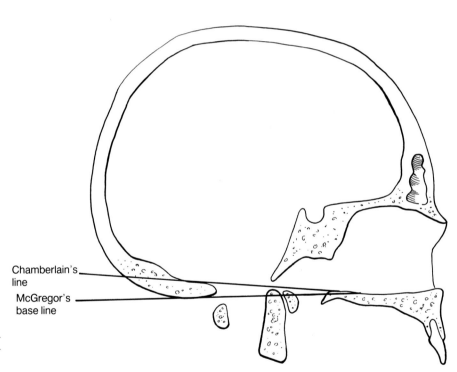

FIGURE 13–3. Measuring basilar invagination using McGregor's and Chamberlain's lines.

lund-Johnell or *Ranawat* methods (Fig. 13-4). Neurologic findings with basilar impression vary from various degrees of weakness to intermittent apnea (Fig. 13-5).

Flexion-extension x-rays of the cervical spine are important for assessing instability and subluxation. Normally, the atlantoaxial distance should not increase between flexion and extension.

Myelograph-enhanced computed tomography (CT) and magnetic resonance imaging (MRI) can be extremely useful in identifying cord compression due to proliferation of pannus in the epidural space (Fig. 13-6).

Because many patients are asymptomatic, it is important to assess the cervical spine in all patients with RA who are going to undergo general endotracheal anesthesia. Presurgical evaluation should include flexion-extension lateral x-rays of the cervical spine. Only half the patients with radiographic progression have a deteriorating neurologic deficit. Progression is unpredictable.

Most patients can be treated nonoperatively. Indications for surgery include intractable pain associated with any neurologic deterioration, progression of myelopathy due to atlantoaxial instability or basilar invagination, and severe weakness resulting in significant functional disability. Some recent work suggests that when the space available for the cord is less than 14 mm, there may be an increased probability for neurologic deterioration. This may influence surgical decision-making.

Surgery, if undertaken, must be directed toward decompression and stabilization. If there is bony compression, preoperative traction may be helpful. An example of this is basilar invagination. A posterior C1–C2 fusion is usually recommended for symptomatic patients with C1–C2 instability. If there is a fixed subluxation of C1 on C2 with spinal cord compression and myelopathy, appropriate treatment would be a C1 laminectomy with an occiput to C3 fusion. Because of the multiorgan involvement that RA can produce, surgery can have significant morbidity and mortality; thus, surgery should be undertaken only by those trained and experienced in this field.

Juvenile Rheumatoid Arthritis

Juvenile rheumatoid arthritis (JRA) is not uncommon and can be categorized into three subtypes: systemic onset, polyarticular, and pauciar-

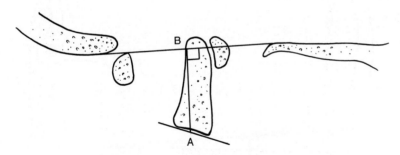

A–B distance is the Redlund-Johnell value (A is the midpoint of the inferior margin of the body of the axis)

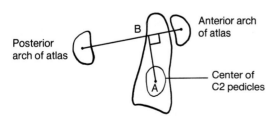

A–B distance is the Ranawat value

FIGURE 13–4. Measuring basilar invagination using Redlund-Johnell and Ranawat methods.

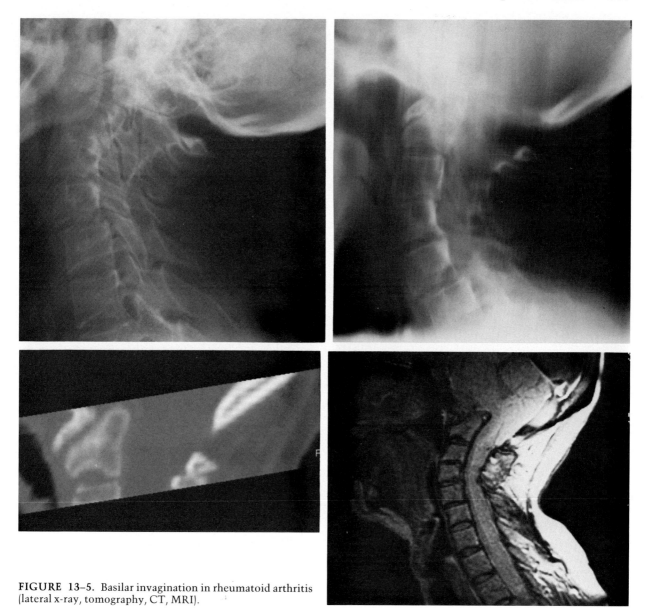

FIGURE 13–5. Basilar invagination in rheumatoid arthritis (lateral x-ray, tomography, CT, MRI).

ticular disease. Polyarticular JRA is the most common syndrome and the one associated most frequently with spine involvement. As with adult rheumatoid disease, involvement of the thoracolumbar spine is infrequent.

CERVICAL SPINE

It is estimated that over half of patients with JRA have involvement of the cervical spine. This may be simply neck pain or stiffness but can be as serious as gross C1–C2 instability. In investigating these patients, it is important to include plain radiographs of the cervical spine, occasionally supplemented with flexion-extension views. Osteoporosis of the cervical vertebrae occurs early in the disease.

In the subaxial region, facet joint involvement can result in ankylosis or fusion, most commonly at the C2–C3 level. Cervical spine involvement

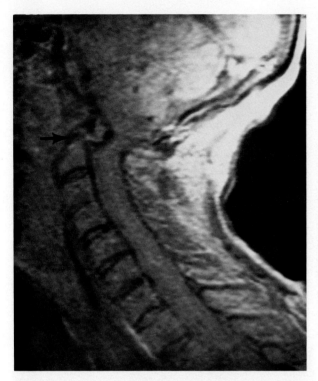

FIGURE 13–6. MRI showing pannus with cord compression in rheumatoid arthritis.

may occur before other peripheral joints are affected.

Systemic Lupus Erythematosus

Systemic lupus erythematosus (SLE) affects many organ systems, but joint involvement is the most common clinical feature. The usual joints affected are those of the hands, wrists, and knees. An autoimmune mechanism is responsible for many of the manifestations of this disease. Deposits of immunoglobulins, fibrinogen, and complement proteins can be found in blood vessels, renal glomeruli, and skin. Mechanical abnormalities of the spine due to SLE are infrequent, but the spinal column can be affected in SLE by an immunoglobulin deposition.

SPINAL CORD

The blood supply to the spinal cord can become jeopardized by deposits in its vascular nutrient pathway. When this occurs, transverse myelitis can result. This causes variable sensory and motor loss below the affected level.

SERONEGATIVE DISEASES

Ankylosing Spondylitis

Ankylosing spondylitis (AS; also called Marie-Strümpell disease or von Bechterew's disease) is associated with the HLA tissue type B27. It is seronegative because no rheumatoid factor can be found in the patient's sera. It is primarily an *enthesopathy*, meaning that there is inflammation at entheses, the sites of ligamentous attachment to bone. The disease always affects the sacroiliac joints and may or may not be associated with uveitis, prostatitis, and cardiac, pulmonary, and peripheral joint involvement.

CLINICAL

Males are more commonly affected than females. Patients may present with vague complaints of stiffness in the low back, but this can be distinguished from mechanical low back pain because it is usually made better, not worse, with exercise. The Rome criteria for AS are given in Table 13-1. Often the diagnosis is not made until late in the disease process. When taking a history from a young adult presenting with nonspecific back pain one must inquire as to family history and involvement of other systems. Physical ex-

TABLE 13–1. **Rome Criteria for Ankylosing Spondylitis**

Clinical Criteria
1. Low back pain and stiffness more than 3 months not relieved by rest
2. Pain and stiffness in the thoracic region
3. Limited motion in the lumbar spine
4. Limited chest expansion
5. History of evidence of iritis or its sequelae

Radiologic Criteria
X-ray showing bilateral sacroiliac changes characteristic of ankylosing spondylitis

Diagnosis
Criterion B + 1 clinical criterion
or
4 clinical criteria in absence of radiologic sacroiliitis

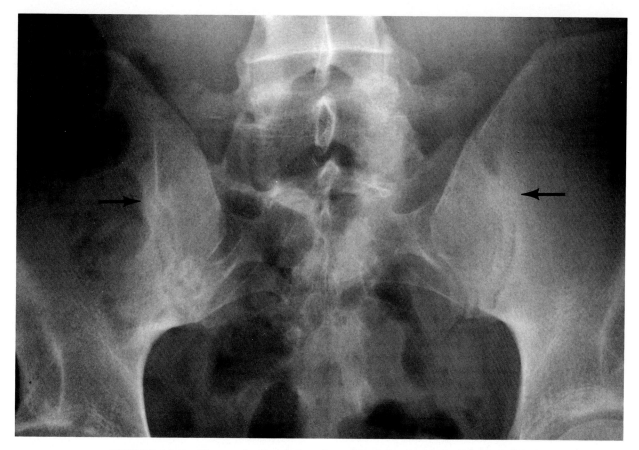

FIGURE 13–7. AP x-ray showing fusion of sacroiliac joints in ankylosing spondylitis.

amination should assess range of motion in the spine, chest expansion, and the sacroiliac joints (see Chap. 3).

X-RAY

The earliest radiographic manifestations of AS are found in the sacroiliac joints. Initially there is blurring, with erosions or sclerosis on either side of the joints. As the disease progresses, the joints become fused and obliterated (Fig. 13-7). Because of the oblique orientation of the sacroiliac joints, they are often difficult to assess on plain radiographs. CT scanning is a much more sensitive method for evaluating early involvement.

AS almost always involves the lumbar spine. Initially, the lumbar vertebrae become squared due to involvement of the enthesis where the fibers of the annulus fibrosus insert into the anterior vertebral surface. As the disease progresses, ossification can be seen in the intervertebral disc,

anterior longitudinal ligament, and posterior longitudinal ligament. Ossification of the ligamentum flavum has been described (Fig. 13-8). The facet joints, like joints elsewhere affected by AS, lose their cartilage space, become ankylosed, and go on to solid fusion (Fig. 13-9).

The term *bamboo spine* is used to describe the appearance of the spinal column when there is confluence of one vertebra to the other because of ossification of the ligaments and vertically oriented lines of calcification of the annulus fibrosus (Fig. 13-10).

CERVICAL SPINE

About half of the patients with AS have involvement of the cervical spine. The radiographic changes are similar to those seen elsewhere in the spinal column. There is calcification of the ligaments and intervertebral discs, leading to ankylosis. Again, it is unclear why in many pa-

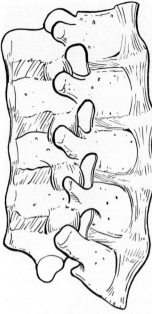

Normal lumbar spine

Loss of lordosis

Ossification of
anterior longitudinal
ligament, posterior
longitudinal ligament,
facet capsules and
interspinous ligaments

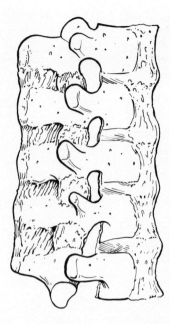

FIGURE 13–8. Changes in lumbar spine associated with ankylosing spondylitis.

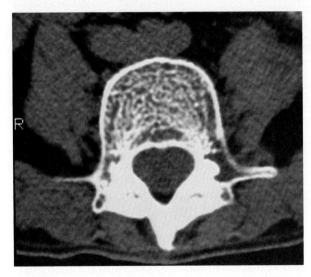

FIGURE 13–9. CT showing fusion of lumbar facet joints in ankylosing spondylitis.

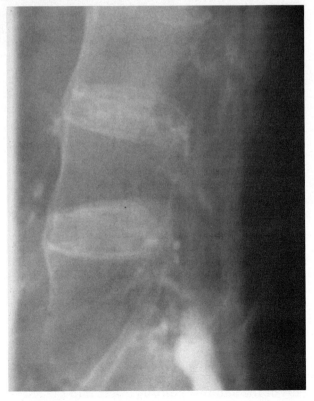

FIGURE 13–10. X-ray showing bamboo spine of ankylosing spondylitis.

tients there is loss of the cervical lordosis and the development of a kyphotic deformity. The deformity can progress to the point that the chin abuts the chest, making it difficult for the patient to eat. It also makes it impossible for the patient to look forward (Fig. 13-11).

With the development of a long rigid spinal column, the cervical spine becomes prone to fracture (Fig. 13-12). This can follow even minimal trauma. The incidence of significant neurologic injury associated with these fractures is high. There is a significant risk of epidural hemorrhage, ascending paralysis, and death. Traction should be used to align the fracture, with halo vest immobilization usually recommended until the fracture heals.

If the cervical spine deformity is large enough to interfere with the patient's inability to see ahead or eat, then surgical correction should be considered. Because the risk of intraoperative spinal cord injury is high, most surgeons perform this procedure under local anesthesia, which allows for sensitive monitoring of spinal cord function and permits the patient to help establish the ideal corrected position of the head.

THORACOLUMBAR SPINE

With progressive ankylosis of the thoracolumbar spine, the range of motion becomes limited. For reasons that are not entirely clear, as the disease progresses, some patients develop a decreasing lordosis in the lumbar spine and increasing kyphosis in the thoracic spine (Fig. 13-13). As fusion ensues, the patient's posture becomes

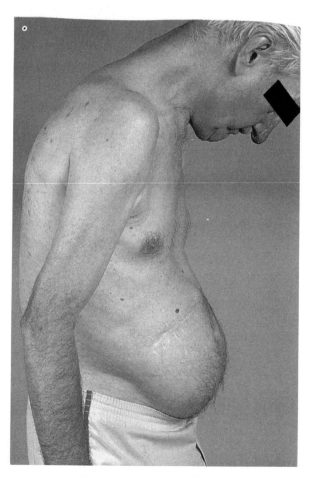

FIGURE 13–11. Cervical kyphosis.

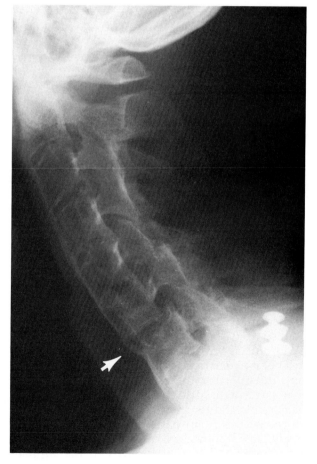

FIGURE 13–12. Cervical spine fracture in ankylosing spondylitis.

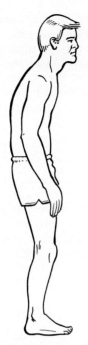

FIGURE 13–13. Stooped posture due to thoracolumbar kyphosis.

stooped (Fig. 13-14). The bone itself becomes osteopenic.

Spondylodiscitis is a complication of AS. The cause is presumed to be either traumatic or inflammatory. The affected disc undergoes destructive changes, and there are reactive sclerotic changes in the adjacent end plates. In many instances, motion can be detected at the level of spondylodiscitis, and it is almost always associated with pain. Although nonoperative treatment, involving immobilization of the affected segment, can be successful in some instances, surgery is usually required.

Ossification of the posterior longitudinal ligament and ligamentum flavum can lead to narrowing of the spinal canal. When this stenosis becomes marked, neurologic deficits can result. Indeed, there have been reports of cauda equina syndrome as the result of AS.

The mainstay of treatment is nonsteroidal anti-inflammatory agents and physical therapy. The latter is used to maintain as much motion as possible and to ensure a reasonable posture if fusion occurs. Many patients are seen late and already have significant hyperkyphosis of the thoracic spine and loss of lordosis of the lumbar region. These patients can be helped by osteotomies to restore normal posture.

Reiter's Syndrome

Reiter's syndrome is a rheumatologic condition that occurs following infection. The infection may be of the urethra or the gastrointestinal tract, causing urethritis or diarrhea. Because the arthritis occurs subsequent to infection, Reiter's syndrome is also called *reactive arthropathy*. It is more prevalent in males than females, and there is a high incidence of the HLA-B27 haplotype in affected patients. Some patients are prone to recurrent attacks, and these patients are most susceptible to sacroiliac joint and spine involvement.

THORACOLUMBAR SPINE

Reiter's syndrome is similar to AS in that there can be involvement of the sacroiliac joints and spine. However, with Reiter's syndrome, sacroiliac joint involvement is almost always asymmetric. In addition, the degree of calcification and ossification about the spine is less with Reiter's disease than with AS. Lateral osteophytes and syndesmophytes can lead to bridging of contiguous vertebrae, especially at the thoracolumbar junction. This ankylosis is less constant in Reiter's syndrome than in AS and often skips vertebral levels. Reiter's syndrome should be included in the differential diagnosis of young adults, especially males, presenting with acute low back pain.

Unlike AS, Reiter's syndrome does not result in appreciable spinal deformity, so treatment is solely medical. Early intervention with anti-inflammatory and immunosuppressive agents may improve the course of the disease.

Psoriatic Arthritis

About 6% of patients suffering from psoriasis have a seronegative polyarthritis, an association termed *psoriatic arthritis*. The risk that a patient with psoriasis will develop the arthritis is significantly increased in patients with specific HLA haplotypes, including B27. In over 80% of patients, the skin disease antecedes the arthritis.

There are many patterns of arthritis, but the most common is an asymmetric erosive process especially affecting the distal interphalangeal joints. Other clinical patterns include arthritis mutilans and asymmetric arthritis involving only a few joints or symmetric arthritis affecting many joints, similar to RA.

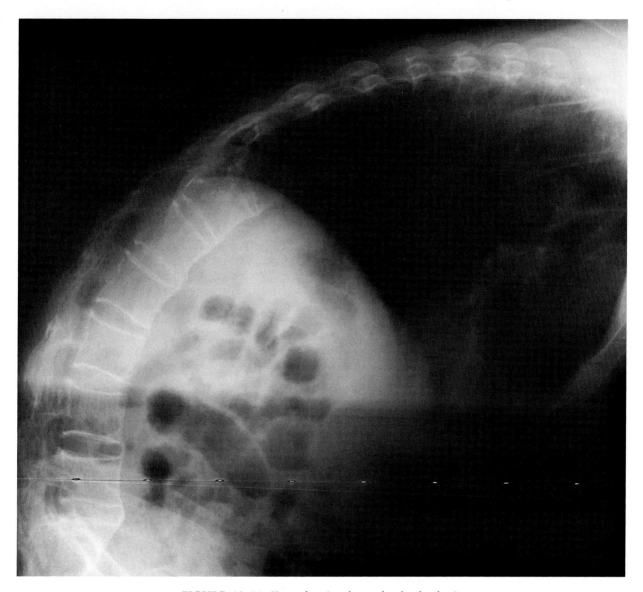

FIGURE 13–14. X-ray showing thoracolumbar kyphosis.

THORACOLUMBAR SPINE

Forty percent of patients with psoriatic arthritis have involvement of the thoracolumbar spine. This is most common in men. The changes are similar to those found in AS. There is paravertebral ossification and syndesmophyte formation. A quarter of patients have involvement of the sacroiliac joints. This, in its early stages, can be distinguished from AS because the iliac side of the joint is much more affected than the sacral side.

CERVICAL SPINE

When psoriatic arthritis affects the cervical spine, there is a tendency toward ankylosis. This is manifested by calcification in the anterior longitudinal ligament, intervertebral disc space narrowing, and spontaneous fusion of the apophyseal joints. Cases of spontaneous atlantoaxial fusion have been reported. This ankylosis is not associated with kyphosis and therefore rarely requires surgical intervention.

OTHER RHEUMATOLOGIC DISORDERS

Diffuse Idiopathic Skeletal Hyperostosis

Diffuse idiopathic skeletal hyperostosis (DISH), which primarily affects middle-aged and older men, is characterized by bone formation about the spine and in the extremities. It is associated with an abnormal glucose tolerance test. An estimated 40% of patients with DISH have diabetes mellitus. It is also more common in patients with gout. The extraspinal manifestations include the formation of large spurs, particularly in the heel and elbow. There is also ligamentous calcification.

THORACOLUMBAR SPINE

The most common area of the spine to be affected by DISH is the lower thoracic region. Large spurs form on the anterolateral side of the

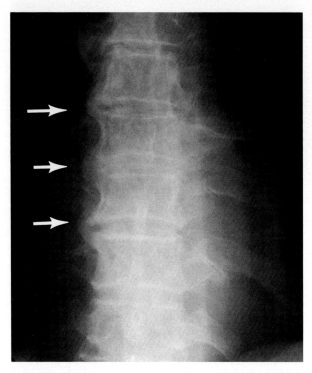

FIGURE 13–15. X-ray showing diffuse idiopathic skeletal hyperostosis (DISH).

vertebral body. At contiguous levels, the spurs flow into one another. This contiguous flowing ossification is most common on the right side of the thoracic spine (Fig. 13-15). Pulsations of the aorta are thought to prevent large osteophytes from forming on the left side.

The disc height is maintained. There is no involvement of the facet joints or the sacroiliac joints. DISH affecting the thoracolumbar spine is almost always asymptomatic. Some patients complain of stiffness, but range of motion is usually almost normal.

CERVICAL SPINE

Because the paravertebral ossification can produce very large excrescences, patients can suffer from dysphagia. Calcification of the posterior longitudinal ligament and ligamentum flavum in the cervical region can cause spinal stenosis and give rise to myelopathy.

Fibromyalgia

Fibromyalgia, also known as *fibrositis*, is a condition classified as a rheumatologic disorder not affecting joints. The underlying cause is still not understood. It has been suggested that disturbances in non-REM sleep can lead to this syndrome. The cardinal feature for diagnosis is the tenderness that can be elicited by palpation at 14 sites (Fig. 13-16). Frequently, these sites are not the areas where the patient complains of pain; indeed, the pain is often poorly localized by the patient and can be widely distributed. In addition, patients complain of stiffness and fatigue.

SPINE

Patients with fibromyalgia often complain of neck and low back pain. Physical examination is unremarkable unless specific attention is directed toward the palpation of the tender points. Radiographs do not show any changes in the spine resulting from this condition. The diagnosis in general is one of exclusion, but at least 12 tender points must be demonstrated.

Patients usually benefit from heat. Nonsteroidal anti-inflammatory agents can be useful in reducing symptoms. In patients who have a history of sleep disturbance, tricyclic antidepressants given in small doses at night can be useful.

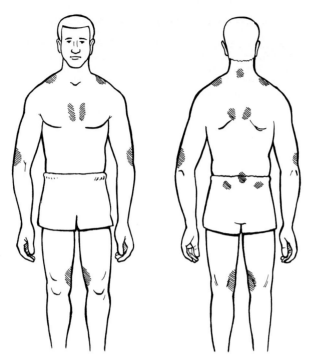

FIGURE 13–16. Sites of tenderness in fibrositis.

Spinal Arachnoiditis

Arachnoiditis is a chronic inflammation of the meninges. The pia and dura mater are extremely vascular and are the sites of the initial inflammatory response. This can progress to fibroblastic proliferation and collagen deposition in the arachnoid and subarachnoid space.

The major causes of arachnoiditis are the introduction of foreign agents into the subarachnoid space, infections (particularly tuberculosis), and trauma to the thecal sac, either from spinal column injuries or surgery. With present surgical techniques and with the use of water-soluble contrast media, the incidence of arachnoiditis has decreased substantially.

The diagnosis is based on clinical, radiographic, and operative findings. Symptoms are not discrete and can often be due to other conditions. In almost all patients, the initial symptom is constant low back or leg pain accentuated by activity. Neurologic symptoms include sensory loss in one or more dermatomes. Bladder disturbance has been reported. The radiographic criteria for arachnoiditis include intradural adhesions involving nerve roots, intradural clumping, nonfilling or distortion of root sheaths, and distortion of the thecal sac. This can be assessed both on MR scanning or myelography and CT scanning. At surgery, arachnoiditis appears as thickening of the dura. The dura may appear whiter and more opaque than usual.

The results of treatment are uniformly poor. In general, treatment is symptomatic and directed toward pain relief.

KEY POINTS

1. When seropositive rheumatic diseases affect the spine, involvement is primarily cervical.
2. Ankylosing spondylitis is primarily an enthesopathy that can affect the entire spinal column. It can result in progressive kyphosis and ankylosis.
3. Fibromyalgia (fibrositis) primarily affects soft tissues. It often gives rise to neck and low back pain.
4. Arachnoiditis, or inflammation of the meninges, can be caused by various agents and circumstances. It can be asymptomatic or give rise to various clinical complaints. It is not easily treated.

BIBLIOGRAPHY

BOOKS

Agur A. Grant's atlas of anatomy. 9th ed. Baltimore: Williams & Wilkins, 1991.
Crock HV, Yoshizawa H. The blood supply of the vertebral column and spinal cord in man. New York: Springer-Verlag, 1977.
Giles LGF. Anatomical basis of low back pain. Baltimore: Williams & Wilkins, 1989.
Hollingshead WH. Anatomy for surgeons. The back and limbs. Vol 3. 3rd ed. New York: Harper & Row, 1982.
Schmorl G, Junghanns H. The human spine in health and disease. New York: Grune and Stratton, 1959.

JOURNALS

Bland JH, Boushey DR. New gross anatomy of the cervical spine. Arthritis Rheum 1989;32(suppl):518.
Kikuchi S, Sato K, Konno S, Hasue M. Anatomic and radiographic study of dorsal root ganglia. Spine 1994;19:6–11.
Luk KD, Ho HC, Leong JCY. The iliolumbar ligament: A study of its anatomy, development and clinical significance. J Bone Joint Surg [Br] 1986;68:197–200.

Macintosh JE, Bogduk N. The morphology of the lumbar erector spinae. Spine 1987;12:658–668.

Macintosh JE, Bogduk N, Pearcy MJ. The effects of flexion on the geometry and actions of the lumbar erector spinae. Spine 1993;18:884–893.

Panjabi MM, Oxland T, Takata K, Goel V, Duranceau J, Krag M. Articular facets of the human spine: Quantitative three-dimensional anatomy. Spine 1993;18:1298–1310.

Schaffler MB, Alson MD, Heller JG, Garfin SR. Morphology of the dens. A quantitative study. Spine 1992;17:738–743.

Smith GA, Aspden RM, Porter RW. Measurement of vertebral foraminal dimensions using three-dimensional computerized tomography. Spine 1993;18:629–636.

Zindrick MR, Wiltse LL, Doornik A, Widell EH, Knight GW, Patwardham AG, Thomas JC, Rothman SL, Fields BT. Analysis of morphometric characteristics of the thoracic and lumbar pedicles. Spine 1987;12:160–166.

Textbook of Spinal Disorders, by Stephen I. Esses.
J. B. Lippincott Company, Philadelphia © 1995.

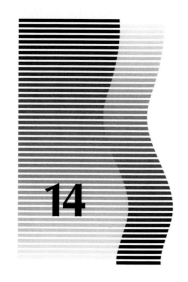

14

Spinal Deformity

Jesse H. Dickson • Wendell D. Erwin • Stephen I. Esses

SCOLIOSIS
 Congenital
  Evaluation
  Treatment
 Neuromuscular
  Evaluation
  Treatment
 Idiopathic
  Etiology
  Natural History
  Types of Curves
  Skeletal Maturity
  Patient Evaluation
  Radiographic
   Evaluation
  Treatment
 Adult
  Evaluation
  Treatment

KYPHOSIS
 Scheuermann's
 Adult
  Evaluation
  Treatment

SCOLIOSIS

Scoliosis is a fixed lateral curvature of the spine. It is considered abnormal when this curvature in the frontal plane exceeds 5°. As discussed in Chapter 5, motion of the vertebra in one plane is associated with motion in another plane. This coupling effect almost always results in rotation of a vertebra within the scoliotic curve. This rotation is important because it leads to significant asymmetry in the paravertebral area of the spine. This prominence in the thoracic region is often referred to as a *rib hump*.

The prevalence of scoliosis varies considerably from publication to publication, due in part to the screening process used. Reasonable estimates of the true prevalence are 7.7% at 5° or more, 2.3% at 10° or more, 0.5% at 20° or more, 0.2% at 30° or more, and 0.1% at 40°. Clearly, most patients with scoliosis have small curves.

In the past, it was thought that curves did not progress after skeletal maturity had been reached, but we now know this is not true. Indeed, about 70% of curves greater than 5° progress after skeletal maturity. It is impossible to predict with certainty which curves will progress and to what degree, but larger curves, curves associated with significant rotation, and curves associated with significant imbalance are more likely to progress in adult life.

There are five categories of scoliosis, divided by cause: metabolic, myopathic, neuropathic, osteogenic, and idiopathic. Metabolic scoliosis is seen in such conditions as rickets, osteogenesis imperfecta, and juvenile osteoporosis. Myopathic curves are those in which the primary etiology is muscular, as in muscular dystrophy and arthrogryposis. Neuropathic curves result from neurologic conditions such as poliomyelitis, spinal muscular atrophy, or cerebral palsy. Osteogenic curves are due to a bony, congenital abnormality. These four categories make up between 10% and 15% of all cases of scoliosis. Idiopathic scoliosis, the etiology of which is unknown, makes up the rest.

Congenital

Congenital scoliosis results from the malformation of vertebral segments, the etiology of which is unknown. It is the result of some insult to the embryo at 6 to 8 weeks of gestation. There is no evidence to suggest that it is a genetic disorder. Congenital scoliosis can be classified as hemivertebra, which is a failure of formation; unsegmented bar, which is a failure of formation; and mixed type, which includes multiple segmentation defects (Fig. 14-1). There are varying degrees of these segmentation defects. A failure of formation can be a small defect with minimal asymmetry of the vertebral body, or there may be an almost complete absence of one side of a

I: Failure of Formation

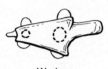

Wedge
formation

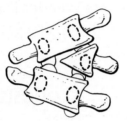

Hemivertebra

II: Failure of Segmentation

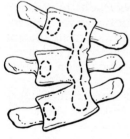

Unilateral bar

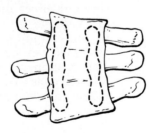

Bilateral bar

III: Mixed

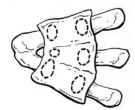

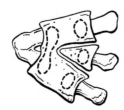

FIGURE 14–1. Classification of congenital scoliosis.

vertebral body, producing a classic hemivertebra. The failure of segmentation form of congenital scoliosis may be unilateral, in which case there is normal growth on one side of the spine, or bilateral, in which case a bloc vertebra is formed.

The natural history of congenital scoliosis depends on the type of deformity and the location of the vertebral abnormality. Some prediction of progressive deformity can be made by studying x-rays. If there is greater growth potential on one side of the spine than the other side, progression is likely. Bloc vertebrae have an excellent prog-nosis and rarely require treatment. A hemivertebra placed near the thoracolumbar junction is likely to show progression, whereas a hemivertebra in the thoracic region is much less likely to produce progressive deformity (Fig. 14-2). Hemivertebrae located at the lumbosacral junction create a pronounced oblique take-off at this level and may or may not cause increasing deformity.

The unilateral unsegmented bar, the most rapidly progressive deformity, may involve two or more segments. When multiple segments are involved and there is a disc space on the segmented

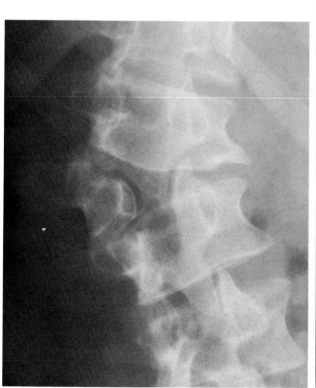
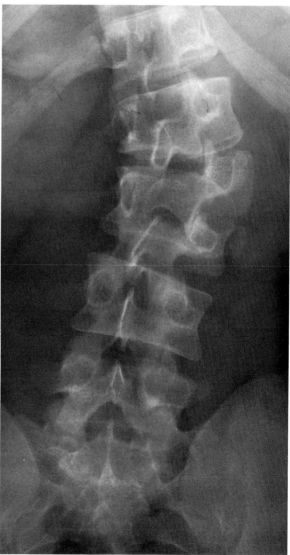

FIGURE 14–2. Hemivertebra causing small congenital scoliosis in an adult (AP and oblique x-ray).

side with normal growth, a rapid deformity can occur (Fig. 14-3).

Hemivertebrae may be discovered early in life when an x-ray is taken for another purpose. A small child or infant who has a noticeable physical deformity will probably have a progressive scoliosis. Many vertebral abnormalities are not discovered until the adolescent growth spurt, when there has been enough growth and change in the ribs and surrounding structures to produce an obvious clinical deformity.

EVALUATION

Evaluation of a patient with congenital scoliosis begins with the history. Inquiry should be made about other organ system involvement, such as renal, cardiac, pulmonary, and neurologic problems. As the spine develops at between 6 to 8 weeks of gestation, so do these organ systems, and an intrauterine insult during this time may cause problems in one or more of these areas. The clinician should determine if there has been obvious progression of the clinical deformity.

In the physical examination, the clinician should carefully look at the alignment of the thoracic area over the pelvis. Cutaneous lesions such as nevi, hairy patches, or dermal sinuses should be sought. These cutaneous lesions are frequently associated with spinal dysraphism or intraspinal abnormalities (Fig. 14-4). Neurologic deficits or abnormal extremity findings such as foot deformity should raise the index of suspicion for intraspinal abnormalities. The most common foot deformity associated with congenital spinal defects is pes cavus.

In evaluating congenital scoliosis, the standing posteroanterior and lateral x-rays should be examined. The lateral x-ray is crucial to determine whether a kyphotic deformity is also present. A posteriorly placed hemivertebra frequently causes a kyphotic deformity (Fig. 14-5). Plain standing x-rays may be supplemented with supine x-rays for bony detail; occasionally, bending x-rays are helpful. The complexity of these deformities requires the observer to compare previous x-rays with current x-rays. No one can merely "eyeball" the x-rays and make intelligent treatment decisions. More specialized x-rays are rarely indicated on initial presentation. If there is widening of the pedicles, cutaneous abnormalities, or foot deformities suggestive of spinal dysraphism, then additional studies such as a magnetic resonance image (MRI) should be obtained. In severely deformed spines, a myelogram is more helpful, followed by a postmyelogram computed tomographic (CT) scan, to delineate intraspinal pathology. Before surgery, all patients with congenital scoliosis should have an MRI or complete myelogram.

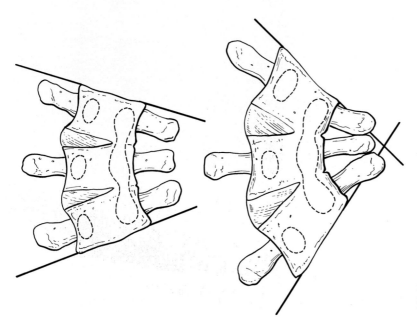

FIGURE 14–3. Rapid progression of spinal deformity in unilateral unsegmented bar.

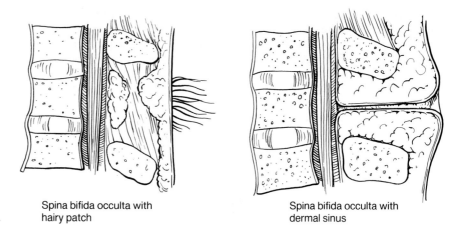

FIGURE 14–4. Spinal dysraphism.

Spina bifida occulta with hairy patch

Spina bifida occulta with dermal sinus

Several associated anomalies have been described with congenital scoliosis. The most common is a renal abnormality. Twenty to thirty percent of patients with congenital scoliosis have urinary tract anomalies, so patients should have an ultrasound study to determine whether two functioning kidneys exist. Additional urologic studies might be indicated if abnormalities are discovered. The incidence of intraspinal anomalies is about 30%. Congenital pulmonary and cardiac deformities have also been described in association with congenital scoliosis. In addition, Klippel-Feil syndrome is frequently associated with congenital scoliosis.

TREATMENT

Treatment of congenital scoliosis is based on the anticipated natural history and follow-up documenting progression or lack thereof based on standing x-rays. Large series of congenital scoliosis have shown that about 25% of patients will have no progression, 25% will have slight progression, and about 50% of patients will have progression greater than 30° and will require surgical intervention.

Treatment consists firstly of observation at 6-month intervals. In an infant, follow-up at 4-month intervals for the first 2 to 3 years of life may be indicated to determine if a rapidly progressive deformity is present. The frequency of observation depends on the type of congenital deformity present and its clinical course. Many of these patients do not need to be seen more frequently than once a year.

Bracing has virtually no role in the treatment of congenital spinal deformities because it is impossible to change the shape of underlying malformed vertebral segments. Occasionally, a centrally placed hemivertebra near the thoracolumbar junction in a long flexible curve can be braced. If a curve is flexible, bracing may be used in a young patient to allow more growth to an older age when surgery can more easily be performed. There is no evidence that physical therapy or manipulation of the spine has any role in treatment. Manipulation can be dangerous, particularly when there are cervical spine congenital abnormalities.

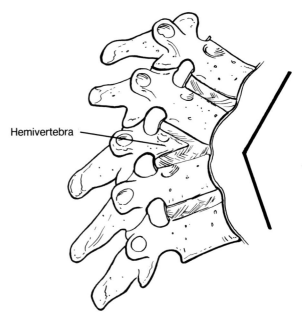

Hemivertebra

FIGURE 14–5. Kyphotic deformity due to a posterior hemivertebra.

Various surgical procedures are used in treating congenital scoliosis. Surgery is indicated when a curve is rapidly progressive during the growth years. The congenital anomalies most likely to require surgery are double hemivertebrae, unilateral unsegmented bars, and unilateral unsegmented bars with a contralateral hemivertebrae. Surgery is almost always required when these anomalies are associated with progression of more than 3° per year. It is unnecessary to wait for the end of growth before proceeding with surgery—it is much better to do a fusion in a young child with a progressive deformity than to allow severe uncorrectable deformities to occur.

The most common surgical procedure done is a posterior in situ fusion of the posterior elements. This stops growth in selected areas. External support in the form of braces or casts is necessary until solid fusion occurs. This is a successful procedure with little associated risk. When a congenital scoliosis is associated with thoracic lordosis and fusion of the ribs on the concave side of the curve, both an anterior and posterior spinal fusion may be necessary. Posterior instrumentation and fusion are commonly done in long flexible curves. Several instrumentation systems are available; the selection depends on the size of the patient and the surgeon's preference. Care must be taken not to overdistract the spine whenever instrumentation is used.

Anterior hemiepiphysiodesis has been done with increasing frequency in recent years. This technique produces a fusion on the convex side of a curve, allowing continued growth on the concave side (Fig. 14-6). This procedure must be done at an early age in a curve that is not too large.

A hemivertebra can be excised with a combination of anterior and posterior procedures. This is most commonly and safely done at the lumbosacral junction. This technically difficult procedure should be done only by an experienced, specially trained surgeon.

Neuromuscular

Neuromuscular scoliosis is, as the name implies, a result of either neurologic or muscular disease. As neurologic and muscular diseases are better defined, there is an increasing number of known diagnoses associated with the development of scoliosis. Neurologic scoliosis can result from either upper motor neuron lesions, such as

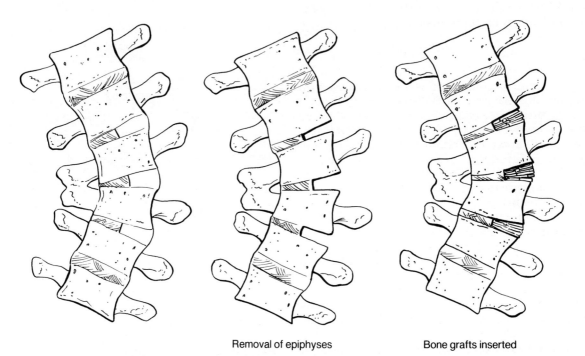

Removal of epiphyses   Bone grafts inserted

FIGURE 14–6. Anterior hemiepiphysiodesis.

in cerebral palsy and Friedreich's ataxia, or lower motor neuron lesions, such as childhood paraplegia, spinal muscular atrophy, and polio (Fig. 14-7). Muscular causes are numerous; the most common is Duchenne muscular dystrophy (Fig. 14-8). Myelomeningocele scoliosis results from impaired neurologic function at the cord level. Commonly, myelomeningocele patients have hydrocephalus and frequently have congenital spinal deformities, resulting in a mixed form of neuromuscular scoliosis.

The incidence of scoliosis varies in neuromuscular disorders. In cerebral palsy, the overall incidence is 20% of patients but may be as high as 60% in institutionalized patients. More severely involved patients with cerebral palsy have a greater incidence of scoliosis. Nearly all patients with Duchenne muscular dystrophy develop scoliosis. Scoliosis occurs in 75% to 80% of myelomeningocele patients. The chance that scoliosis will develop after a spinal cord injury in a child approaches 95%.

EVALUATION

Evaluation of neuromuscular scoliosis involves the same x-rays as in other forms of scoliosis. However, because many of these patients cannot stand, x-rays are obtained in a sitting position.

TREATMENT

Decision-making in the treatment of neuromuscular scoliosis is much more complicated than in other forms of scoliosis. Neuromuscular scoliosis patients frequently have either mental retardation or other organ system involvement, such as cardiac and pulmonary, that makes their management much more difficult and challenging. Patients with severely diminished pulmonary function and swallowing difficulties are extremely high-risk surgical candidates. Shortened life expectancy in many of the neuromuscular disorders makes treatment decisions more difficult as well.

Indications for treatment in neuromuscular scoliosis are to prevent severe deformity and to prevent progressive impairment of pulmonary function. Progressive deformity decreases functional activities that require sitting balance. As sitting balance is lost, patients cannot effectively use their upper extremities to perform tasks with lap boards, communication devices, and electric wheelchairs. Other common problems are decubitus ulcers, back pain, and hip dislocation associated with pelvic obliquity.

The impairment of pulmonary function in neuromuscular scoliosis in children is not merely a result of the curve but also of the impaired muscular function. Correction of spinal deformity does not necessarily improve pulmonary function, because the respiratory muscles remain weak. Patients whose life expectancy extends into and beyond the second decade may have pulmonary compromise resulting from severe scoliosis.

Treatment options remain the same in these patients: observation, bracing, or surgery. Observation is indicated early in the diagnosis of neuromuscular disorders, and these patients can usually be seen every 6 or 12 months. Neuromuscular scoliosis continues to progress even in adulthood. Adults should be followed at 2- to 5-year intervals to monitor progression. If treatment is not indicated, then monitoring by x-ray should not be done. Most of these curves remain very flexible, and treatment can be delayed until early adolescence if surgery is indicated.

Bracing has little or no role in treating neuromuscular disorders; in fact, bracing can have a deleterious impact on these patients. Their functional activities such as walking and upper extremity use can be impaired with extreme bracing. Bracing muscles that are seldom used can create additional weakness due to lack of use. Wheelchair modifications using pads, reclining backs, and seating systems are helpful for positioning but do not stop progression of the scoliosis.

Surgery is used for severe progressive deformities. The indications for surgery vary with the various diagnostic categories. For patients with Duchenne muscular dystrophy, a posterior spinal fusion should be considered early on, because pulmonary function may deteriorate and preclude surgery. In general, operative stabilization with instrumentation should be considered as soon as the child stops walking, even if the curve is less than 35°. The principles for surgical treatment remain the same as in all scoliosis: correction of the curve and stabilization of the curve by fusion. The one factor that distinguishes neuromuscular scoliosis from other types is the frequent involvement of musculature about the pelvis, creating an oblique pelvis or an elevation of the pelvis to one side. This pelvic obliquity may impair sitting balance and make hip dislocation more likely.

(text continues on page 266)

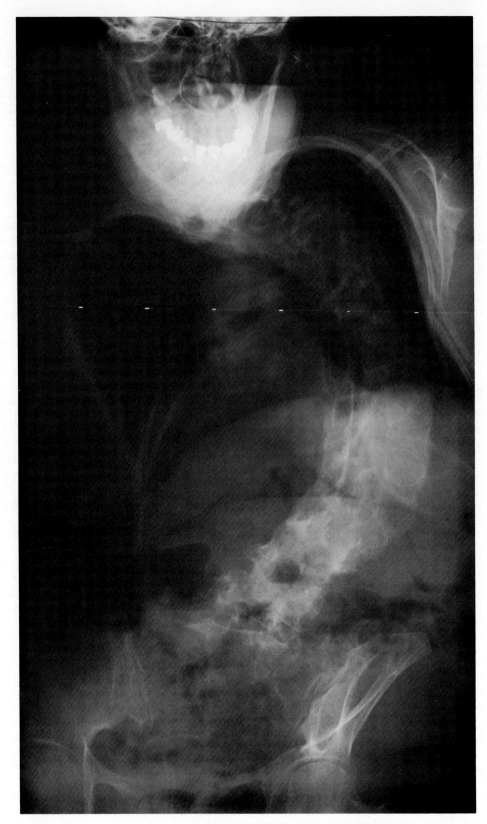

FIGURE 14–7. Neuromuscular scoliosis after polio.

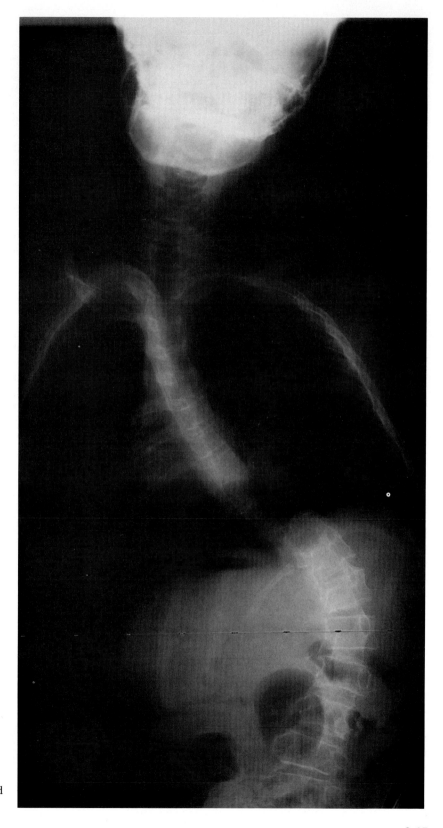

FIGURE 14–8. Scoliosis associated with muscular dystrophy.

Instrumentation and fusion in neuromuscular scoliosis requires more vertebral segments to be fused than in idiopathic scoliosis. Fusion must extend from the upper thoracic area to the fifth lumbar segment. Fusion to the sacrum is commonly carried out when there is pelvic obliquity. Recent studies have shown that the fusion can usually end at the fifth lumbar segment.

Anterior spinal surgery with release of rigid segments is performed before posterior instrumentation and fusion in severe curves, particularly in the lumbar area. In myelomeningocele patients, the deficient posterior elements frequently necessitate anterior and posterior fusions. These are difficult procedures that require specialized training.

Idiopathic

There are three types of idiopathic scoliosis, depending on the age of onset. *Infantile* scoliosis occurs within the first 3 years of life, *juvenile* scoliosis between ages 3 and 10, and *adolescent* idiopathic scoliosis after age 10. These divisions are important because the scoliosis has different characteristics in the different age groups.

Infantile scoliosis occurs primarily in boys; about 80% to 85% of cases spontaneously resolve. Of those that do not improve, progression is significant. These curves can become severe, life-threatening deformities.

In juvenile idiopathic scoliosis, the incidence in boys and girls is equal when the onset is between ages 4 and 6. As the age of onset reaches 7 to 8, it begins to occur more in girls than in boys. Progression is extremely variable. Some spontaneously disappear, and some remain the same for several years, only to progress at the time of the adolescent growth spurt. Others remain the same throughout the time the child is growing. There is some evidence that 10% to 15% percent of children who have the onset of their scoliosis between ages 3 and 10 have some spinal cord abnormality, such as syringomyelia, hydromyelia, or Arnold-Chiari syndrome. Therefore, in these children, MRIs of the cervical, thoracic, and lumbar spine should be considered as part of the initial work-up, especially if any neurologic abnormality is noted.

Although we use age to classify idiopathic curves, adolescent idiopathic scoliosis is strictly defined as a curve manifesting itself after the onset of puberty. It is seen more often in girls than in boys, particularly with curves greater than 20°.

ETIOLOGY

The following abnormalities have been associated with idiopathic scoliosis: vestibular and cerebellar abnormalities, posterior spinal column reflex abnormalities, abnormal intervertebral discs, and abnormal skeletal muscle histology. However, it is impossible to determine whether the scoliosis caused these abnormalities or whether these abnormalities played some role in the cause of the scoliosis. Family studies have shown an increased risk of scoliosis in first-degree relatives of a patient with idiopathic scoliosis. Current research is directed at elucidating the molecular basis for this deformity.

NATURAL HISTORY

Most cases of infantile scoliosis resolve spontaneously, but a few progress and become severe. The progression in juvenile idiopathic scoliosis is variable; there are no good prognostic features to help determine whether a specific curve will progress. In adolescent idiopathic scoliosis, there are some indicators to help determine which curves will progress, and these indicators are useful for children who are still growing. They are the sex of the patient, the severity of the curve, skeletal immaturity, and curve type.

Females have a much greater chance of curve progression than do males. Although there are conflicting reports, it is generally agreed that curves in females are two to three times more likely to progress than similar curves in males. The greater the degree of curvature, the more likely it is that progression will occur. Curves that measure 20° or less progress in 15% to 20% of patients. Curves measuring between 20° and 30° progress 30% to 50% of the time.

The greater the amount of growth remaining after the onset of the curve, the more likely it is that progression will occur. Thus, determination of skeletal immaturity is important in deciding whether curve progression is likely. Progression is much more probable in a patient who has 4 or 5 years of growth remaining than in a patient with only 1 year of growth remaining.

Different curve patterns have different probabilities of progression. Lumbar curves tend to progress less often than do thoracic curves. Double curves are more likely to progress than thoracolumbar curves.

TYPES OF CURVES

Curves can be classified in a variety of ways. The apex and extent of the curve, the magnitude of the curve, and the presence of other curves are all important features. The site of the scoliosis is also important: a *thoracic curve* occurs in the thoracic spine and has its apex from T2 to T11; a *lumbar curve* has its apex between the L1–2 disc space and the L4–L5 disc space; and a *thoraco-lumbar curve* has its apex at T12 or L1 or the intervening disc. A *structural curve* is a fixed curve that does not completely correct with lateral bending or in the supine position. A *minor curve* is compensatory to a *major curve*, is more flexible than the major curve, and is at least 10° smaller than the major curve.

There are many classification systems for idiopathic curves. A popular curve classification developed by King and associates is given in Table 14-1.

SKELETAL MATURITY

The determination of skeletal maturity is important because of its relevance to the probability of curve progression. However, determining skeletal maturity is difficult, particularly in preteens and young teenagers. This is due, in part, to the wide age range at which youths reach sexual maturity. In females, the greatest risk of progression of scoliosis is from the time they begin breast budding and the onset of menses. Thus, a girl whose scoliosis begins 1 year after the onset of her menses has a much lower chance of progression than if she had just started breast budding.

The *Risser sign* (Fig. 14-9), in some cases a reliable indicator of remaining growth, refers to ossification of the iliac crest apophysis. It initially starts at the anterior-superior iliac spine and progresses posteriorly to the posterior-superior iliac spine, with the wing of the ilium being divided into four equal areas. Patients who have a Risser 0, 1, or 2 have a greater chance of progression of a curve than patients who have a Risser sign 3 or 4.

Skeletal maturity can also be determined by Gruelich-Pyle bone age films. An x-ray of the wrist and hand is obtained and compared to those in the Gruelich-Pyle atlas. Skeletal age is thus determined. In general, girls cease growing at a bone age of 16 years, boys at a bone age of 18 years. Girls generally start menstruating between a bone age of 13 years and 13 years, 6 months.

PATIENT EVALUATION

The first step in patient evaluation is obtaining a clear history. It is important to obtain the date of onset of the deformity and what actually was detected (eg, whether it was a prominence of the hip, elevation of the shoulder, or a hump on the back). It is important to find out whether the patient, family, or friends noticed any progression of the abnormality. It is also important to determine if and how fast the child is growing.

The elicitation of pain is important. In general, idiopathic scoliosis does not cause back pain. If the patient complains of pain, the clinician should attempt to obtain a more thorough description from the patient. It is not unusual for young people to complain of back pain, particularly those who are extremely active. This type of back pain usually does not show consistency—that is, it does not occur at any one time or after doing only one or two types of activities. In general, this type of pain is probably normal. However, there is cause for concern if pain is present at night or if pain is persistent, recurring, and in a specific area. Indeed, these symptoms can sig-

TABLE 14–1. **Curve Classification**

Type	Primary Curve	Secondary Curve
IA	Left lumbar	Flexible right thoracic
IB	Left lumbar	Rigid right thoracic
IIA	Right thoracic	Flexible left lumbar
IIB	Right thoracic	Rigid left lumbar
III	Right thoracic	None
IV	Long right thoracolumbar (includes L4)	None
VA	Right thoracic	High flexible left thoracic
VB	Right thoracic	High rigid left thoracic

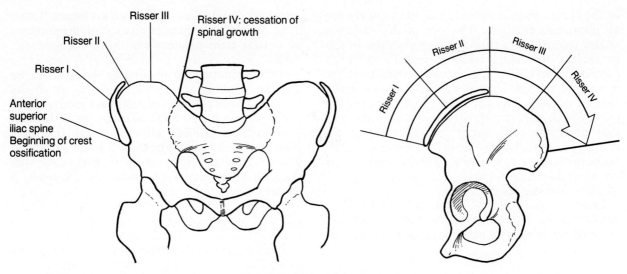

FIGURE 14–9. Risser sign.

nify a bone tumor as the underlying etiology of the scoliotic curve.

The physical examination begins with the patient standing and facing away from the examiner (Fig. 14-10). The position of the shoulders is noted, as well as whether the pelvis is level. Any prominence of the scapulae is assessed. It is noted whether the arms are an equal distance from the side. By dropping a plumb line from the occiput or C7, it is possible to determine whether the head, shoulders, and midtrunk are centered over the pelvis. Any cutaneous abnormalities on

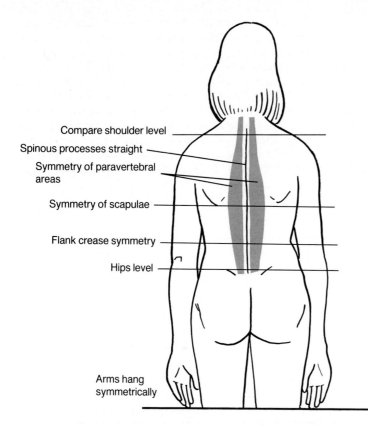

FIGURE 14–10. Physical examination for scoliosis.

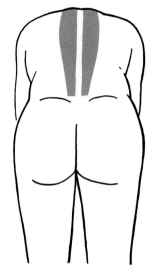

Paravertebral symmetry in forward flexion

FIGURE 14–11. Forward-bending test.

the back such as a hairy patch, birthmark, or sinus tract are noted because they may indicate underlying spinal cord abnormality.

The patient is then asked to bend forward, and any asymmetry in the paravertebral muscle area is noted, both in the thoracic and lumbar regions (Fig. 14-11). Right and left side bending is done to determine the flexibility of the curve. Patients with idiopathic scoliosis do not usually have any restriction of forward flexion and lateral bending. If there is restriction of motion, especially in forward flexion, the scoliosis is considered to be a reactive phenomenon, as seen with spinal cord or bone tumors. Figures 14-12 and 14-13 show the typical appearance of a right thoracic curve. Other curve pattern appearances are shown in Figure 14-14.

A thorough neurologic examination of the upper and lower extremities is done. Deep tendon reflexes are elicited. Leg lengths are measured. The feet are examined to determine whether there is any abnormality, such as pes cavus or difference in size.

(text continues on page 272)

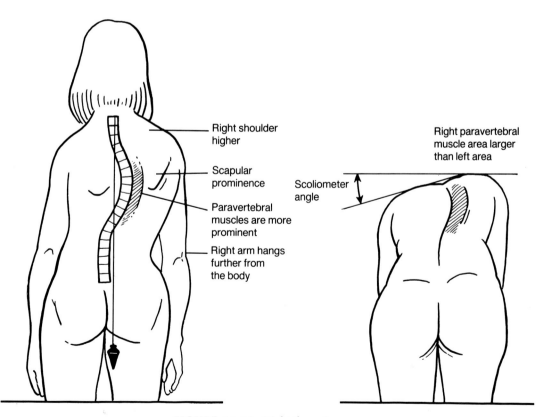

Right shoulder higher

Scapular prominence

Paravertebral muscles are more prominent

Right arm hangs further from the body

Right paravertebral muscle area larger than left area

Scoliometer angle

FIGURE 14–12. Right thoracic curve.

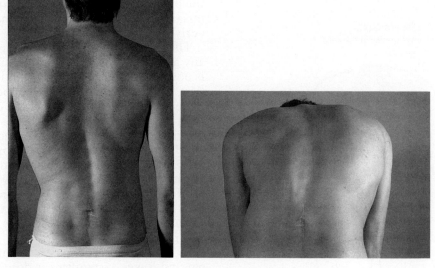

FIGURE 14–13. Right thoracic curve.

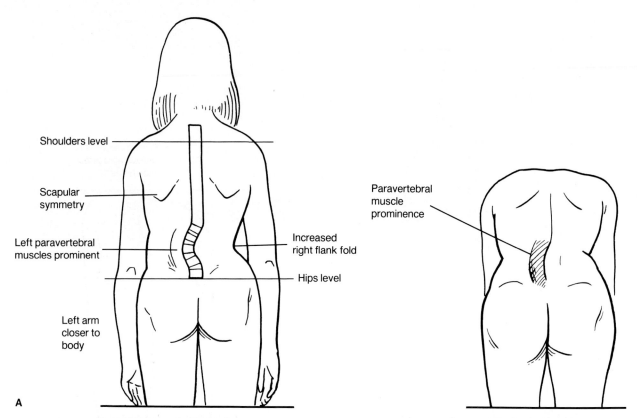

FIGURE 14–14. (**A**) Left lumbar, (**B**) right thoracolumbar, and (**C**) double major right thoracic and left lumbar curves.

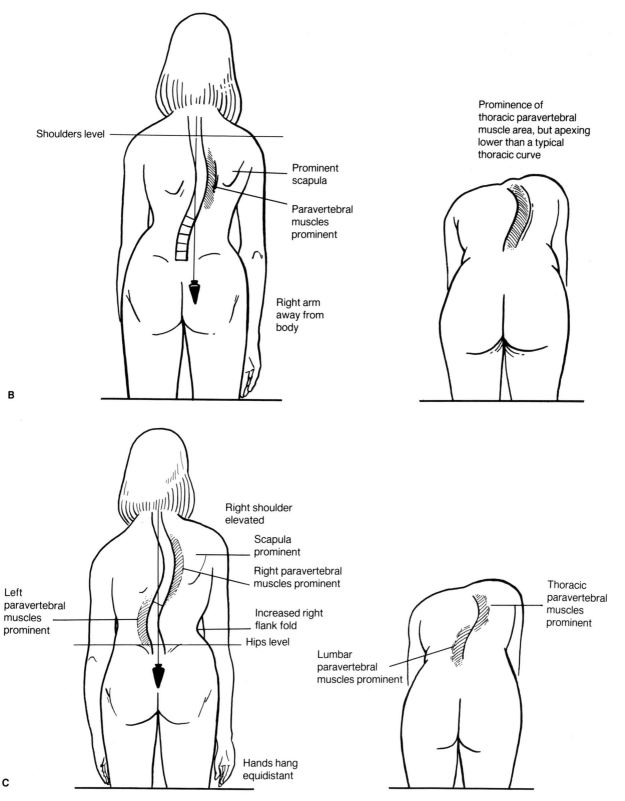

Shoulders level

Prominent scapula

Paravertebral muscles prominent

Right arm away from body

B

Prominence of thoracic paravertebral muscle area, but apexing lower than a typical thoracic curve

Left paravertebral muscles prominent

Right shoulder elevated

Scapula prominent

Right paravertebral muscles prominent

Increased right flank fold

Hips level

Hands hang equidistant

Lumbar paravertebral muscles prominent

Thoracic paravertebral muscles prominent

C

FIGURE 14–14. *(Continued)*

Throughout the examination, the clinician should remember that idiopathic scoliosis is a diagnosis of exclusion, so he or she must look for any signs of a causative agent.

RADIOGRAPHIC EVALUATION

Radiographs of the spine should be taken in the standing position, preferably with the entire spine seen on a single x-ray film. If this type of x-ray cassette holder is unavailable, one can obtain two separate standing x-rays, one in the thoracic area and one in the lumbar area. If bony abnormalities are seen on these standing x-rays, such as an abnormal-shaped vertebra or widening of the interpedicular distances, then specific x-rays of those regions should be obtained. Because scoliosis is a multidimensional deformity, it is important to obtain lateral views as well. If necessary, additional x-rays of the lumbosacral junction should be obtained in the lateral projection to rule out a spondylolysis or spondylolisthesis. X-rays of the wrist can be obtained for determination of bone age.

The curve measurement by x-ray is determined by the *Cobb technique*. The two end vertebrae are selected, defined as the last vertebrae tilted into the concavity of the curve. The disc spaces in the curve are always wider on the convexity of the curve than on the corresponding concave side. When the disc spaces begin to be wider on the opposite side, the vertebra is then beginning to angle into the opposite direction, and thus the vertebra is not in the curve being measured. Once the end vertebrae have been selected, a line is drawn across the vertebral end plates and a right angle is drawn from these lines. The intersection of the two lines creates an angle, which is the angle of the curvature (Fig. 14-15). The Cobb measurement is really the angle between the upper and lower end vertebrae. This technique of measurement is used only because lines drawn from the end plates of the end vertebrae would intersect at a great distance, usually off the x-ray film; thus, right angles are created to make measurement technically easier. In severe cases these right angles are unnecessary.

Vertebral rotation is more difficult to measure. The *Nash technique* determines rotation by visualizing the position of the pedicles or the spinous processes (Fig. 14-16). The techniques used to measure rotation all have large errors in accuracy. It is usually not possible to determine whether there has been progression of rotation using these techniques.

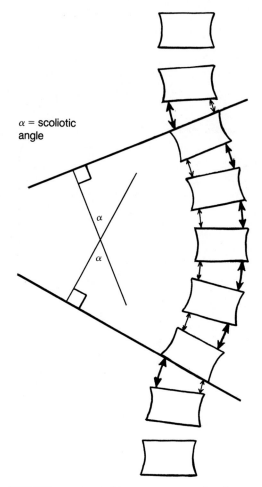

α = scoliotic angle

FIGURE 14-15. Cobb measurement of scoliosis.

TREATMENT

There are three basic treatment options available for idiopathic scoliosis: observation, nonoperative treatment such as bracing, or surgical intervention. Observation is always used in a growing child with a mild curve. Growing children who have curves less than 20° are observed for progression. They are usually examined at 4- to 6-month intervals. Children who when first seen have curves in the 20° range are observed an additional 4 to 6 months. They should show 5° of progression before bracing is instituted. If a child who is growing presents with a curve of greater than 30°, a brace is immediately prescribed, and there would be no observation period.

The mainstay of nonoperative treatment is bracing. The original successful brace treatment for scoliosis was a standard Milwaukee brace or cervical thoracic lumbosacral orthosis (CTLSO) (Fig. 14-17). The basic concept of bracing is prevention of curve progression rather than correction of the curve. It will only prevent curves from progressing as the child continues to grow. Thus, braces are applied when a curve is progressing and is between 20° and 40°. In addition, a brace is usually prescribed in premenarchal girls if their curve measures greater than 30° at the time of first evaluation. Rarely does a brace work after a curve is 40° or greater.

Since the development of the original Milwaukee brace, other orthoses have been developed. These are primarily underarm braces or what is called a thoracolumbosacral orthosis (TLSO). There are numerous types of these braces, such as the underarm Milwaukee brace, the DuPont brace, the Boston brace, and the Risser brace. All are basically similar to the standard Milwaukee brace but cosmetically are much more appealing. They are usually as effective as the standard Milwaukee brace.

There is considerable controversy as to the effectiveness of brace treatment. The most recent prospective study suggests that bracing has some effect, at least short-term, on the natural history of idiopathic scoliosis. Curves reduced to less than 50% by the brace during the first year of treatment have a good chance of obtaining significant permanent correction. Twenty-five percent of patients who wear a brace will continue to show a progression of the curve, and about half of these progress to the point where surgery is indicated.

Three factors are essential to successful bracing. First, someone must manage the brace and know when it is and is not to be used. Second, the brace must be well-fitting, comfortable, and effective. Third, the patient must be willing to wear the brace conscientiously. It is difficult to wear a brace during adolescence. A great deal of time and effort should be expended to teach the patient the goals and rationale of the brace.

In the 1940s and 1950s, when the Milwaukee brace was first applied, it was prescribed for 24 hours a day. It has now been shown that the brace works equally well if the patient is allowed out of the brace for an 8-hour period during any particular day. Thus, the patient can go to school without wearing the brace as long as he or she uses it before and after school and while sleeping.

Night braces have been developed that hold the patient in an overcorrected position. Advocates suggest that they need to be worn only at night. Initial results show that this type of brace is as effective as a regular TLSO, but this brace is not as effective as a TLSO when dealing with double major curves.

The use of electric stimulation for the treatment of scoliosis has been investigated for decades. The most active investigation occurred in the late 1970s and early 1980s. The rationale for electric stimulation was that contraction of the paravertebral muscles on the convex side of the curve would cause straightening of the spine and strengthening of those muscle groups. Although initially there was some suggestion that electric stimulation was as effective as brace treatment, this does not seem to be the case. Indeed, the most recent studies suggest that electric stimulation has no place in the treatment of spinal deformity (Fig. 14-18).

Two surgical approaches are used in treating idiopathic curves: posterior spinal instrumentation and fusion, and anterior spinal instrumentation and fusion. The objective is the same: to partially correct the deformity and to permanently stabilize that area of the spine. Partial correction

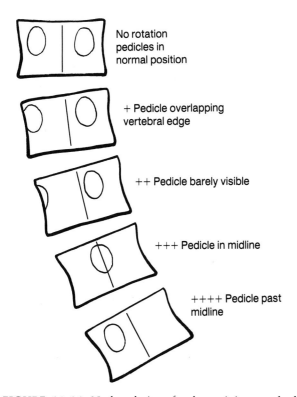

No rotation
pedicles in
normal position

\+ Pedicle overlapping
vertebral edge

\++ Pedicle barely visible

\+++ Pedicle in midline

\++++ Pedicle past
midline

FIGURE 14–16. Nash technique for determining vertebral rotation.

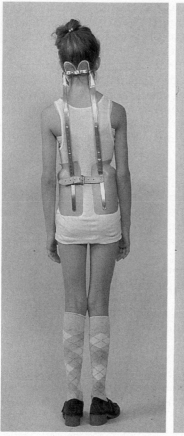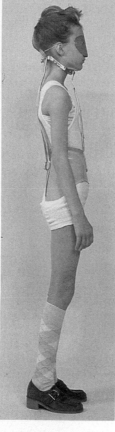

FIGURE 14–17. The Milwaukee brace.

use techniques that stabilize multiple individual vertebrae throughout the curve. The Luque technique consists of placing two rods along the posterior elements of the spine and passing wires beneath the lamina and tying them to the rod. This procedure has a certain risk factor, because passing the wires under the lamina into the spinal canal can cause neurologic deficits. Other segmental techniques have been developed using hooks; these techniques include the Cotrel-Dubousset, Texas Scottish Rite Hospital, Isola, and Mod-U-Lock systems. All have the same basic principle: segmental fixation with hooks (Fig. 14-20). Some surgeons think that these systems not only correct the frontal plane deformity but also help restore the normal sagittal contour of the spine.

The results of the segmental fixation systems and the Harrington system are probably not much different in regard to the degree of correction of the curve. There is some suggestion that the segmental systems allow better restoration of normal thoracic kyphosis and lumbar lordosis. The major difference between the two systems is that with segmental fixation, no postoperative immobilization is needed, and thus the patient does not need to wear a body jacket postoperatively. With the Harrington procedure, a body jacket is usually used for 6 to 9 months.

One problem with posterior fusions for scoliosis is due to the *crankshaft phenomenon*. Because of rotation, the posterior fusion involves more of the convex than of the concave deformity. In patients who undergo posterior spinal fusion before the adolescent growth spurt, the vertebral bodies will continue to grow. The anterior growth coupled with the slightly asymmetric fusion posteriorly can lead to loss of correction, increased vertebral rotation, and recurrence of the rib hump.

Two major instrumentation systems are used for anterior spinal instrumentation and fusion, the Dwyer and Zielke systems. A thoracoabdominal approach is used for both. The approach is made on the convex side of the spine. The intervertebral discs are removed and screws are placed in the vertebral bodies as fixation points (Fig. 14-21). In the Dwyer procedure, a cable is threaded through the screw heads, and as the cable is tightened the vertebral bodies approach each other because the discs have been removed. Thus, partial correction of the curve can be obtained. With the Zielke procedure, a threaded rod is used instead of a cable (Fig. 14-22). This allows better positioning of the vertebrae as the rod is tightened.

is obtained using metal implants; permanent stabilization is accomplished by bony fusion.

The first successful surgical correction and stabilization of scoliosis was accomplished using a technique described by Paul Harrington in which two hooks were inserted at either end of a scoliotic curve and a metal rod was placed between these hooks. Distraction was then accomplished similar to the way one would jack up a car. This would partially correct the deformity. The hook and rod system was used to hold the curve in the corrected position until a bony fusion had developed. This technique has been used in thousands of cases and has been shown to be very reliable and safe (Fig. 14-19).

The second group of posterior spinal instrumentation techniques has been classified as segmental fixation. The difference between these techniques and the Harrington procedure is that the latter does not stabilize any of the vertebrae within the curve. Segmental instrumentations

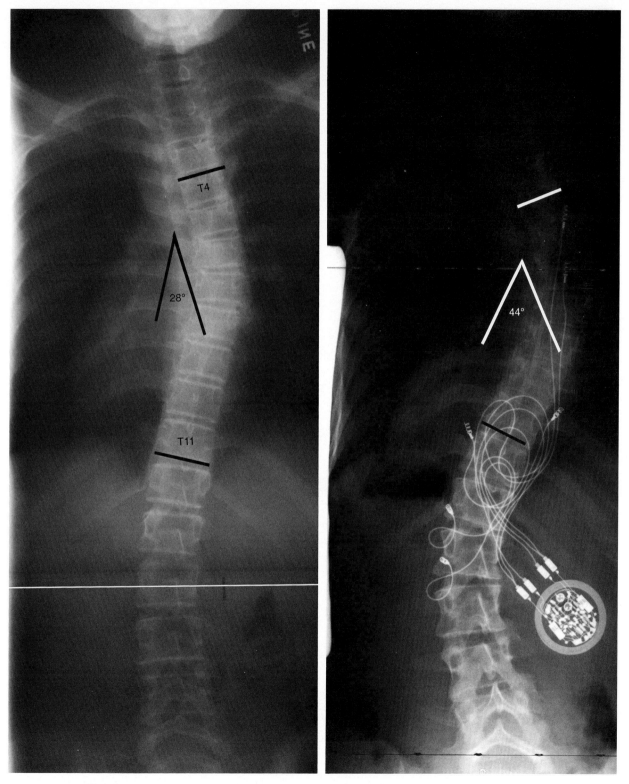

FIGURE 14–18. Progression of idiopathic adolescent scoliosis despite implanted electronic stimulator.

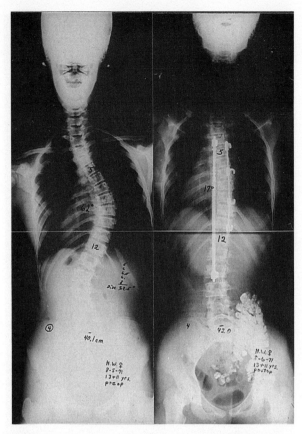

FIGURE 14–19. X-ray showing Harrington instrumentation for scoliosis.

Adult

The incidence of scoliosis in adults is between 2% and 4%. Adults with scoliosis can be divided into two main groups: those who had scoliosis before skeletal maturity, and those whose onset was after skeletal maturity. There are several contributing risk factors in the latter group, including osteoporosis, prior back surgery, trauma, and degenerative disease. Indeed, these curves are sometimes referred to as *degenerative* scoliosis. It is occasionally difficult to distinguish between adult-onset curves and curves that began as idiopathic adolescent deformities. Degenerative curves are usually lumbar, have fewer vertebrae in the curve, and are associated with a loss of lordosis (Fig. 14-23).

It was formerly thought that once patients with idiopathic adolescent scoliosis reached skeletal maturity, their curves would not progress; we now know this is not true (Fig. 14-24). Many

studies have attempted to identify which curves are most likely to progress in adult life, but there is a wide discrepancy in the results. Any curve, large or small, thoracic or lumbar, has the potential for progression in adulthood. Single major thoracic curves measuring between 60° and 80° have the greatest likelihood of continued progression in adult life.

EVALUATION

A careful history is the first step in evaluating an adult with scoliosis. The clinician should ascertain when the deformity was first noted and whether the patient has felt any progression of the curve. This may be manifest by a feeling of imbalance or a feeling of getting shorter. The clinician should ask whether recent alterations have been necessary in clothes. It is important to

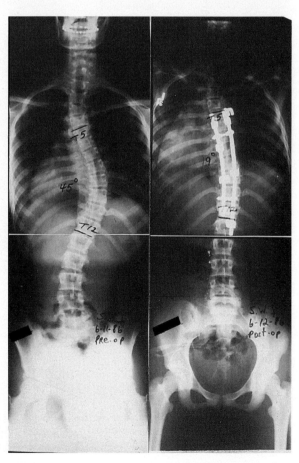

FIGURE 14–20. X-ray showing Cotrel-Dubousset instrumentation for scoliosis.

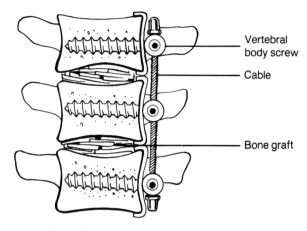

Dwyer Cable System

- Vertebral body screw
- Cable
- Bone graft

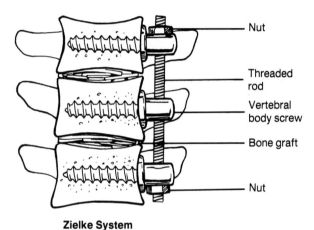

Zielke System

- Nut
- Threaded rod
- Vertebral body screw
- Bone graft
- Nut

FIGURE 14–21. Anterior spinal instrumentation and fusion for scoliosis.

Three-foot standing AP and lateral radiographs should be obtained. If surgical intervention is being considered, right- and left-bending x-rays can be used to assess the curve flexibility. If a patient has any neurologic symptoms or findings, then MR scanning should be considered. However, when spinal deformity is present, it is often very difficult to assess the spinal cord, cauda equina, and nerve root with MRI. This can usually be done more effectively with myelography followed by CT scanning.

TREATMENT

Because any curve has the potential for progression, the first part of treatment should be pe-

document whether pain is present and where that pain is perceived. Idiopathic adolescent scoliosis is not painful, but scoliosis in the adult can cause local discomfort because of the development of degenerative disease, particularly at the apex of the curve. In addition, with the development of degenerative disease, spinal stenosis can cause leg pain or weakness. Pulmonary function is not usually affected by curves less than 60°, and significant pulmonary compromise is unusual in curves less than 90°.

Physical examination should include not only an evaluation of the back but also a thorough neurologic examination, especially of the lower extremities, to ascertain whether there is any spinal cord or nerve root impairment.

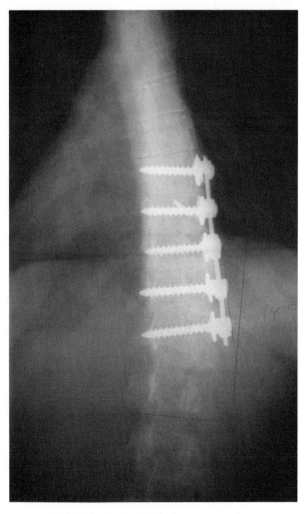

FIGURE 14–22. Zielke instrumentation.

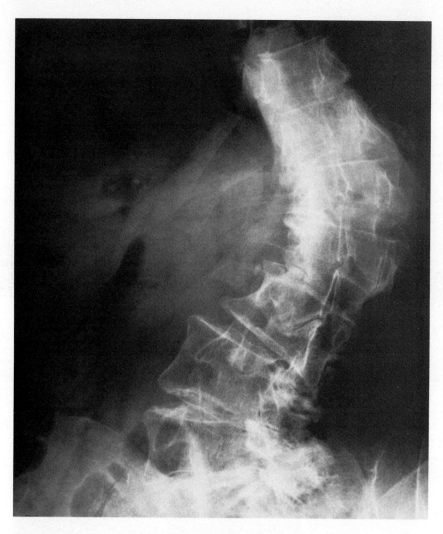

FIGURE 14–23. Degenerative lumbar scoliosis in the adult.

riodic evaluation to determine whether progression is occurring. It is prudent to evaluate patients once every 2 or 3 years. Patients should be told that if they develop pain or have an increased amount of discomfort, they should return sooner.

For patients with back pain, symptomatic treatment includes analgesics, nonsteroidal anti-inflammatory agents, and bracing. Occasionally, soft molded orthoses can control pain, but they do not correct or prevent progression of deformity.

Very few patients with adult scoliosis require surgery. The presence of a curve, by itself, no matter what the magnitude, is not sufficient indication for operative intervention. The main reason for recommending surgery to a patient is the presence of neurologic symptoms severe

enough to restrict activities. Surgery is undertaken to decompress the symptomatic stenotic areas. A concomitant fusion is necessary; otherwise, the deformity will progress postoperatively. Other indications for surgery include unremitting back pain that does not respond to nonoperative measures, documented progression of the curve, and, very rarely, pulmonary compromise due to thoracic curves of great magnitude. Some authors have suggested that cosmesis is a relative indication for surgical intervention. We do not agree: the role of surgery is to prevent progression, not to correct the deformity, and the incidence of complications is reported to be as high as 60% even in expert hands.

The leading cause of failure is pseudarthrosis. This is particularly common when the fusion is extended to the sacrum. Attempts have been

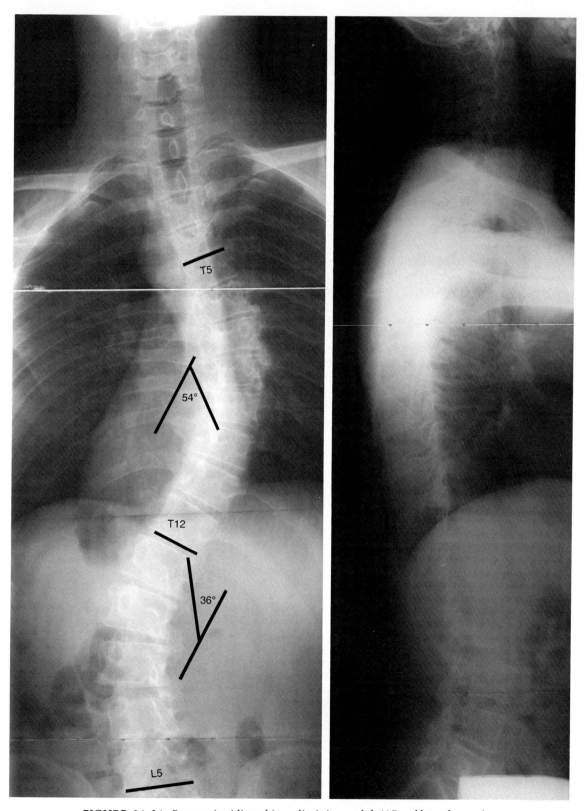

FIGURE 14–24. Progressive idiopathic scoliosis in an adult (AP and lateral x-rays).

made to improve results by avoiding fusion to the sacrum whenever possible or by performing a supplemental anterior fusion when the sacrum must be included.

KYPHOSIS

When looking at a person from the side, there are three curvatures in the spine: a curving inward in the neck area (lordosis), a rounding of the thoracic spine (kyphosis), and a curving inward of the lumbar spine (lordosis). The normal amount of kyphosis in the thoracic spine varies from about 20° to 40°.

There are two major reasons for excessive kyphosis: postural and structural. Excessive kyphosis due to poor posture is a result of the person not holding himself or herself straight. The patient can consciously correct this. There is no intrinsic pathology in the muscles, nerves, bones, discs, or ligaments, so direct treatment to one of these areas is not beneficial. Exercises may be recommended to strengthen the paravertebral muscles, but emphasis must be directed toward the patient consciously holding himself or herself straight.

Structural excessive kyphosis is due to intrin-

sic pathology in the spinal column. Congenital kyphosis has the same underlying pathology as congenital scoliosis. There is a high association with renal and cardiac anomalies, and significant association with other intraspinal pathology has been documented.

Scheuermann's

Scheuermann's disease, first described in 1920, is excessive fixed kyphosis in which at least three contiguous involved vertebrae are wedged anteriorly more than 5° (Fig. 14-25). Normally, on the sagittal view of the vertebral column, the vertebrae are rectangular. The curvature of the thoracic spine is due to angulation through the disc spaces rather than the vertebrae themselves.

A condition called thoracic hyperkyphosis acts and presents exactly as Scheuermann's kyphosis. In the former condition, however, there is no wedging of the vertebral bodies. In general, this condition is treated the same as Scheuermann's disease.

The etiology of Scheuermann's kyphosis is unknown. Abnormalities in the cartilaginous vertebral ring apophyses, herniation of the nucleus pulposus into the vertebral bodies, disturbance

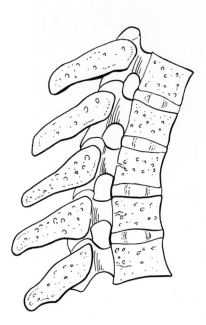

Normal kyphosis

Square bodies in the sagittal plane

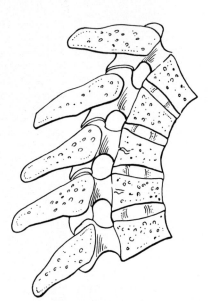

Scheuermann's disease

At least three contiguous vertebrae wedged anteriorly >5°

FIGURE 14–25. Scheuermann's kyphosis.

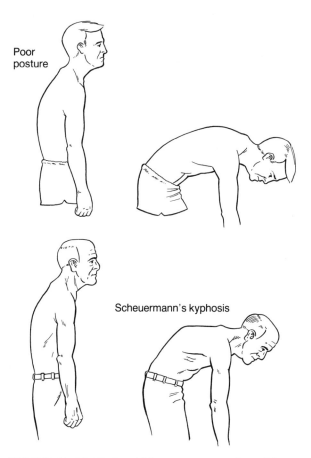

FIGURE 14–26. Distinguishing poor posture from Scheuermann's kyphosis.

of enchondral growth, mechanical factors, muscular contractures, and poor posture have all been said to cause the kyphosis, but none of these have been proven to be the etiologic agent.

The prevalence of Scheuermann's kyphosis is reported to be 0.5% to 8%, depending on whether x-rays are used to diagnose the condition. It is probably more frequent in females than males and has its onset between ages 12 and 15 years. Pain occurs in 20% to 50% of cases. Pain is more frequent in patients who have the apex of the kyphosis at the thoracolumbar junction. Pain is uncommon in patients who have the apex of the kyphosis in the middle or upper thoracic spine.

The physical examination of a patient with Scheuermann's kyphosis shows that the increased kyphosis is rigid (Fig. 14-26). Using the Cobb method, the amount of thoracic kyphosis can be measured on lateral x-rays (Fig. 14-27).

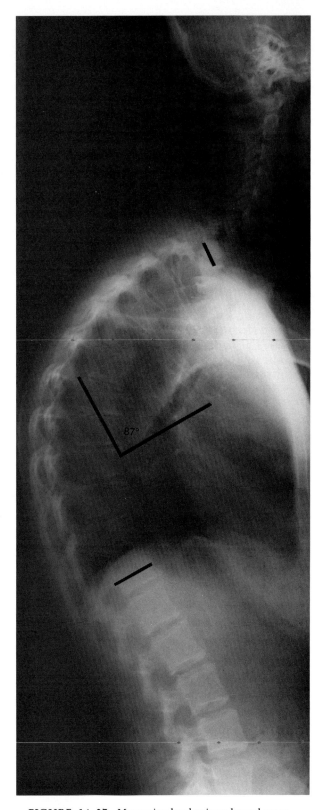

FIGURE 14–27. Measuring kyphosis on lateral x-ray.

The primary treatment for thoracic hyperkyphosis and Scheuermann's disease is a Milwaukee brace (CTLSO). An underarm brace is insufficient to control the upper half of the kyphotic curve. In addition, Scheuermann's kyphosis is usually associated with a forward translation of the head and neck, which can be corrected only with a full Milwaukee brace. It is worn 24 hours a day for 1 year. The patient is then weaned out of the brace over 6 months until he or she only sleeps in the brace. This stage may last an additional 1 to 3 years. As brace treatment is discontinued, the patient must be made aware of his or her posture. Braces are used in patients who have curves greater than 60° and who have some skeletal growth remaining or show excessive unevenness of the vertebral apical end plates. Once the patient is 16 or 17 years old, a brace will not provide any permanent benefit.

Surgery is reserved for patients with persistent unrelenting symptoms despite adequate conservative treatment, and those with a significant kyphosis. The degree of kyphosis for which surgery is indicated varies according to the apex of the deformity. A 60° kyphosis with the apex at T10 is much worse than a 60° kyphosis with the apex at T6. Most physicians agree that curves of less than 60° do not require surgery, but curves greater than 90° probably do.

Adult

The most common cause of increased thoracic kyphosis in adults is osteoporosis, discussed in Chapter 17. Other causes include Scheuermann's disease and posttraumatic kyphosis. Ankylosing spondylitis, although rare, is often accompanied by increasing kyphotic deformity in adulthood. Kyphotic deformities may be divided into two groups: an acute angular kyphosis, and a kyphotic deformity that extends over multiple levels (Fig. 14-28). As the kyphotic deformity increases, the moment arm on the apex of the deformity similarly increases (Fig. 14-29). There is, therefore, an increased tendency to progression with larger deformities. Table 14-2 lists the common curves of increased thoracic kyphosis in the adult.

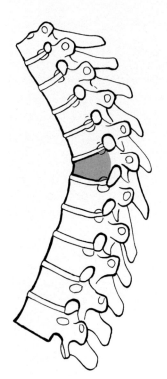

Acute angular kyphosis

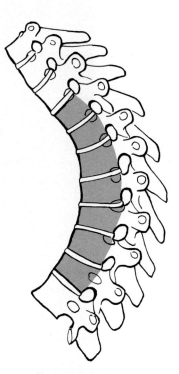

Kyphotic deformity over
multiple levels

FIGURE 14–28. Types of kyphotic deformity.

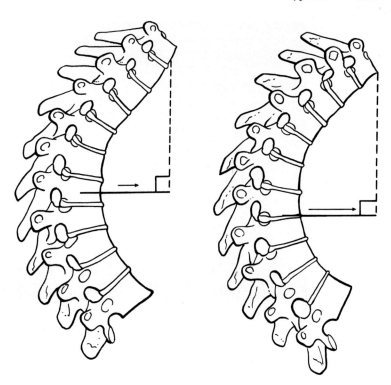

FIGURE 14–29. Increasing moment arm with increasing kyphosis.

EVALUATION

The history usually identifies the underlying cause of the kyphotic deformity (Fig. 14-30). Physical examination should include a neurologic evaluation. Kyphotic deformities are more likely to be associated with neurologic deficits than are deformities in the frontal plane. Standing x-rays are used to measure the degree of deformity (Fig. 14-31). X-rays taken with the patient supine indicate the degree of flexibility of the curve. MR scanning is extremely useful in identifying the degree of spinal cord compromise, if present.

TREATMENT

As with adult scoliosis, routine follow-up is important to identify progressive deformities. Symptomatic treatment for pain includes analgesics, nonsteroidal anti-inflammatory agents, and padded orthoses. These orthoses may provide some pain relief but do not control progression of the deformity to any extent.

Indications for surgery include neurologic symptoms, progressive deformity, and pain that does not respond to the above measures. Various surgical approaches have been used, but in general anterior fusion and posterior fusion with instrumentation is the procedure of choice. The risk of causing neurologic injury at the time of operation is greater than with the surgical management of most other spinal disorders.

(text continues on page 286)

TABLE 14–2. Classification of Adult Thoracic Kyphosis

Congenital
Scheuermann's
Postinfective
Metabolic
Ankylosing spondylitis
Posttraumatic
Postsurgical
Osteoporosis

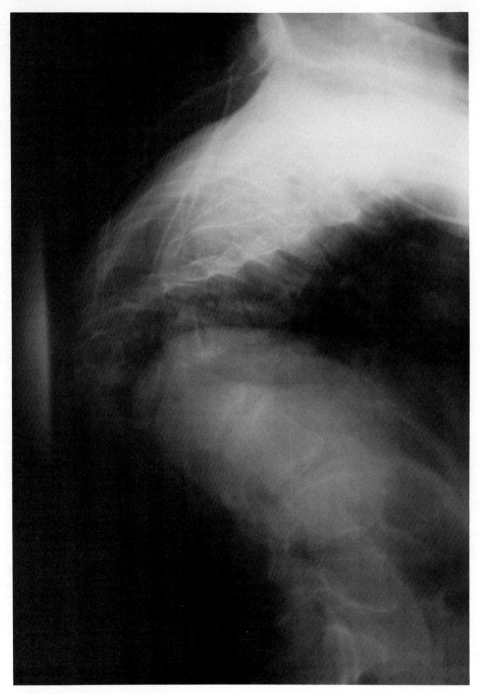

FIGURE 14–30. Lateral x-ray showing major thoracic kyphosis. The patient had a history of tuberculosis of the spine.

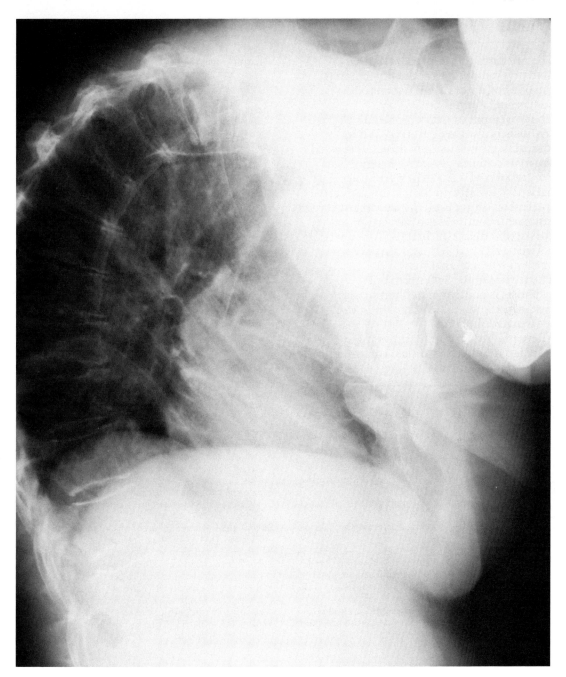

FIGURE 14–31. Neuromuscular thoracic kyphosis with measurements.

KEY POINTS

1. The presence of a congenital spinal deformity should alert the physician to the possibility of other associated congenital anomalies.
2. The treatment of neuromuscular scoliosis is always operative. When undertaken, it is usually directed toward the maintenance of sitting balance.
3. Progression of a curve in a growing patient is usually an indication for active treatment. In general, the treatment for idiopathic scoliosis is observation for curves less than 20°, bracing for curves between 20° and 40°, and surgery for curves greater than 40°.
4. The treatment of Scheuermann's kyphosis is controversial, but bracing has been shown to be effective in the growing adolescent.
5. There is a high complication rate associated with the surgical treatment of adult spinal deformities.

BIBLIOGRAPHY

BOOKS

Bradford DS, Lonstein JE, Moe JH, Ogilvie JW, Winter RB. Moe's textbook of scoliosis and other spinal deformities. 2nd ed. Philadelphia: WB Saunders, 1987.

Cailliet R. Scoliosis: Diagnosis and management. Philadelphia: FA Davis, 1975.

Stagnara P. Spinal deformity. London: Butterworths, 1988.

JOURNALS

Boachie-Adjei O, Lonstein JE, Winter RB, Koop S, Vanden Brink K, Denis F. Management of neuromuscular spinal deformities with Luque segmental instrumentation. J Bone Joint Surg [Am] 1989;71:548–562.

Bradford DS, Boachie-Adjei O. One-stage anterior and posterior hemivertebral resection and arthrodesis for congenital scoliosis. J Bone Joint Surg [Am] 1990;72:536–540.

Bridwell KH. Surgical treatment of adolescent idiopathic scoliosis: The basics and the controversies. Spine 1994;19:1095–1100.

Dhar S, Dangerfield PH, Dorgan JC, Klenerman L. Correlation between bone age and Risser's sign in adolescent idiopathic scoliosis. Spine 1993;18:14–19.

Goldberg CJ, Dowling FE, Hall JE, Emans JB. A statistical comparison between natural history of idiopathic scoliosis and brace treatment in skeletally immature adolescent girls. Spine 1993;18:902–908.

Jeng CL, Sponseller PD, Tolo VT. Outcome of Wisconsin instrumentation in idiopathic scoliosis: minimum 5-year follow-up. Spine 1993;18:1584–1590.

Karol LA, Johnston CE II, Browne RH, Madison M. Progression of the curve in boys who have idiopathic scoliosis. J Bone Joint Surg [Am] 1993;75:1804–1810.

Kostuik JP. Decision making in adult scoliosis. Spine 1979;4:521–525.

Lenke LG, Bridwell KH, Baldus C, Blanke K, Schoenecker PL. Cotrel-Dubousset instrumentation for adolescent idiopathic scoliosis. J Bone Joint Surg [Am] 1992;74:1056–1067.

Martin J Jr, Kumar SJ, Guille JT, Ger D, Gibbs M. Congenital kyphosis in myelomeningocele: Results following operative and nonoperative treatment. J Pediatr Orthop 1994;14:323–328.

Moskowitz A, Trommanhauser S. Surgical and clinical results of scoliosis surgery using Zielke instrumentation. Spine 1993;18:2444–2451.

Müller EB, Nordwall A, Oden A. Progression of scoliosis in children with myelomeningocele. Spine 1994;19:147–150.

Murray PM, Weinstein SL, Spratt KF. The natural history and long-term follow-up of Scheuermann kyphosis. J Bone Joint Surg [Am] 1993;75:236–248.

Pritchett JW, Bortel DT. Degenerative symptomatic lumbar scoliosis. Spine 1993;18:700–703.

Simmons ED Jr, Kowalski JM, Simmons EH. The results of surgical treatment for adult scoliosis. Spine 1993;18:718–724.

Sturm PF, Dobson JC, Armstrong GWD. The surgical management of Scheuermann's disease. Spine 1993;18:685–691.

Swank SM. The management of scoliosis in the adult. Orthop Clin North Am 1979;10:891–904.

Willers U, Hedlund R, Aaro S, Normelli H, Westman L. Long-term results of Harrington instrumentation in idiopathic scoliosis. Spine 1993;18:713–717.

Willers U, Normelli H, Aaro S, Svensson O, Hedlund R. Long-term results of Boston brace treatment on vertebral rotation in idiopathic scoliosis. Spine 1993;18:432–435.

Winter RB, Moe JH. Congenital kyphosis. J Bone Joint Surg [Am] 1973;55:223–256.

Textbook of Spinal Disorders, by Stephen I. Esses.
J. B. Lippincott Company, Philadelphia © 1995.

15 Spinal Trauma

ACUTE
  MANAGEMENT
    Clinical Evaluation
    Imaging
CERVICAL SPINE
    Occipitocervical
    Junction
    Atlas
    Axis
    Lower Cervical Spine

THORACOLUMBAR
  SPINE
    Classification
    Minor Fractures
    Major Fractures
SACRAL SPINE
REHABILITATION

ACUTE MANAGEMENT

Almost 50% of patients who sustain spinal trauma have other associated injuries. Patient management begins at the accident site. The key to appropriate patient care is to suspect spinal column injury in any patient who has multiple trauma or a head injury or who is comatose. The most common spine injuries occur as the result of motor vehicle accidents, falls, and sports injuries. These patients should not be moved until the spine has been temporarily immobilized. This is usually achieved with a rigid spine board. The head is secured with tape or by placing sandbags on either side. A hard collar is usually carefully applied. This ensures that there is no inadvertent motion of the cervical spine. Any turning or transfer of the patient must be done with gentle in-line traction and log-rolling. Appropriate maintenance of airway, breathing, and circulation must be initiated before further attention to the spine is given.

Clinical Evaluation

Once the patient has been stabilized according to trauma care principles, patient history can be reviewed. Details of the mechanism of injury can arouse or confirm suspicion of trauma to the spinal column. The patient's symptoms at the time of injury may provide important information in the assessment of neurologic impairment. Transient paresis or paresthesias at the time of the accident suggest a major fracture pattern. The physical examination should include palpation of the spine from head to sacrum. Any areas of tenderness and bruising are noted. Occasionally, a gap is felt between two contiguous spinous processes, suggesting a major ligamentous disruption. A careful neurologic evaluation is done. If any neurologic deficit exists, a spinal injury flowsheet is started to document any fluctuations in neurologic status over time; the neurologic evaluation is repeated every 10 to 15 minutes.

Various spinal cord syndromes were discussed in Chapter 3. The Brown-Séquard syndrome, due to injury to half the spinal cord, results in ipsilateral muscle paralysis and contralateral loss of pain and temperature sensation. The central cord syndrome results in flaccid paralysis of the upper extremities and spastic paralysis of the lower extremities. Perianal sensation is usually preserved due to sacral sparing. The anterior cord syndrome results in complete motor and sensory anesthesia, except for preservation of deep pressure sensation and proprioception. The posterior cord syndrome is manifest by the loss of deep pressure, deep pain, and proprioceptive sensation. The patient continues to have pain and temperature sensation along with full motor power.

The rectal examination is important for several reasons. Perianal sensation is provided by the lower sacral roots and may be spared even in major spinal cord injuries. The patient's ability to contract the sphincter voluntarily indicates sacral root motor function. Assessment of the bulbocavernosus reflex determines whether the patient is in spinal shock or whether a permanent complete lesion exists.

Imaging

The clinician should use an organized approach when imaging the cervical and thoracolumbar spine. If a neck injury is suspected, this should take precedence over evaluating the rest of the spinal column. A lateral x-ray is taken. This x-ray must show the cervicothoracic junction because this is a common site of spinal injury. If the initial lateral film does not show down to the C7–T1 interspace, it may be repeated while pulling down on the patient's arms. If this

is unsuccessful, a swimmer's view may be obtained (Fig. 15-1). If this is inadequate in showing the cervicothoracic junction, then tomography or computed tomographic (CT) scanning should be considered.

If the lateral x-ray is normal, then a complete cervical spine series should be obtained, including AP, oblique, and through-mouth views. If these do not show a cervical injury but there is continuing concern that one exists, supervised flexion-extension x-rays can be obtained. A "stretch" x-ray can also be obtained by applying 20 pounds of traction to the head. This should be done only under direct supervision and with careful monitoring of the patient. Instability is present if disc space height increases by more than 1.7 mm or if there is a change in neurologic function. Traction can be incrementally increased to about 30% of body weight.

CT scanning and magnetic resonance imaging (MRI) provide valuable information about a cervical injury. MRI should also be used to investigate patients with neurologic injury at the cervical level without radiographic abnormalities. Myelography is rarely indicated in the assessment of acute trauma.

Because about 15% of patients with a spine fracture have another noncontiguous spinal column injury, the entire spine should be evaluated in patients who have an identified spinal injury. An algorithm for imaging the cervical spine is given in Table 15-1. It is very similar to that for the thoracolumbar spine (Table 15-2). With the spine temporarily immobilized, a shoot-through lateral radiograph of the thoracolumbar spine is obtained. If this is normal, AP and oblique x-rays are obtained. Injudicious spinal movement should be avoided when performing the latter views: the x-ray tube should be tilted rather than turning the patient. If these x-rays are also interpreted as normal, then the patient's history and physical examination should be repeated. If the clinician still suspects a thoracolumbar injury, further investigation is necessary. Flexion-extension x-rays, stress views, CT, and MRI are all useful in this regard.

The spine must remain immobilized until spinal column injury has been ruled out. Plain radiographs are essentially used as a screening tool. CT scanning is especially useful for identifying the nature and extent of bony injury. MRI is most useful for assessing neural anatomy and intervertebral disc pathology.

Many patients present days to weeks after trauma to the neck with persisting pain. For

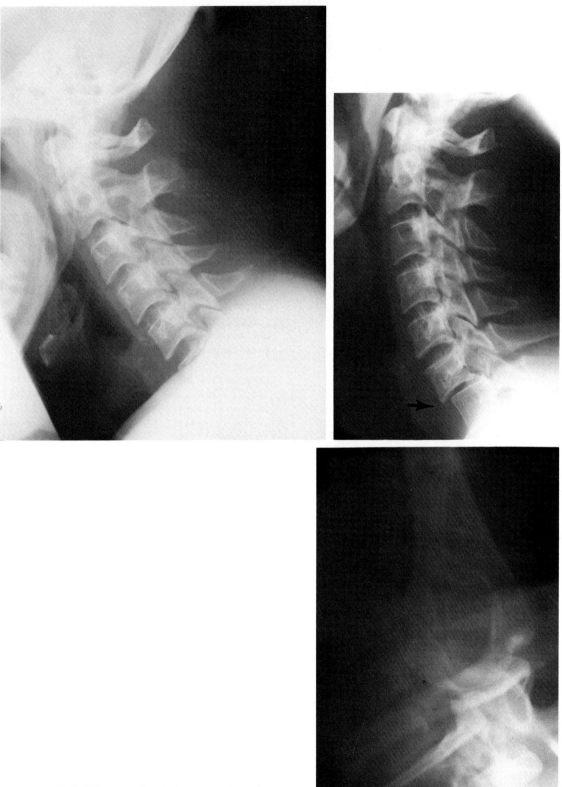

FIGURE 15–1. Cervical x-rays to show fracture.

TABLE 15–1. **Imaging The Cervical Spine**

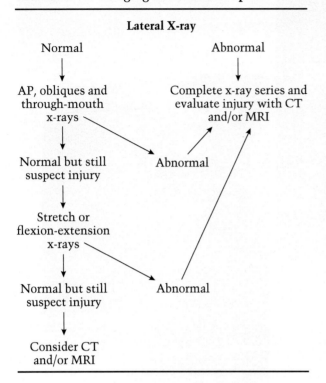

Lateral X-ray

injury is suspected, tomograms or CT scanning should be done.

Atlas

Fractures can occur anywhere in the ring of the atlas. Isolated posterior arch fractures are not uncommon and usually result from a hyperextension force. These injuries can usually be recognized on a lateral x-ray. Axial compression can result in a bursting injury of the atlas, referred to as a *Jefferson fracture*. This type of injury is best identified on the through-mouth x-ray (Fig. 15-2). There is lateral translation of one or both lateral masses. Because these injuries result in an increased space for the spinal cord, they are usually not associated with neurologic injury.

When the overhang of the lateral masses on both sides together measures more than 7 mm, there is usually a concomitant rupture of the transverse ligament (see Fig. 5-24). This further destabilizes the C1–C2 complex. CT scanning is extremely useful for defining injuries of the ring of the atlas. Fractures of the atlas are frequently associated with other cervical spine injuries (Fig. 15-3). The entire cervical spine should be carefully evaluated in any patient with a C1 injury.

The transverse ligament can become attenuated and is susceptible to rupture in elderly patients. This may result from a fall with no bony

these patients, a supervised lateral flexion-extension set of radiographs is the best way to detect previously unrecognized soft tissue injury.

CERVICAL SPINE

Occipitocervical Junction

The inherent stability of the occipitocervical junction renders it susceptible to injury only when extremely violent force occurs, and usually this degree of trauma results in death. Occipitocervical dislocation has been proposed as one of the most common causes of death from motor vehicle accidents.

Rotatory forces between the occiput and atlas can result in either a dislocation of one articular process on the lateral mass of the atlas or an avulsion fracture of an occipital condyle. These injuries often go undiagnosed, primarily because the AP and lateral x-rays are insufficient in showing the underlying pathology. If an occipitocervical

TABLE 15–2. **Imaging The Thoracolumbar Spine**

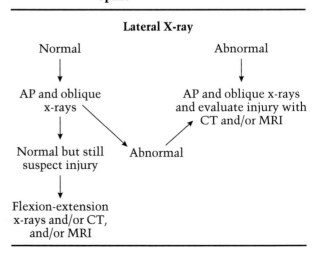

Lateral X-ray

fracture. The only radiographic finding may be instability of the C1–C2 complex demonstrated on flexion-extension x-rays.

Axis

Fractures of the odontoid process make up a large percentage of all cervical injuries. Anderson and D'Alonzo classified odontoid fractures into three types (Fig. 15-4). *Type I* occurs through the upper part of the odontoid process, probably as a result of an avulsion at the insertion of the alar ligament. *Type II* fractures occur at the junction of the odontoid process with the vertebral body. *Type III* extends down into the body of the atlas (Fig. 15-5).

Type I and III injuries are considered stable and do not require surgical treatment, but the most appropriate treatment for type II injuries is controversial. Management depends on various factors, including the amount and type of displacement, age of the patient, degree of associated instability, and neurologic status. In undisplaced type II fractures in patients under age 40, halo immobilization is usually recommended and is successful in over 60% of cases. When there is significant displacement or angulation of the fracture, particularly in older patients, surgery may be recommended.

Traumatic spondylolisthesis of the axis usually results from forceful hyperextension. Fractures occur through the pedicles, or pars lateralis, of C2. There may be varying degrees of associ-

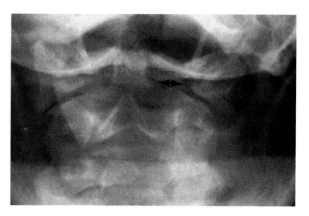

FIGURE 15–2. Jefferson fracture.

ated spondylolisthesis of C2 on C3. This injury is often called the *hangman's fracture* because it was thought to be the type of injury induced by hanging. These injuries can be classified into three types (Fig. 15-6). Type I, nondisplaced fractures, can be treated with an orthosis. Type II fractures have variable degrees of angulation, displacement, or both, but the anterior longitudinal ligament and the C2–C3 intervertebral disc remain intact (Fig. 15-7). If reduction can be achieved using skeletal traction, then a halo vest may be used to allow ambulation with posttraction immobilization. Type III injuries are associated with unilateral or bilateral facet dislocations at C2–C3. Type III injuries are the most unstable and can be associated with neurologic injury. They generally require surgical management.

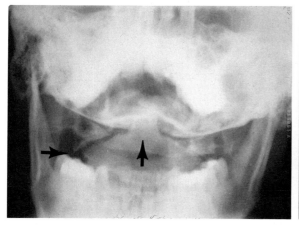
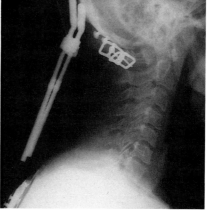

FIGURE 15–3. Jefferson fracture associated with odontoid fracture.

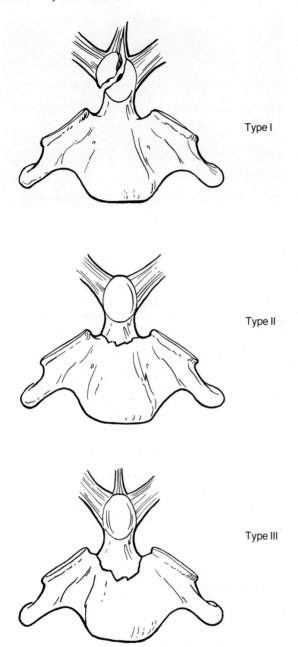

Type I

Type II

Type III

FIGURE 15–4. Classification of odontoid fractures.

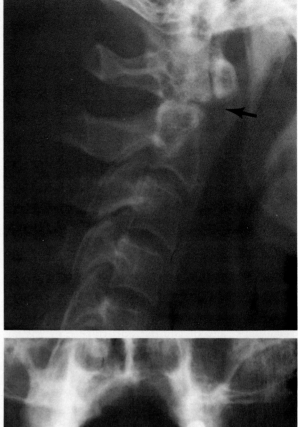

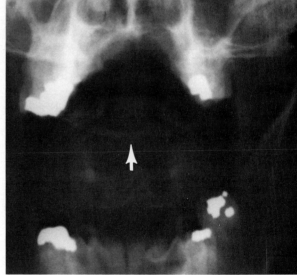

FIGURE 15–5. Displaced odontoid fracture (lateral x-ray and through-mouth x-ray).

Lower Cervical Spine

Various classification systems have been proposed for traumatic injuries to the lower cervical spine. Some divide the fractures and dislocations according to the mechanism of injury. Although it is valuable to determine the forces and vectors that resulted in a cervical spine injury, in many cases the mechanism is unclear. For this reason, a morphologic classification is preferable. After analyzing the imaging studies, an injury can be classified according to failure of the posterior, anterior, or lateral elements. The structures that can be damaged posteriorly are the facet joints,

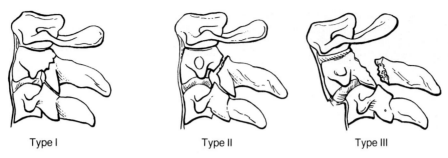

Type I   Type II   Type III

FIGURE 15–6. Classification of hangman's fractures.

spinous processes, and laminae. Anteriorly, there may be injury to the vertebral body or intervertebral disc. Laterally, injury may occur to the pars lateralis or pedicles.

Facet dislocations may be unilateral or bilateral. Unilateral facet dislocations occur as the result of flexion and rotation force. Bilateral facet dislocations usually result from significant flexion forces. Unilateral facet dislocations are identified on the AP x-ray by rotation of the spinous processes. On the lateral x-ray, there may be forward displacement of the superior vertebral body by up to 30% (Fig. 15-8). Oblique x-rays show the facet dislocation (Fig. 15-9). Bilateral facet dislocations may not be associated with any rotation; thus, the spinous processes may continue to be aligned on the AP x-ray. The lateral x-ray shows at least 50% displacement of the superior vertebra (Fig. 15-10). The unilateral facet dislocation may be associated with radicular symptoms due to compression of the neural foramen on the dislocated side. Bilateral facet dislocations are usually associated with significant neurologic deficit due to spinal cord compression.

The key to initial treatment of a unilateral or bilateral facet dislocation is gentle traction to effect reduction. Traction is applied either with skull tongs or a halo. Traction should begin with 15 pounds and be increased in 5-pound increments every 20 to 30 minutes. X-rays are taken after each increase and the patient's neurologic status is carefully monitored. A maximum of 40 pounds is used. Once closed reduction is achieved, a decision should be made as to whether the patient can be treated with a halo jacket or whether a posterior fusion should be recommended. Factors that should be considered are the degree of neurologic injury and whether there is posterior element fracture. Pure soft tissue injuries do not heal well and have a high inci-

dence of recurrent subluxation or dislocation. Early posterior fusion should be considered for dislocations that are purely ligamentous.

If reduction cannot be achieved through closed traction, an open posterior reduction and fusion is recommended. Recently, increased neurologic deficits have been reported in patients undergoing open posterior reduction. This is thought to be due to the intervertebral disc at the level of injury being pushed back into the canal at the time of reduction. Therefore, MR scanning should be done before reduction to assess the status and position of the disc. If there is disc material in the canal, an anterior discectomy may be needed before reduction.

Facet subluxation may occur without complete dislocation. This injury may be recognized by widening of the interspinous distance or angulation at the injured level on the lateral x-ray. The oblique x-ray is useful in determining the

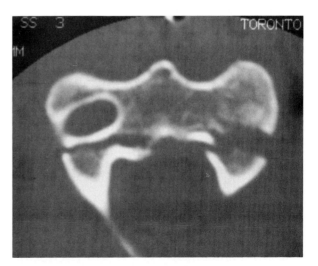

FIGURE 15–7. Hangman's fracture (axial CT).

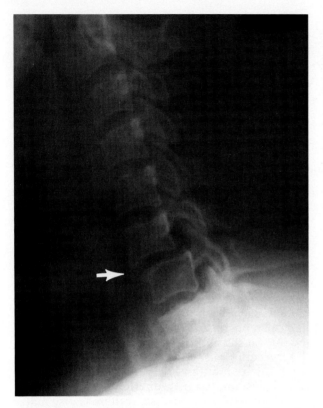

FIGURE 15–8. Unilateral facet dislocation (lateral x-ray).

tive treatment may be recommended. If there is significant displacement, particularly retropulsion of bone into the canal, surgical decompression and stabilization provides the best chance for recovery of incomplete neurologic deficits and restoration of spinal stability (Fig. 15-12).

Extension injuries may result in a simple avulsion of the anterior vertebral body where the anterior longitudinal ligament inserts. In older patients with cervical spondylosis, this may result in a central cord syndrome. With increased extension force, there may be complete disruption of the intervertebral disc with marked instability.

Fractures of the lateral elements usually result from lateral flexion forces. When there is both a pedicle and laminar fracture on the same side, the entire lateral mass becomes detached. This floating lateral mass fracture is extremely unstable and is best treated with internal fixation.

An isolated spinous process fracture, usually at C7, is called *clay shoveler's injury*. It is caused by avulsion of the spinous process due to sudden

amount of subluxation. Most of these injuries can be treated with an orthosis. At 3 months, flexion-extension x-rays are used to determine whether any instability persists.

The vertebral body may be injured from forward flexion, extension, or axial compression. Forward flexion injuries are usually stable. They result in a wedging of the vertebral body (Fig. 15-11). If the posterior structures are intact, then there is usually no neurologic deficit and the injury can be treated with an orthosis. More than 50% of anterior compression of the vertebral body and an intact posterior vertebral body wall suggest posterior element disruption. When there is concomitant posterior element damage, the injury is much more unstable and may be associated with spinal cord injury.

Axial loading results in comminution of the vertebral body. Part of the posterior half of the vertebral body may be displaced into the spinal canal, and there may be significant spinal cord injury. For comminuted vertebral body fractures in which there is minimal displacement, nonopera-

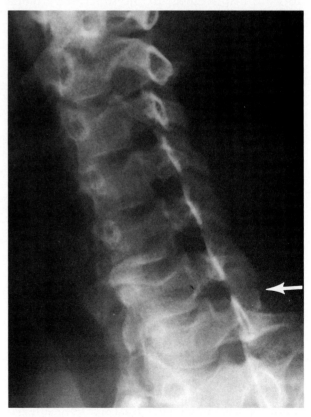

FIGURE 15–9. Unilateral facet dislocation (oblique x-ray).

contraction of the spine extensor and scapular elevator muscles.

THORACOLUMBAR SPINE

Classification

Over the past 50 years various classification systems have been proposed for thoracolumbar injuries, and controversy continues over which is the most accurate and practical. Most clinicians use a classification based on a three-column conceptualization of the spine (see Fig. 5-40). The anterior column is formed by the anterior half of the vertebral body, together with the anterior longitudinal ligament and the anterior fibers of the annulus fibrosus. The middle column is formed by the posterior fibers of the annulus fibrosus, together with the posterior wall of the vertebral body and posterior longitudinal ligament. The posterior column is formed by the posterior ligamentous complex (supraspinous and interspinous ligaments, facet joint capsule, and ligamentum flavum) and the posterior bony arch.

Thoracolumbar spinal injuries can be classified as either minor or major. Minor injuries include minimal wedge compression fractures, articular

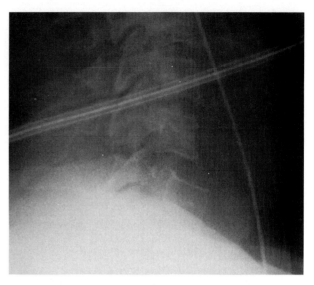

FIGURE 15–10. Bilateral facet dislocation (lateral x-ray).

process fractures, transverse process fractures, spinous process fractures, and fractures of the pars interarticularis. There are four major types of spinal injuries. These are major wedge compression fractures, flexion-distraction injuries, burst fractures, and fracture dislocations.

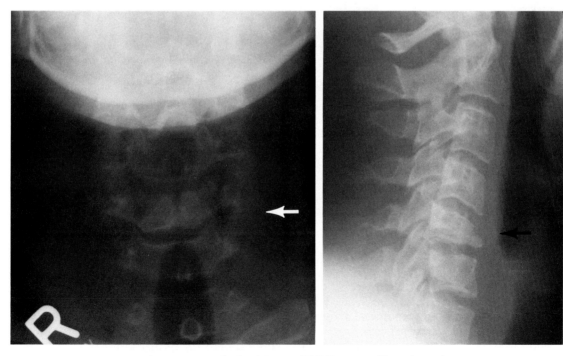

FIGURE 15–11. Flexion injury at C5 (AP x-ray and lateral x-ray).

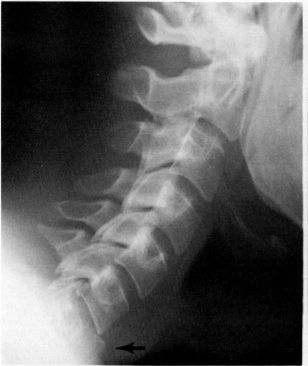

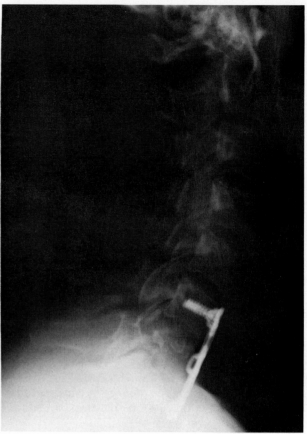

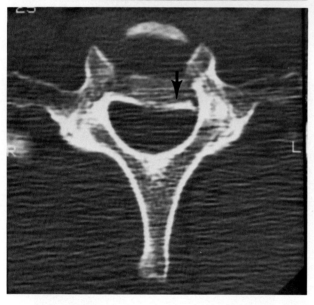

FIGURE 15–12. Comminuted cervical fracture with retropulsion, preoperative and postoperative.

Minor Fractures

There are five minor fracture pattern types: minimal wedge compression fractures, articular process fractures, transverse process fractures, spinous process fractures, and fractures of the pars interarticularis. After making a diagnosis of a minor fracture, the patient's history, physical examination, and imaging studies should be thoroughly reviewed because these fractures are occasionally associated with occult major fracture patterns. Rarely, a minor fracture may be the only remaining indication that a true dislocation of the spine occurred at the time of injury.

Fractures of the transverse processes, articular processes, and minimal wedge compression fractures can be treated by rest and gradual ambulation (Figs. 15-13 and 15-14). An orthosis is occasionally useful in making the patient more comfortable while being mobilized. Isolated fractures of the spinous process can be treated in a similar fashion. However, avulsion fractures of the spinous process occasionally occur as the result of a flexion-distraction injury. For this reason, it is worthwhile to do a CT and MR scan of these injuries to exclude associated fractures and to assess ligamentous damage.

Acute fractures of the pars interarticularis, unilateral or bilateral, have been described after hyperextension injuries. It is frequently difficult to determine whether a defect in the pars interarticularis identified on x-ray is old or the result of an acute injury. The history and physical examination are important in distinguishing between the two. Sometimes a technetium bone scan and a CT scan are necessary to confidently assess the

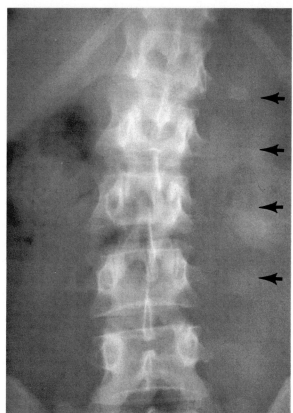

FIGURE 15–14. Lumbar transverse process fractures (AP x-ray).

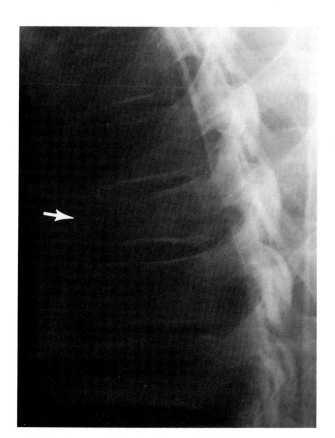

FIGURE 15–13. Thoracic compression fracture (lateral x-ray).

age of the defect. Immobilization, either with a body cast or a well-fitted orthosis, has been recommended in young patients with an acute fracture of the pars interarticularis. A neutral position is recommended. Very occasionally, traumatic fractures of the pars interarticularis do not heal with immobilization alone. In those cases, surgical repair may be indicated if the patient is symptomatic. Surgery consists of bone-grafting the defect, usually in association with internal fixation.

Major Fractures

The four major types of spinal injuries are major wedge compression fractures, flexion-distraction injuries, burst fractures, and fracture-dislocations. With the advent of CT scanning, our ability to image spine fractures has increased significantly, resulting in a better appreciation of the anatomic disruption of these injuries. One distinguishing feature between these major injuries is the mode of failure of the middle column. Even in major compression fractures, the middle column is not injured. In burst fractures, however, the middle column fails in compression. In flexion-distraction injuries, the middle column fails in distraction. In fracture-dislocations, the middle column may fail in distraction, rotation, or shear.

In a burst fracture, the anterior and middle columns are both injured from a compressive force, and in most cases there is also a failure of the posterior column, usually in the form of a vertical laminar fracture. Because the entire vertebral ring is disrupted, the pedicles become splayed, and an increased interpedicular distance is seen on the AP radiograph. An important feature of the burst fracture is retropulsion of bony fragments from the posterior vertebral body into the spinal canal. The most common site for these bony fragments to become retropulsed is from the posterosuperior aspect of the involved vertebral body. Dural impingement by these fragments can cause the neurologic deficits frequently associated with burst fractures (Fig. 15-15). In patients with lumbar burst fractures with neurologic deficit, there is a high incidence of dural tear and nerve root entrapment by the laminar fracture.

There is considerable controversy as to whether these burst injuries are best treated operatively or nonoperatively. Proponents of surgery argue that decompression of the canal leads to better neurologic recovery. They further argue that surgical stabilization prevents the development of symptomatic kyphosis in some bursting injuries. Obviously, each fracture must be assessed individually. Most burst fractures can be treated nonoperatively. Bracing is usually recommended to prevent any progression of deformity at the injury site. Clinical evaluation should be done at regular intervals to document neurologic recovery and to detect any late neurologic symptoms or signs.

It is important to distinguish between major wedge compression injuries and burst fractures. As mentioned above, the significant difference between the two is that the middle column is intact in a wedge compression injury but is disrupted in a burst fracture. This may be difficult to distinguish on x-rays, so CT scanning is recommended. Because the posterior cortex of the vertebral body is intact in a major wedge compression fracture, there are no retropulsed fragments impinging on the dural sac. A major wedge compression fracture is rarely associated with neurologic injury; if neurologic damage is present, it is thought to be due to the acute kyphotic deformity at the fracture site. Most of these injuries occur in older, sedentary patients and are associated with osteoporosis. Treatment with a hyperextension brace is usually recommended. In young, active patients with significant compression associated with significant angular deformity, operative intervention may be considered. Operative intervention is also indicated in those rare instances in which a major wedge compression fracture is associated with neurologic injury.

In flexion-distraction injuries, all three columns fail in distraction. These injuries can be classified as to whether the injury is primarily bony or ligamentous (Fig. 15-16). Purely ligamentous injuries do not heal well and consideration should be given to a primary posterolateral fusion with instrumentation. Bony injuries, known as *Chance fractures*, have a good prognosis, and patients are usually treated with an extension orthosis while bony union occurs.

Fracture-dislocations of the thoracolumbar spine involve a complete disruption of all three columns. In most instances, radiographs show displacement or complete dislocation of the spinal column (Fig. 15-17). CT scanning is useful in assessing the integrity of the facet joints. In cases of dislocation, only half the joint is seen, giving rise to the "empty nest sign" (Fig. 15-18). Occasionally the spinal column may appear aligned, if there was a spontaneous reduction of the fracture-dislocation. In these instances, recognition of the fracture pattern, together with an assessment of the patient's neurologic function, ensures accurate assessment of the extent of displacement that occurred at the time of injury. Most fracture-dislocations are associated with a major neurologic deficit that is related to the level of injury as well as the injury pattern. These injuries are extremely unstable. Surgical fusion with instrumentation provides a reliable means of obtaining stability and preventing progression of deformity. Although some clinicians continue to advocate postural reduction and stabilization with orthoses, conservative techniques often fail to reduce the deformity, particularly when it is large.

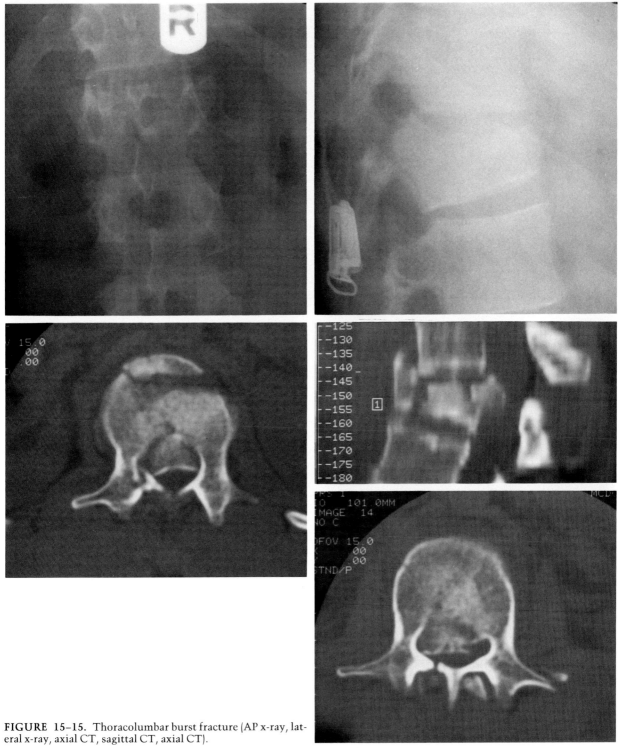

FIGURE 15–15. Thoracolumbar burst fracture (AP x-ray, lateral x-ray, axial CT, sagittal CT, axial CT).

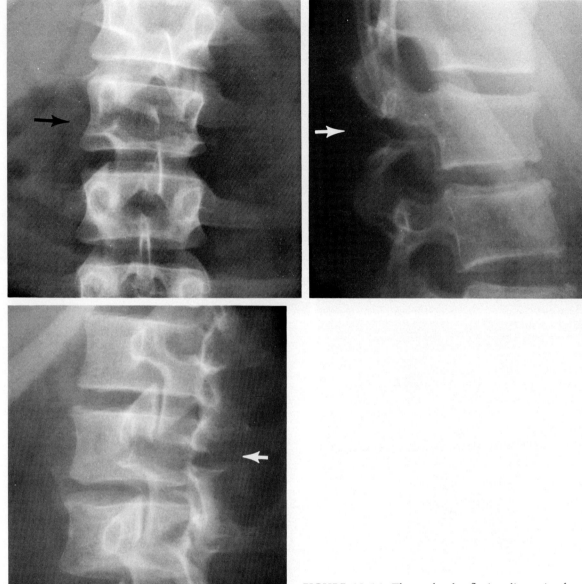

FIGURE 15–16. Thoracolumbar flexion-distraction fracture (AP x-ray, lateral x-ray, oblique x-ray).

SACRAL SPINE

Many classifications have been proposed for sacral injuries, but one of the most useful divides fractures according to location (Fig. 15-19). Zone I injuries involve a fracture through the ala without damage to the foramina or central canal. Zone II injuries involve one or more foramina but not the sacral canal. Zone III injuries involve the sacral canal and are usually transverse. Neu-

rologic injury is rarely associated with zone I injuries. Zone II injuries are associated with nerve root injury, particularly when displacement is present. Most zone III fractures are associated with significant neurologic deficits.

Major sacral injuries are usually associated with disruption of the pelvis. In these instances, treatment of the sacral injury is determined by management of the pelvic disruption. Most sacral fractures that occur as isolated injuries can

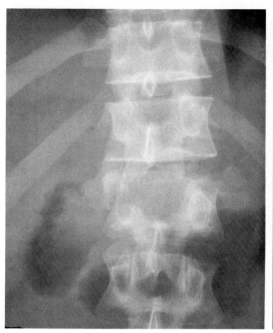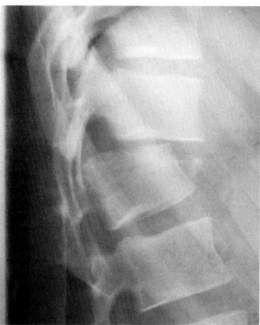

FIGURE 15–17. Thoracolumbar fracture-dislocation (AP x-ray and lateral x-ray).

be treated nonoperatively. Only if displacement is associated with neurologic deficit or if the fracture is markedly displaced should surgery be contemplated.

REHABILITATION

The establishment of spinal cord injury centers has resulted in a significant improvement in the rehabilitation of these patients. Rehabilitation begins at the time of hospitalization and involves not just the treatment of problems but also their prevention.

Spinal cord lesions above the T10 level result in decreased pulmonary function. Attention must be paid to clearing secretions so as to avoid atelectasis and pneumonia. Deep vein thrombosis is extremely common after spinal cord injury, and some consideration should be given to prophylactic anticoagulation. Lesions above the T4 level may be associated with autonomic dysreflexia, which presents as acute headache, hypertension, and bradycardia. The usual cause is distention of the bladder or bowel. Particular attention must be given to skin care in patients with insensate areas. Physical therapy should include active and passive range of motion of the joints to prevent contractures. A bowel program should be initiated early.

It is customary to define the level of spinal cord injury as the lowest spinal cord segment with intact motor and sensory function. Thus, C4 quadriplegics continue to have function of the diaphragm and shoulder elevators. Although they cannot transfer independently, they can use a

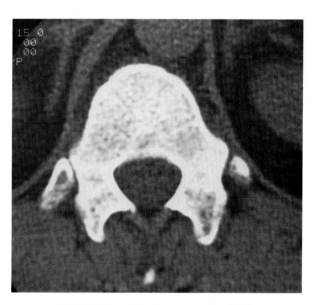

FIGURE 15–18. Empty nest sign (CT).

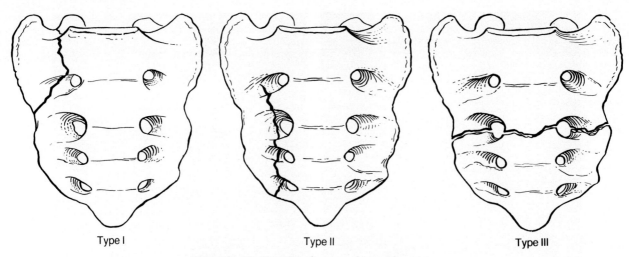

Type I Type II Type III

FIGURE 15–19. Classification of sacral fractures.

mouth-controlled wheelchair. A C5 quadriplegic has limited arm function and can use a wheelchair with hand controls. A C6 functional level allows independence in wheelchair transfers, personal dressing, and prehension if fitted with a flexor hand splint. The highest level at which functional ambulation is possible is L2; bilateral long leg braces are necessary in conjunction with a walker or crutches.

There is a high mortality rate associated with spinal cord injury early on, but patients who survive beyond 3 months after their injury have a good prognosis. The age at time of injury is an important determinant of survival—younger patients have a better prognosis than older patients. Renal failure is the most common fatal complication in spine-injured patients.

KEY POINTS

1. The spinal column must be protected and immobilized in multitraumatized, comatose, or head-injured patients.
2. A careful history and physical examination will help identify patients who may have sustained a spinal injury. An organized approach to imaging the spinal column should be used.
3. Unstable injuries may be stabilized by an orthosis or surgery. Management decisions depend on many considerations, and each fracture should be individually assessed.

BIBLIOGRAPHY

BOOKS

Errico TJ, Bauer RD, Waugh T, eds. Spinal trauma. Philadelphia: JB Lippincott, 1991.
Floman Y, Farcy JPC, Argenson C, eds. Thoracolumbar spine fractures. New York: Raven, 1993.
Lorenz MA, ed. Spine. Spinal fracture-dislocations. State of the Art Reviews. Vol 7, no. 2. Philadelphia: Hanley and Belfus, 1993.

JOURNALS

Beyer CA, Cabanela ME, Berquist TH. Unilateral facet dislocations and fracture-dislocations of cervical spine. J Bone Joint Surg 1991;73:977–981.
Cantor JB, Lebwohl NH, Garvey T, Eismont FJ. Non-operative management of stable thoracolumbar burst fractures with early ambulation and bracing. Spine 1993;18:971–976.
Dekutoski MB, Conlan ES, Salciccioli GG. Spinal mobility and deformity after Harrington rod stabilization and limited arthrodesis of thoracolumbar fractures. J Bone Joint Surg [Am] 1993;75:168–176.
Gurwitz GS, Dawson JM, McNamara MJ, Federspiel CF, Spengler DM. Biomechanical analysis of three surgical approaches for lumbar burst fractures using short-segment instrumentation. Spine 1993;18:977–982.
McBride GG. Cotrel-Dubousset rods in surgical stabilization of spinal fractures. Spine 1993;18:466–473.
McGrory BJ, Klassen RA, Chao EY, Staeheli JW, Weaver AL. Acute fractures and dislocations of the cervical spine in children and adolescents. J Bone Joint Surg [Am] 1993;75:988–995.
McLain RF, Sparling E, Benson DR. Early failure of short-segment pedicle instrumentation for thoracolumbar fractures. J Bone Joint Surg [Am] 1993;75:162–167.
Mumford J, Weinstein JN, Spratt KF, Goel VK. Thoracolum-

bar burst fractures: The clinical efficacy and outcome of nonoperative management. Spine 1993;18:955–970.

Riebel GD, Yoo JU, Fredrickson BE, Yuan HA. Review of Harrington rod treatment of spinal trauma. Spine 1993;18: 479–491.

Sasso RC, Cotler HB. Posterior instrumentation and fusion for unstable fractures and fracture-dislocations of the thoracic and lumbar spine: A comparative study of three fixation devices in 70 patients. Spine 1993;18:450–460.

Textbook of Spinal Disorders, by Stephen I. Esses.
J. B. Lippincott Company, Philadelphia © 1995.

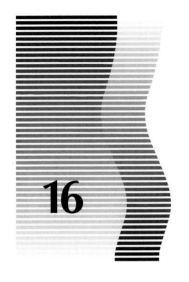

16 Tumors of the Spine

PRIMARY TUMORS
  Clinical Presentation
  Investigation and
    Staging
  Benign Primary
    Tumors
  Malignant Primary
    Tumors
  Treatment

METASTATIC
  TUMORS
  Patient Evaluation
  Nonoperative
    Treatment
  Operative Treatment

Tumors of the spine, both primary and secondary, present a diagnostic and therapeutic challenge. In most cases a multidisciplinary approach is needed for optimal patient care. Technological advances have increased our ability to deal with these neoplasms more effectively, resulting in better patient evaluation and care. By using an array of specialists, every facet of patient management can be improved. An effective spinal tumor team consists of a neuroradiologist, pathologist, angiographer, oncologist, and spinal surgeon. Only by a coordinated effort can these physicians ensure successful patient outcome. Scrupulous attention to treatment goals is essential to quality patient care.

PRIMARY TUMORS

As with musculoskeletal tumors elsewhere, the classification is based on the cell origin or differentiation. Sometimes the cytology is difficult to identify, but some matrix is produced by the proliferating cells, and this is used to infer the tumor origin. These neoplasms can have their origin in cartilage cell lines, bone cell lines, marrow elements, fibrous cell lines, vascular cell lines, and notochordal cell lines. The resultant

TABLE 16–1. **Benign and Malignant Neoplasms**

Cell of Origin	Benign Tumor	Malignant Tumor
Fibrous tissue	Fibroma	Fibrosarcoma
Cartilage tissue	Chondroblastoma, osteochondroma	Chondrosarcoma
Bone tissue	Osteoid osteoma, osteoblastoma	Osteosarcoma
Notochordal tissue		Chordoma
Vascular tissue	Hemangioma	Hemangiosarcoma
Hematopoietic tissue		Myeloma, plasmacytoma
Lymphatic tissue		Lymphoma
Unknown	Aneurysmal bone cyst	Giant cell tumor, Ewing's tumor

benign and malignant neoplasms are listed in Table 16-1.

Clinical Presentation

Back pain, with or without sciatica, is a common symptom. Unless the clinician maintains a high index of suspicion for underlying neoplasm, this diagnosis is often overlooked. Indeed, many patients with primary bone tumors affecting the spine have undergone laminectomy based on a preoperative diagnosis of a herniated intervertebral disc. Every patient must be asked specifically about pain at night, pain unrelated to activity, and systemic malaise. The presence of any or all of these features should caution the physician and warrants further investigation. It is unusual for patients under the age of 25 to have prolonged neck or back pain due to a mechanical disorder. Thus, a tumor should be suspected in patients in this age group who complain of significant neck or back discomfort. Scoliosis associated with pain is usually due to an irritative focus, and often this indicates an underlying neoplasm.

The usual age of patients afflicted with primary spinal malignancies is about 50. The mean age of patients with benign spinal tumors is about 20. Only by taking a complete history and performing a thorough physical examination will the clinician be able to identify patients who warrant further investigation.

Investigation and Staging

In almost all primary tumors, plain radiographs demonstrate the lesion. Every patient with a suspected spinal column tumor must have a complete set of high-quality x-rays. These roentgenograms should be carefully scrutinized, paying particular attention to the pedicles, cortical vertebral shell, and posterior elements. Most tumors affecting the posterior elements are benign, and most lesions in the vertebral body are malignant. The distribution of tumors by location is shown in Figure 16-1.

The lesion can be further assessed using tomography, computed tomography (CT), and magnetic resonance imaging (MRI). The latter has essentially obviated the need for myelography (Fig. 16-2). Angiography, by providing infor-

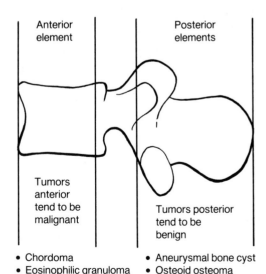

FIGURE 16–1. Anatomic distribution of primary spine tumors.

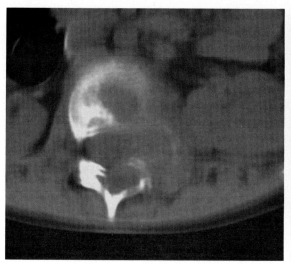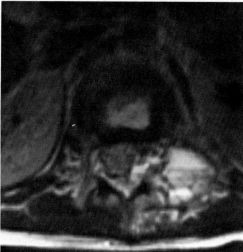

FIGURE 16–2. CT and MRI of aneurysmal bone cyst.

mation about tumor vascularity, can often assist with formulating an accurate differential diagnosis. It also occasionally helps with preoperative surgical planning by demonstrating large feeding vessels.

Local staging of these tumors cannot be undertaken using standard guidelines that are applied to tumors of other parts of the musculoskeletal system. Staging must address three important issues: the site of bony involvement, spinal canal intrusion, and soft tissue involvement. The clinician must know whether the lesion involves the anterior column, the posterior column, or both; whether there has been invasion into the spinal canal, with or without dural sac compression; and whether there has been any other soft tissue extension. Information about these three items will allow a rational decision as to the optimal surgical approach.

Staging requires a whole body technetium 99 bone scan, a chest x-ray, and a CT scan of the lungs. Sometimes a CT scan of the abdomen and an intravenous pyelogram are indicated. These studies may show metastases elsewhere and thus provide information about the malignancy of the neoplasm.

Benign Primary Tumors

Although any benign primary tumor of bone can occur in the vertebral column, the four most common tumor types encountered are *hemangi-*

oma, osteoid osteoma, osteoblastoma, and *giant cell tumor.*

A hemangioma can usually be differentiated from other lesions with plain radiographs. These neoplasms exhibit a typical honeycomb appearance due to linear reactive ossification about the radiolucent vascular tissue (Fig. 16-3). They involve primarily the vertebral body but occasionally extend into the posterior elements via the pedicles. An associated compression fracture or vertebral body collapse is unusual. If there is doubt about the diagnosis, angiography can usually confirm the nature of the lesion; more recently, MRI has been useful in this regard (Fig. 16-4). This is particularly important to prevent unanticipated hemorrhage if surgery is done.

Osteoid osteomas and osteoblastomas are tumors of young patients: more than 90% of cases involving the spinal column have been found in patients under age 30. These tumors may cause sufficient irritation to result in a scoliosis. They characteristically cause pain, which is significantly relieved by aspirin. Size is the primary distinguishing characteristic between the two lesions. Osteoid osteomas are less than 2 cm in diameter, whereas osteoblastomas are larger (Figs. 16-5 and 16-6). Both lesions usually occur within the posterior elements of the vertebra, especially the lamina. CT scanning may demonstrate the core, or *nidus*, of these tumors, which is usually surrounded by marked reactive bone formation (Fig. 16-7). They are characteristically

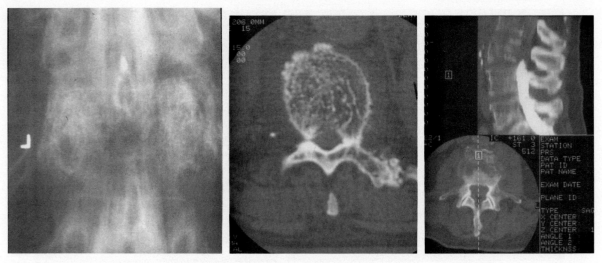

FIGURE 16-3. Hemangioma (AP myelogram, axial CT, sagittal CT myelography).

expansive lesions, and a thin shell of new bone can be detected at the tumor margins. Treatment is usually surgical excision. If the nidus is removed, there is immediate symptomatic relief without recurrence.

Giant cell tumors usually grow rapidly, so they often present with cortical expansion and neurologic disturbances. Most lesions are in the vertebral body (Fig. 16-8). Patients are usually in the third or fourth decade of life. The overall prognosis of these benign tumors is poor because they are very aggressive and recur locally unless tumor removal is complete. Some authors have suggested excision, not curettage, of these lesions so as to avoid local recurrence, with its subsequent morbidity and mortality. Recurrence rates of up to 50% have been reported.

Malignant Primary Tumors

The most common primary malignant tumors affecting the spinal column are *myeloma, plasmacytoma, malignant lymphoma, Ewing's sarcoma,* and *chordoma.*

Myeloma is the most common of all these neoplasms; indeed, it is the most common neoplasm of bone in adults. It commonly affects patients in the sixth and seventh decades of life. The diagnosis can often be made on the basis of an abnormal immunoglobulin detected on serum immunoelectrophoresis. Other associated blood findings are an increased erythrocyte sedimentation rate,

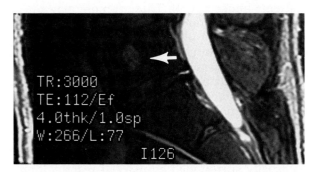

FIGURE 16-4. Hemangioma (MRI).

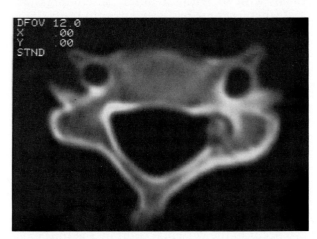

FIGURE 16-5. Osteoid osteoma (axial CT).

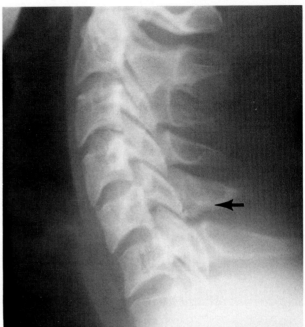

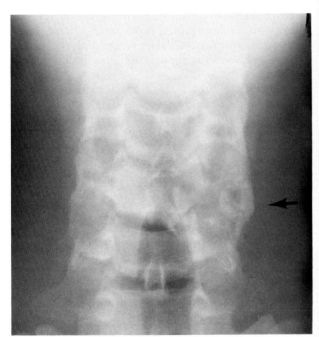

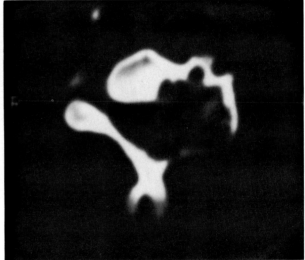

FIGURE 16–6. Osteoblastoma (AP x-ray, lateral x-ray, axial CT).

hypercalcemia, a normochromic normocytic anemia, and amyloidosis. The radiographic findings are typically osteolytic "punched-out" lesions (Fig. 16-9). There is little periosteal reaction, indicating the aggressive nature of these lesions. Occasionally, diffuse spinal column disease can present radiographically with osteopenia. Thus, it is crucial to keep this entity in mind before diagnosing osteoporosis as the cause of diffuse osteopenia. If the histology of a lesion is identical to that of multiple myeloma but a complete skeletal survey rules out the presence of other lesions, the bone marrow examination is negative, and there is no evidence of dysproteinemia, then the lesion can safely be referred to as a solitary plasmacytoma.

The histogenesis and cell of origin of Ewing's sarcoma are uncertain. The tumor cells are probably derived from the connective tissue framework of the bone marrow. Typically, this tumor

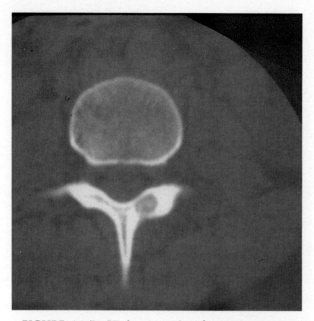

FIGURE 16–7. CT showing nidus of osteoid osteoma.

affects patients in the second decade of life. These patients present with fever, anemia, and a leukocytosis. Radiographs usually show a mottled, moth-eaten lesion with very poorly defined margins. Although long-term survival of patients with this tumor has improved using newer chemotherapeutic regimens, the overall prognosis is poor.

Lymphomas can present with a radiographic picture similar to that of Ewing's. Based on histology, there are various types, each with a characteristic prognosis. Patients tend to be older than those with Ewing's, and the overall outlook is better.

Chordomas, which develop from notochordal remnants, primarily affect the base of the skull and sacrum, although they can occur anywhere along the spinal column. They are almost always in the midline and radiolucent. Patients are usually in their fifth or sixth decade of life. These tumors are very slow-growing and thus can be very large at presentation. Radiographs are help-

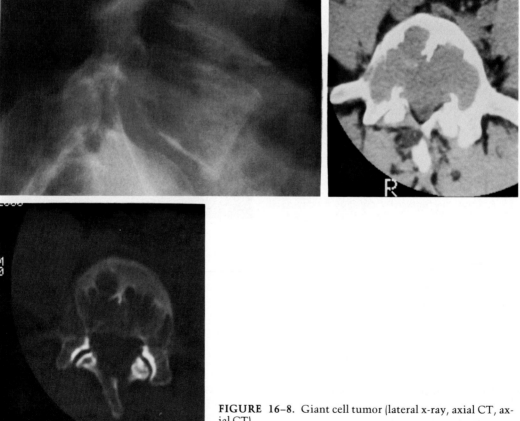

FIGURE 16–8. Giant cell tumor (lateral x-ray, axial CT, axial CT).

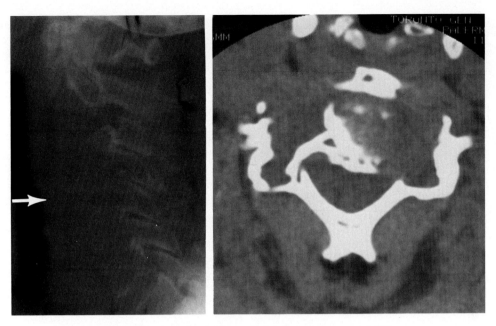

FIGURE 16–9. Multiple myeloma (lateral x-ray, axial CT).

ful but often not diagnostic; MRI is usually the best way of investigating these patients (Fig. 16-10).

Treatment

A prerequisite for treatment is a clear understanding of the management goals. In tumors such as osteoid osteoma and osteoblastoma, the goal is to cure the patient of disease, and this can be accomplished by surgical excision. For giant cell tumors, the goal is also to cure the patient of tumor, and again excision is indicated. Because these tumors are often locally recurrent, a complete excision should be done whenever possible. In patients with hemangioma, the goal is not tumor eradication, but the treatment of cord compression. Occasionally this can be done by embolization or radiation therapy. In resistant cases, surgical decompression of the dural sac is indicated.

The prognosis for patients with a solitary plasmacytoma is much better than for those with multiple myeloma. Treatment is usually radiation therapy in a dose of 3000 to 4000 rads. Progression of disease has been reported even after a 10-year disease-free interval, so regular reevaluation is necessary.

Malignant tumors such as multiple myeloma, lymphoma, and Ewing's require a different approach. The goal of treatment is not tumor extirpation, but rather tumor control and the alleviation of any spinal cord compression. Usually this can be done effectively by a combination of chemotherapy and radiation therapy. Indications for surgery include solitary lesions and spinal cord compression unresponsive to nonoperative treatment. Surgery may also be done in patients who have already received the maximum dose of radiation or to stabilize a pathological fracture.

METASTATIC TUMORS

Advances in treatment have resulted in prolonged life expectancy for cancer patients, which means that more patients will present with spinal epidural tumor deposits. The most common primary tumors to metastasize to the spinal column are bronchogenic, breast, prostatic, and renal carcinomas; occasionally, thyroid and colon cancers spread to the spine. As with metastases elsewhere, the usual route of spread is hematogenous. It has been hypothesized that tumors such as prostatic carcinoma spread to the thoracolumbar spine by means of Batson's plexus. Occasionally, spread occurs by direct extension of tumor,

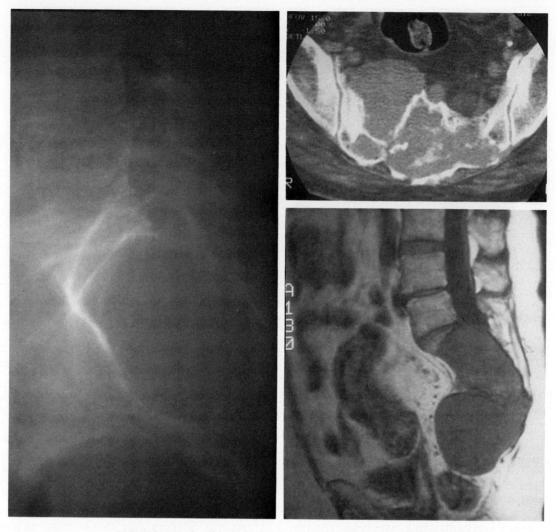

FIGURE 16–10. Chordoma (lateral x-ray, axial CT, sagittal MRI).

such as from lymphomatous involvement of retroperitoneal nodes or from direct tumor invasion of bronchogenic carcinoma.

Patient Evaluation

Some authors have tried to develop staging systems for metastatic disease of the spine. The role of any staging system is to provide guidelines for treatment, and in this regard the staging systems suggested fall short of their goal. Therefore, it is probably reasonable not to depend on these simplified staging systems but to consider specific factors that will influence treatment. Each patient must be evaluated individually, giving thought to the variables listed in Table 16-2.

The tumor type, if known, offers some information about sensitivity to radiation therapy and chemotherapy and may give some indication as to life expectancy. From a surgical standpoint, the tumor type can indicate vascularity and forewarn the surgeon as to intraoperative blood loss. Each patient's neurologic deficit must be carefully documented. The better the patient's neurologic status before treatment, the more hopeful the prognosis after surgery. Patients with complete paraplegia preoperatively have a poor prognosis and rarely regain the ability to ambulate in-

TABLE 16–2. **Treatment Considerations**

Tumor type
Neurologic deficit
Deformity
Stability
Bony involvement
Prior treatment
Medical status
Pain
Life expectancy

dependently. The rate of onset and progression of the deficit is also important to document. A rapid onset and progression of neurologic deficit often indicates that the etiology is ischemia to the spinal cord, not mechanical compression. This holds a worse prognosis from any treatment modality.

Spinal deformity and stability should be assessed. Treatment regimens such as chemotherapy and radiation therapy may cause tumor shrinkage and may result in pain relief, but they often do nothing to improve the stability of the spinal column. If all stability has been lost, the primary treatment is surgical.

Metastatic tumors can result in both osteoblastic and osteolytic areas (Fig. 16-11). Although

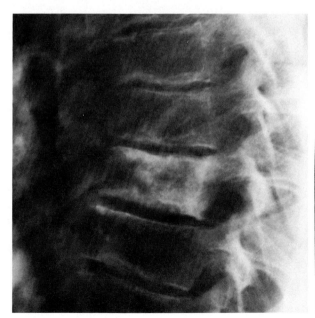
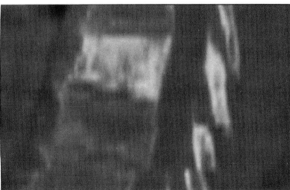

FIGURE 16–11. Osteoblastic lesion due to metastatic breast carcinoma (lateral x-ray, sagittal CT).

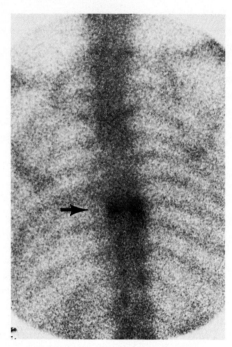

FIGURE 16–12. Technetium 99 bone scan showing metastatic breast disease.

The clinician should assess each patient's life expectancy before determining treatment options. The most important factor is tumor type. If a patient is thought to have less than 6 weeks to live, it is probably unreasonable to subject him or her to major surgery. Palliative treatment and pain control should be strongly considered.

Nonoperative Treatment

The vast majority of patients with spinal epidural metastatic disease do not require treatment. Many patients with back or neck pain due to metastatic disease can be treated simply with analgesics. If the tumor has resulted in some mechanical instability that is causing pain, patients may be treated with external orthoses.

Radiation therapy and chemotherapy have

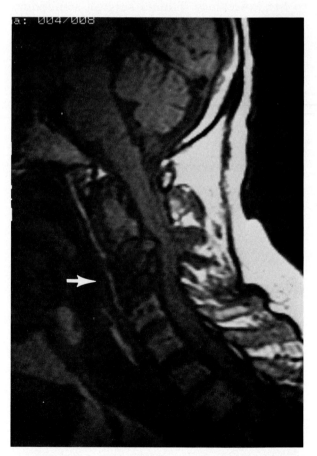

FIGURE 16–13. MRI showing cervical spine involvement by metastatic prostate carcinoma.

plain x-rays may be useful, 30% of the bone mass must be lost before any plain radiographic changes become evident. Technetium 99 bone scanning is a much more sensitive test for detecting occult neoplastic deposits (Fig. 16-12). In the past, myelography and CT scanning were used to determine the presence and extent of spinal cord compression, but MRI is becoming more popular for this purpose (Fig. 16-13).

The patient's overall medical status may determine the treatment by precluding surgical intervention. Complete blood work must be done lest potentially serious conditions such as hypercalcemia, thrombocytopenia, coagulopathy, or hypoproteinemia be overlooked.

Pain is almost always the predominant symptom of spinal metastases. Usually the pain is due to vertebral involvement by the tumor. This pain is not related to activity, occurs even at rest, and is often worse at night. However, the pain may be due to the destabilizing effect of the tumor on the spinal column. This pain is related to activity and can be relieved by limiting activity. It is important to distinguish between these two sources of pain in order to provide optimal treatment.

been effective in the treatment of many patients. The goal of radiation therapy is to shrink the tumor; thus, it is ideal when there is concern about impending spinal cord compression. The decision to use radiation treatment depends in large part on the specific tumor type, the stability of the vertebral column, and the presence of neurologic deficit. Radiation treatment is very effective for metastatic breast disease.

In the last decade there have been major advances in the chemotherapeutic management of many malignancies. Specific chemotherapeutic regimens are still being modified to obtain maximal benefit for each particular carcinoma.

High-dose steroids can be effective in reducing edema around tumors, so steroids can be used to relieve symptoms of spinal cord compression if it is due in part to edema. High-dose steroids have also been shown to have an oncolytic effect.

Operative Treatment

Indications for surgery include spinal instability, neural compression by bone, failure to respond to radiation therapy, and an uncertain diagnosis.

Once the surgeon has decided to operate on a patient with metastatic disease of the spine, the goals of surgery must be clear. In almost all instances, there are only two aims of surgery. The first is to decompress the compressed dural sac. In patient terms, this means an attempt to improve neurologic status if a neurologic deficit exists. The second goal is to stabilize an unstable spine. In patient terms, this means reducing the pain caused by underlying instability.

If the goal of surgery is to decompress, the site of compression must be clearly delineated and exposed at the time of surgery. Many studies in the past documenting the results of surgery have been based mainly on laminectomies. As the sole surgical procedure, a laminectomy is clearly insufficient to decompress the dural sac if the site of compression is anterior.

Stabilization can be surgically undertaken in many ways. The use of polymethylmethacrylate (bone cement) is recommended if the patient's life expectancy is less than 1 year, but because cement does not provide long-lasting stability, the use of bone graft is suggested if the patient is expected to live more than 1 year.

KEY POINTS

1. Primary tumors of the spine are uncommon. Even benign primary tumors are dangerous because of the possibility of spinal cord compression.
2. Metastatic tumors of the spine are common. The primary tumor is usually bronchogenic, breast, prostatic, or renal carcinoma.
3. Most metastatic tumors to the spine do not require surgical treatment.
4. Goals of surgery for metastatic tumors of the spine include decompression of compressed neural elements and stabilization of an unstable spinal segment.

BIBLIOGRAPHY

BOOKS

Harrington KD, ed. Orthopaedic management of metastatic bone disease. St. Louis: CV Mosby, 1988.
Mirra JM. Bone tumors: Diagnosis and treatment. Philadelphia: JB Lippincott, 1980.
Sundaresan N, Schmidek HH, Schiller A, Rosenthal DI, eds. Tumors of the spine: Diagnosis and clinical management. Philadelphia: WB Saunders, 1990.

JOURNALS

An HS, Vaccaro AR, Dolinskas CA, Cotler JM, Balderston AA, Bauerle WB. Differentiation between spinal tumors and infections with magnetic resonance imaging. Spine 1991;16(vol 8 suppl):S334–S338.
Barwick KW, Huvos AG, Smith J. Primary osteogenic sarcoma of the vertebral column: A cliniopathologic correlation of ten patients. Cancer 1980;46:595–604.
Biagini R, DeCristofaro R, Ruggieri P, Boriani S. Giant-cell tumor of the spine. A case report. J Bone Joint Surg [Am] 1990;72:1102–1107.
Bohlman HH, Sachs BL, Carter JR, Riley L, Robinson RA. Primary neoplasms of the cervical spine. Diagnosis and treatment of twenty-three patients. J Bone Joint Surg [Am] 1986;68:483–494.
Harrington KD. Anterior decompression and stabilization of the spine as a treatment for vertebral collapse and spinal cord compression from metastatic malignancy. Clin Orthop 1988;233:177–194.
Manabe S, Tateishi A, Abe M, Ohno T. Surgical treatment of metastatic tumors of the spine. Spine 1989;14:41–47.
Samson IR, Springfield DS, Suit HD, Mankin HJ. Operative treatment of sacrococcygeal chordoma. A review of twenty-one cases. J Bone Joint Surg [Am] 1993;75:1476–1484.
Weinstein JN. Surgical approach to spine tumors. Orthopaedics 1989;12:897–905.
Weinstein JN, McLain RF. Primary tumors of the spine. Spine 1987;12:843–851.

Textbook of Spinal Disorders, by Stephen I. Esses.
J. B. Lippincott Company, Philadelphia © 1995.

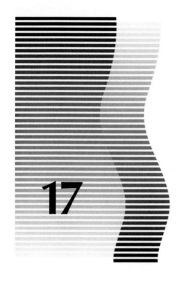

17 Osteoporosis

Michael H. Heggeness • Stephen I. Esses

MEASUREMENT OF
  BONE MASS
  Radiographic
    Methods
  Photon
    Absorbtometry
  Dual Energy X-ray
    Absorbtometry
  Quantitative
    Computed
    Tomography
  Biopsy
FRACTURES
  Spine
    *Diagnosis and
    Classification*
    Patient Management

TREATMENT OF
  OSTEOPOROSIS
  Calcium
  Vitamin D
  Estrogen
    Replacement
  Exercise
  Calcitonin
  Investigational
    Methods
PREVENTION

Osteoporosis is a clinical condition characterized by a decrease in the skeletal bone mass in which the biochemical and histologic characteristics of the bone are normal. It differs from *osteomalacia*, a clinical condition in which the bone mass is diminished as a result of an identifiable metabolic abnormality. *Osteopenia* is used to describe the condition of any patient in whom diminished bone mass has been observed and may be used when referring to patients with either osteomalacia or osteoporosis.

The most common form of osteoporosis is that associated with aging. Humans reach their peak bone mass during the third decade of life, and after that most people lose a small portion of skeletal bone mass each year. As a result, clinically significant osteoporosis is very common in elderly patients.

Women rapidly lose additional skeletal bone mass in the years immediately after ovarian function stops. Immediately after oophorectomy or menopause, women lose up to 5% of their cancellous bone mass and 1% to 2% of their cortical bone mass each year in the initial 2 or 3 years. This postmenopausal bone loss gradually diminishes over the ensuing 5 years. The rapid period of postmenopausal bone loss significantly increases the risk of clinical osteoporosis in women.

An additional epidemiologic factor is the patient's initial peak bone mass. Males on average acquire a significantly higher peak bone mass during young adulthood than females. The patient's race is also important, because blacks acquire significantly higher bone mass than do Asians and Caucasians. Thus, white women are at the highest risk for osteoporosis, black men at the lowest.

Several other epidemiologic factors have been identified and are discussed below.

Scientific study of osteoporosis has been hampered by the obvious fact that this is a continuum of disease. The major clinical consequences of osteoporosis involve fracture of the weakened bones. Fracture risk depends not only on the density of the bone but on its size and shape. The patient's environment, physical demands, and propensity to fall are also critical factors. In addition, skeletal bone loss is not uniform throughout the body. For example, some patients may have markedly diminished bone mass in the proximal femur but satisfactory bone mass in the vertebral column; the reverse is also true. Thus, a clinical diagnosis of osteoporosis is by definition somewhat subjective.

The prevalence of vertebral fracture and the incidence of hip fracture are clearly inversely proportional to the measured bone mineral densities at these sites. The risk of subsequent fracture is also increased after the documentation of any osteoporosis-related fracture.

Genetic risk factors for the development of osteoporosis were discussed above. Environmental, nutritional, and lifestyle factors are also associated with this problem. A low calcium intake is known to increase the risks of osteoporosis and fracture. An association has been made with a vegetarian diet. A history of anorexia nervosa is strongly correlated with adult osteoporosis. Smoking and excessive alcohol intake are also recognized risk factors. Multiparity, late menarche, early menopause (surgical or natural) without estrogen replacement, and an inactive lifestyle also increase the risk of osteoporosis. Other causes of osteopenia need to be excluded before a diagnosis of osteoporosis is made (Fig. 17-1).

Medical conditions associated with osteoporosis include Cushing's syndrome, hyperthyroidism, and hyperparathyroidism. There is evidence that excessive thyroid replacement can be a risk factor for osteoporosis in some hypothyroid patients.

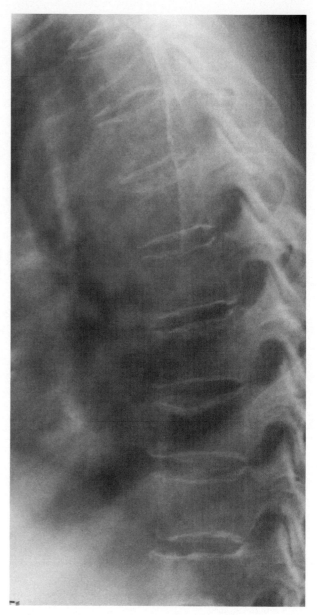

FIGURE 17–1. Lateral thoracic x-ray showing osteopenia due to multiple myeloma.

The use of chronic anticoagulants, glucocorticoids, lithium, and certain anticonvulsants is a significant risk factor for decreased mineral density. Osteoporosis may also be associated with gastrointestinal problems causing decreased absorption of calcium. A history of gastrointestinal or hepatobiliary problems or surgery may be significant.

MEASUREMENT OF BONE MASS

Radiographic Methods

Several methods are currently used to assess skeletal bone mass: radiographic methods, neutron activation analysis, photon absorbtometry, dual energy x-ray absorbtometry, and quantitative CT. Quantitative estimates of bone mineral density can also be made from bone biopsies.

Direct radiographic methods for assessing bone mass use conventional radiographs and a standardized technique to measure cortical thickness and photodensitometry. The clinical usefulness of these techniques is limited by problems of variable film-processing conditions, and error induced by varying layers of soft tissue overlying the bone of interest.

Photon Absorbtometry

Photon absorbtometry involves the use of a highly collimated radionuclide beam, assessed by a scintillation detection system. Particles of a single energy are used, and with the quantitative detection mechanisms currently available, very precise data can be obtained. In single-photon technique, a single beam of a single energy is used. The disadvantage of this method is that the total thickness of soft tissue must be constant over the scanning path. Dual-photon technique can overcome this problem by using two beams of different photon energies. Simultaneous transmission is made at both energies, and the thickness of soft tissue and bone mineral density in the beam path are then computed. Using this technique, bone mineral densities at different points can be precisely measured. This technique has been very effective for assessing the densities in individual vertebrae and in different regions of the hip.

Dual Energy X-ray Absorbtometry

Dual energy x-ray absorbtometry is similar in concept to dual-photon absorbtometry, but an x-ray source is used instead of a radionuclide source. This allows a much higher flux than the gadolinium source conventionally used in dual-photon absorbtometry and allows the creation of precise data using shortened scanning times.

Quantitative Computed Tomography

Quantitative computed tomography (CT) involves the use of a standard CT scanner to obtain a digitized image of the spine. The density calculated for the bones on the CT image is compared to standardized, phantom density standards present in the same scanning field placed under the patient.

All the above techniques are clinically useful, although each has relative advantages and disadvantages in regard to cost, error, and physician preference.

Biopsy

Bone biopsy is a well-established, extremely useful technique in evaluating the osteoporotic patient. Biopsy of virtually any bone is possible and occasionally indicated. Standardized evaluation, coupled with ease of access, has made the anterior iliac crest the site of choice for most routine biopsies. A 6- to 8-mm core is obtained through both cortices of the anterior ilium, and the bone is processed for sectioning in plastic embedding medium without decalcification. This allows histologic assessment of the cellular activity in the specimen, as well as assessment of the structure of the bone itself.

Before biopsy, the bone can be prelabeled with tetracycline. This commonly used antibiotic binds preferentially to mineralizing osteoid and becomes incorporated into the bone. Two short courses of oral tetracycline are given, separated by about 10 days, before the biopsy. At the time of biopsy, this results in two distinct bands of fluorescence visible under the microscope, corresponding to the bone that was being made when the doses were given. The distance between these lines can be used to calculate the rate of bone synthesis. Various quantitative methods are also applied that allow the pathologist to calculate the rate of bone turnover. The absolute amount of cortical and cancellous bone in the specimens can also be measured. These biopsies are occasionally quite useful in the management of patients with osteoporosis, although the detailed histomorphometric measurements are also of great importance in research in this area.

One of the principal values of the bone biopsy applied clinically is to rule out other treatable causes of osteopenia. A biopsy may reveal

previously undiagnosed osteomalacia, masto-
cytosis, or multiple myeloma, for example.

FRACTURES

The incidence of clinical fracture in all socie-
ties is bimodal. Fracture rates peak in late childhood and adolescence and diminish through subsequent adult life. Fracture rates begin to rise
again quite dramatically in the sixth decade and,
in all studies published thus far, continue to rise.
The initial peak is due to the trauma so commonly sustained by younger patients whereas osteoporosis is thought to be the overwhelming
cause of the fractures of the elderly.

Fractures of the hip are the most morbid and
are perhaps the most common fracture associated with osteoporosis. About 300,000 hip fractures occur in the United States each year. The
acute care of these fractures alone accounts for
about $10 billion per year. A more significant
and often forgotten observation is the high mortality rate associated with these injuries. Mortality rates from 24% to 50% have been reported for
the year after hip fracture.

Colles' fracture of the distal radius is the third
most common type of fracture associated with
osteoporosis. The incidence of Colles' fracture
does not increase past age 60; this may be because
many elderly patients cannot extend their arms
during a fall.

Spine

Vertebral fractures associated with osteoporosis are the second most common fracture
type in the elderly. The decrease in vertebral
compressive stiffness in osteoporosis is caused
by a loss of the horizontal trabeculae. In osteoporosis, these horizontal trabeculae are the first
to be lost and do so to a greater degree than the
vertical trabeculae.

Prevalence and incidence rates are difficult to
estimate because of the difficulty in defining precise diagnostic criteria. It is thought that about a
third of vertebral fractures are asymptomatic, so
many such fractures remain undiagnosed. Minor
degrees of end plate collapse can be difficult to
identify on x-rays, particularly in the thoracic
spine, where overlying rib shadows and projec-
tional artifacts contribute to the problem. Prevalence rates reported in the literature have, there-

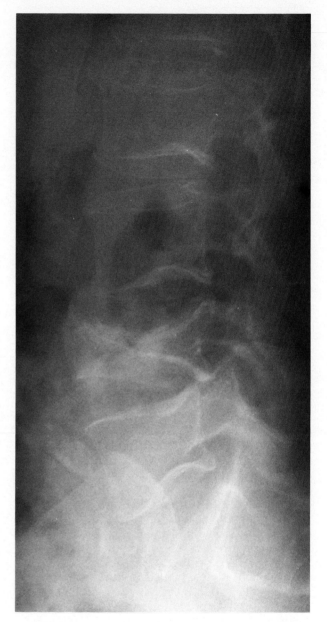

FIGURE 17–2. Lumbar fracture due to osteoporosis.

fore, ranged from 2.9% to 27% in women age 65
or older.

Even though a precise estimate of incidence is
difficult, vertebral fractures are clearly a major
source of morbidity in the elderly. Patients with
multiple thoracic compression fractures commonly have severe acquired thoracic kyphotic

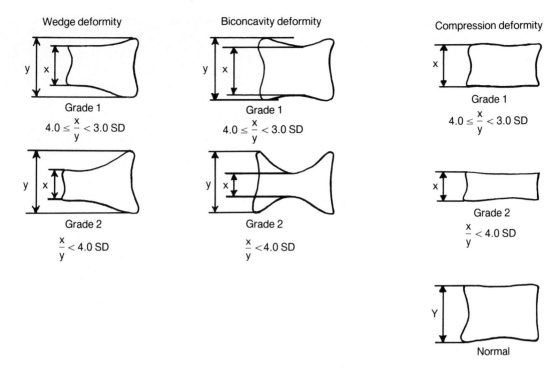

FIGURE 17–3. Classification of osteoporotic vertebral fractures as described by Riggs and Melton.

deformity, frequently associated with chronic disabling pain that is distinct from the pain of an acute fracture.

DIAGNOSIS AND CLASSIFICATION

Only a few osteoporotic vertebral fractures are evaluated acutely by a physician. Patients most frequently present with a history of abrupt onset of pain in the thoracic or thoracolumbar spine. This may or may not be associated with mild trauma, falls, or bending and reaching events. Many patients present with severe, incapacitating pain, although milder degrees of pain are also seen. It is a mystery how such radiographically similar events can have such widely disparate clinical consequences.

Fractures can usually be diagnosed by plain radiographic technique (Fig. 17-2). Very small fractures without substantial compression of the vertebrae may cause severe pain. Indeed, it is not uncommon to identify a patient with the acute onset of back pain and no initial radiographic evidence of a fracture. These fractures can be documented by bone scan. Follow-up x-rays usually show evidence of vertebral collapse, which pro-

gresses over 2 to 3 weeks. This illustrates an important point about osteoporotic compression fractures: the vertebrae often demonstrate insidious progressive collapse over weeks or months to a degree not seen in younger patients. Most osteoporotic vertebral fractures are the result of failure under axial load. Although commonly called compression fractures, they quite often involve the posterior cortex of the vertebral body; thus, many such fractures are technically true burst injuries. Because so few of these fractures are imaged using CT or magnetic resonance imaging (MRI), the incidence of middle column injury is unknown. However, Schmorl's classic autopsy work showed that this is a common feature of these fractures.

Most attempts to classify these injuries have been based on plain radiographic criteria. Riggs and Melton's classification system is shown in Figure 17-3. Vertebral fractures are classified by their gross morphology as *biconcave*, or codfish, fractures, *wedge* fractures, or *crush* fractures. The crush fracture is a gross failure of both anterior and middle columns. It is unknown how many biconcave or wedge fractures also have some posterior cortex involvement. Indeed, as mentioned above, it is not infrequent to see an end plate fracture undergo progressive collapse to a wedge and subsequently a crush fracture appearance. Rarely this leads to late neurologic dysfunction.

In the past it was thought that neurologic compromise from osteoporotic compression fractures was exceedingly rare, but recent reports have indicated that this phenomenon may be more common than previously appreciated. A unique feature of these osteoporotic burst fractures is that the neurologic signs and symptoms usually manifest weeks or months after the initial fracture and are thought to result from insidious collapse of the fractured vertebra. Rarely, profound neurologic deficit, including frank paraplegia, can occur. Patients with such injuries have been successfully managed by both operative and nonoperative means.

PATIENT MANAGEMENT

Management of an osteoporotic compression fracture includes careful patient evaluation, careful diagnostic studies, including investigation of other possible causes of fracture such as metastatic disease, and then, in the vast majority of cases, nonoperative care.

Patient history should include specific reference to risk factors for osteoporosis. A history of any trauma is also important (why the patient fell, for example). A history of weight loss may suggest a tumor. A history of smoking may support the diagnosis of either tumor or osteoporosis. The possibility of multiple myeloma must always be kept in mind (Fig. 17-4).

Radiographs are carefully examined for fracture morphology. Does the location of the pain correspond to the radiographically documented fracture(s)? Is there a history of previous fracture?

A laboratory screen should be routinely performed, including complete blood count, sedimentation rate, serum protein electrophoresis, urinalysis, and thyroid function tests. With no evidence of other contributing history, if this workup is negative, a tentative diagnosis of idiopathic osteoporosis may be entertained.

A general physical examination, including a breast examination and palpation of the thyroid and prostate, is encouraged. A careful neurologic examination, especially of the lower extremities, is mandatory. The presence of objective neurologic dysfunction is a strong indication for CT or MR imaging.

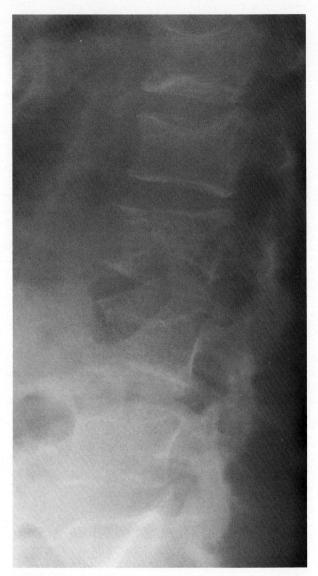

FIGURE 17–4. Lumbar compression fractures due to multiple myeloma.

The initial phase of management is patient education. The patient needs to understand the diagnosis and its implications. It is wise on initial evaluation to inform the patient about the possibility of future fractures, although it is important to stress that these vertebral fractures heal successfully, and spontaneous resolution of pain may be expected in 2 to 10 weeks. The patient is told to seek prompt reevaluation should neurologic signs or symptoms develop, and routine follow-up to assess possible neurologic compromise is needed.

Pain management is a prime concern in these patients. When pain is inadequately addressed, many such patients become limited to bed rest, which places them at risk for venous thrombosis, pulmonary problems, and a worsening of their osteoporosis on the basis of inactivity. A short course of oral narcotics is often indicated to allow the patient a reasonable level of activity.

The use of braces is controversial because many elderly patients, despite their pain, often cannot tolerate brace wear. Attempts to brace fractures in the upper thoracic spine are rarely successful for pain management. Braces such as a canvas corset can be extremely useful for lumbar fractures. Braces of thoracolumbar and midthoracic fractures are less successful. A lumbosacral corset often does not provide adequate support to this region. Many patients find significant relief with the use of a molded soft-foam brace.

There is also controversy about the use of braces for these problems because of the theoretic possibility of stress shielding of the spine with brace use. Stress shielding, it is argued, will exacerbate the osteoporosis. Because patients will use the brace only as long as it is useful for severe pain management, the benefits of keeping the patient ambulatory may far outweigh the theoretic disadvantage of subsequent stress shielding. However, there are no scientific data by which to form a firm conclusion on this issue.

Rarely, a patient experiences such severe pain and physical limitation that hospitalization may be required for supportive care and parenteral pain medication. Mobilization of these patients, even when hospitalized, is encouraged.

The use of parenteral calcitonin is gaining popularity in the acute management of vertebral compression fractures. This polypeptide hormone has a natural action to downregulate osteoclast function. For unknown reasons, in many patients with vertebral compression fractures, the use of calcitonin affords dramatic analgesia. The basis for this phenomenon may lie in central nervous system receptors for this hormone, although the mode of action remains obscure. Parenteral daily doses of about 100 IU of calcitonin are extremely effective for some patients. However, hypersensitivity reactions have been described, and GI side effects of nausea and vomiting are common during the initial days of therapy. For this reason, small doses are usually given initially and are increased over 3 to 5 days into the therapeutic range. Calcitonin treatment and external bracing can usually be discontinued within 4 to 10 weeks of the fracture event.

Progressive bone loss is inevitable for all of us. Some patients experience relentless fractures of multiple vertebrae through their sixth, seventh, and eighth decades. This often results in a dramatic kyphotic deformity and severe postural problems (Fig. 17-5). The progression of the kyphosis usually stops when the ribs begin to impinge on the iliac wings. This phenomenon is frequently associated with local pain from irritation

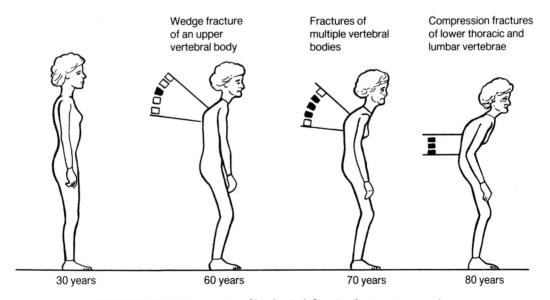

FIGURE 17-5. Progression of kyphotic deformity due to osteoporosis.

of the costal nerves. Spinal osteotomy, or rib resection, is strongly contraindicated. In rare cases of severe intractable pain, costal nerve blocks or nerve ablation procedures may be considered.

TREATMENT OF OSTEOPOROSIS

Calcium

Dietary calcium deficiency has been documented as a risk factor for osteoporosis. Evaluating an individual patient is difficult, however, because of variation in the calcium balance of each person. At present, the recommended oral intake for adults is 1200 mg a day. Women at risk for osteoporosis are recommended to consume 1500 mg a day. These recommendations are useful but must be considered in light of the fact that calcium absorption is strongly influenced by the form in which it is ingested. Calcium is absorbed much more efficiently from dairy products than from vegetable matter, for example. Some commercially available calcium supplements deliver calcium in a form that is all but unabsorbable. Nonetheless, calcium supplementation from 500 to 1000 mg a day (depending on dietary history) for patients at risk is recommended. These recommendations apply particularly to patients in their third, fourth, and fifth decades, because once a substantial amount of bone mineral density is lost, there is no effective means of replacing it.

Vitamin D

Some investigators have found vitamin D to be slightly effective in the treatment of osteoporosis. The basis of this effect may be on those patients with a mild dietary deficiency. Daily supplementation with 25 to 50 IU of vitamin D may be useful and at present is recommended for nearly all patients with osteoporosis. Doses in this range are present in many over-the-counter multivitamins, so the separate prescription of vitamin D preparations often is unnecessary.

Estrogen Replacement

Estrogen replacement following menopause is the most effective treatment available to date for the prevention of osteoporosis. The abrupt loss of bone mineral normally seen following meno-pause or oophorectomy is all but eliminated with estrogen supplementation. This treatment, however, does not usually affect the slower (0.5%) per year bone mineral loss common to all patients. Certain patients cannot tolerate estrogen because of its side effects, and estrogen supplementation has been associated with increased rates of endometrial malignancy. This risk is significantly diminished (and perhaps eliminated) by interval treatment with progestin. Many investigators have also reported a small but significant increase in the incidence of endometrial cancer, cerebrovascular accident, dysfunctional uterine bleeding, and thrombophlebitis in patients using estrogen supplementation. Other possibly deleterious effects of this therapy include an increased incidence of gallstone and atrophic changes in the genitourinary system.

In general, estrogen and progesterone therapy is recommended for all postmenopausal women under age 60 for osteoporosis prophylaxis, provided there are no contraindications. A recommendation for estrogen supplementation in any patient must be made in concert with her treating internist, gynecologist, and endocrinologist.

Exercise

Physical activity is known to stimulate bony hypertrophy, and there is good evidence that physically active patients have a diminished risk for osteoporosis. Regular exercise of 20 minutes' duration, four times a week, for at least 10 years premenopausally, is the best means of preventing postmenopausal osteoporosis. On this basis, judicious exercise is encouraged for all female patients. However, no clear studies have emerged showing that any enforced exercise regimens imposed by physicians have a significant clinical effect. The type of exercise should also be carefully considered for each patient. Elderly patients often have a short gait pattern and balance problems. It is an unpleasant experience to interview a patient who has suffered a fracture by falling off a prescribed treadmill.

Calcitonin

Parenteral calcitonin is approved for the treatment of osteoporosis in the United States. Its value in affecting bone mass is controversial, but some studies indicate small but statistically significant changes in bone mineral content with prolonged use. The controversy surrounding its effectiveness in treating bone mineral content, coupled with the inconvenience of the obligatory injectable administration, has made this form of chronic treatment less popular in recent years. The use of calcitonin for acute pain management is gaining popularity, however.

Investigational Methods

Bisphosphonates such as sodium etidronate are powerful inhibitors of osteoclast action. Their mode of action is not completely understood but may involve some frank toxicity to the osteoclast. They are generally used in intermittent pulses separated by several weeks. Initial reports on the use of these medications were extremely encouraging, but more recent, longer-term studies have raised questions about their effectiveness. More research is needed. The high cost of these investigational medications should also be considered before initiating the treatment. Second- and third-generation bisphosphonates are under investigation and hold great promise.

Modified androgens and other *anabolic steroids* are under investigation as possible agents in the treatment of osteoporosis. This area of research has great potential, but at present no clinically useful preparations have become available.

Sodium fluoride supplementation has been found useful for dental applications at doses believed to be insufficient to affect the bony skeleton. At higher doses (50 mg/day), significant increases in skeletal bone density have been documented. However, no clear decrease in fracture rates was demonstrated in these studies; indeed, there was some suggestion that hip fracture rates might actually increase. This is believed to be due to the effect of fluoride iron in creating larger hydroxyapatite crystals, making the bone more brittle. At present fluoride, at least at these dosage ranges, is not recommended for the treatment of osteoporosis. A lower dose may yet prove beneficial, and clinical studies on this issue are continuing.

PREVENTION

The treatment of vertebral osteoporosis and fracture can be very frustrating for the physician. It is likely that a solution for this problem will result not from its cure but from its prevention.

Lifestyle modification (increased exercise), postmenopausal estrogen supplementation, and adequate calcium and vitamin D intake together may significantly decrease the magnitude of this problem. Patients must be identified and treated in their early and middle adult years, however, for these approaches to be effective.

Once osteoporosis is established, acute treatment of fractures can significantly decrease the patient's suffering. Home safety and fall prevention can also be very useful. Patients at risk and their families should strenuously avoid activities where falls are likely. Icy sidewalks and an obstacle-strewn living environment (eg, throw rugs and lamp cords) are preventable causes of fracture. A discussion of these issues should be part of the treatment of any patient with osteoporosis.

KEY POINTS

1. Osteoporosis is a clinical condition in which skeletal bone mass is decreased although the bone itself is biochemically normal.
2. Humans reach their peak bone mass in early adulthood and slowly and steadily lose bone mass thereafter. Women rapidly lose bone mass for 5 to 7 years after menopause if estrogen supplementation is not given.
3. The clinical consequences of osteoporotic vertebral fracture vary. Some fractures are asymptomatic; others are severely painful. Neurologic compromise from true fractures is possible.
4. Treatment of patients with vertebral fracture secondary to osteoporosis includes investigation of the cause of the mineral density problem, symptomatic treatment of the fracture, and patient education, including fall prevention.

BIBLIOGRAPHY

BOOKS

Avioli LV, ed. The osteoporosis syndrome: Detection, prevention, and treatment. 2nd ed. Orlando: Grune and Stratton, 1987.

Avioli LV, Krane SM, eds. Metabolic bone diseases and clinically related disorders. 2nd ed. Philadelphia: WB Saunders, 1990.

Boden SD, Wiesel SW, Laws ER Jr, Rothman RH. The aging spine: Essentials of pathophysiology, diagnosis and treatment. Philadelphia: WB Saunders, 1991.

Coe FL, Favus MJ, eds. Disorders of bone and mineral metabolism. New York: Raven, 1992.

JOURNALS

Aaron JE, Makins NB, Sagreiya K. The microanatomy of trabecular bone loss in normal and aging men and women. Clin Orthop 1987;215:260–271.

Charnley RM, Bickerstaff DR, Wallace WA, Stevens A. The measurement of osteoporosis in clinical practice. J Bone Joint Surg [Br] 1989;71:661–663.

Eastell R, Cedel SL, Wahner HW, Riggs BL, Melton LJ III. Classification of vertebral fractures. J Bone Miner Res 1991;6:207–215.

Heggeness MH. Spine fracture with neurological deficit in osteoporosis. Osteoporosis International 1993;3:215–221.

Kanis JA, Pitt FA. Epidemiology of osteoporosis. Bone 1992;13(suppl 1):S7–S15.

Mizrah J, Silva MJ, Keaveny TM, Edwards WT, Hayes WC. Finite-element stress analysis of the normal and osteoporotic lumbar vertebral body. Spine 1993;18:2088–2096.

Ryan PJ. Fracture thresholds in osteoporosis: implications for hormone replacement treatment. Ann Rheum Dis 1992;51:1063–1065.

Textbook of Spinal Disorders, by Stephen I. Esses.
J. B. Lippincott Company, Philadelphia © 1995.

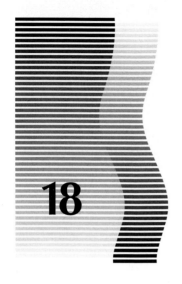

18

The Future

OUTCOMES
RESEARCH
BASIC SCIENCE
RESEARCH
CLINICAL RESEARCH

OUTCOMES RESEARCH

As health costs increase and as the population becomes better educated, there is more and more pressure for scientific validation of the treatment modalities being used. The direct costs of spinal problems in the United States are estimated to exceed $20 billion annually; indirect costs are thought to be about three times this amount. It is no wonder, therefore, that a critical analysis of treatments is being called for.

Outcomes research aims to assess the effect of a specific intervention on the natural history of the disease process. It is critically important to know what the natural history is of the disorder to measure the influence of a specific treatment. Unfortunately we lack adequate information in this regard. Until recently, most of the literature concerning spinal disorders consisted of a retrospective analysis of patients or prospective but uncontrolled patient groups. These studies are grossly inadequate. Optimal study design is prospective and randomized. Furthermore, the instrument used to assess patient outcome must reflect what is important to the patient. For example, whether a surgical technique for low back pain results in a solid fusion is unimportant. Whether it results in an improved quality of life for the patient and whether the patient's expectations have been met are much more important. We all have a responsibility to patients to critically assess how we practice medicine and participate in outcomes research.

BASIC SCIENCE RESEARCH

For most things, prevention is the best medicine. Basic science research aims to elucidate the underlying cause of disease and then, with this knowledge, strives to develop means by which that sequence of events can be changed. No matter how elegant techniques become for the surgical management of scoliosis, they will pale compared to the knowledge of why scoliosis occurs and how it can be prevented. Similarly, although many surgical and nonsurgical modalities are used to treat neck and low back pain, we do not, in most instances, understand why the pain exists. Recently, it has been shown that certain afferent neurons produce substances that may mediate the perception of pain. These neuropeptides include *substance P*, shown to be present in the dorsal root ganglion.

Much research has been directed at improving our ability to stimulate bone formation. We have known for some time that the molecules associated with bone induction and osteogenesis are the *bone morphogenic proteins* (BMPs). Recent work has been done in an attempt to synthesize bone graft substitutes, including hydroxyapatite and tricalcium phosphate. It is hoped that with further research we will no longer need to harvest a patient's own bone to perform a successful spinal fusion.

As we gradually come to understand the cellular and molecular basis for the structure and function of the spinal column, ideally we will be able to prevent many of the pathologic conditions discussed in this text. This is why basic research must continue to be an important component of the academic spine community.

CLINICAL RESEARCH

Biomedical advances have led to the development of multiple new techniques in the spine surgeon's armamentarium. As in other surgical fields, there has been a trend toward minimally invasive, percutaneous procedures. Under endoscopic control, discectomies and fusions are now

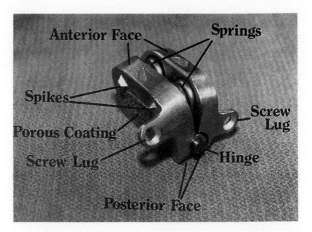

FIGURE 18–1. Artificial intervertebral disc.

possible. This area of surgery will probably continue to expand rapidly.

Although they are not in general clinical use, artificial intravertebral discs (Fig. 18-1) and ligaments have been developed. As better materials become available, these will become refined. At present, stabilization of a spinal motion unit is synonymous with fusion. It may be possible in the future to functionally stabilize an abnormal level by using implants without performing a fusion.

KEY POINTS

1. There is an urgent need for outcomes research to validate the usefulness, or lack thereof, of surgical and nonsurgical treatment modalities used for spinal disorders.
2. Basic science research is being directed at discovering the molecular basis for spinal disorders such as scoliosis and degenerative disease.
3. Surgical techniques are being developed to obviate the need for bone grafting and arthrodesis.

BIBLIOGRAPHY

JOURNALS

Amadio PC. Editorial. Outcomes Measurements. More questions: Some Answers. J Bone Joint Surg [Am] 1993;75: 1583–1584.

Bridge JA. Cytogenetic and molecular cytogenetic techniques in orthopaedic surgery. J Bone Joint Surg [Am] 1993;75:606–614.

Burstein AH, Cohen J. Editorial. Measurements in the conduct of research. J Bone Joint Surg [Am] 1993;75:319–320.

Frymoyer JW. Quality. An international challenge to the diagnosis and treatment of disorders of the lumbar spine. Spine 1993;18:2147–2152.

Keller RB, Rudicel SA, Liang MH. Instructional Course Lecture. American Academy of Orthopaedic Surgeons. Outcomes Research in orthopaedics. J Bone Joint Surg [Am] 1993;75:1562–1574.

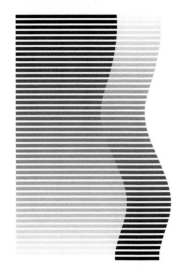

Index

Page numbers followed by *f* indicate figures;
page numbers followed by *t* indicate tables.

A

Abdomen
  superficial skin reflexes, 58, 59f
  thoracolumbar kinetics and,
      127–128
Abscess
  epidural, 238–239
  psoas, in spinal tuberculosis,
      234, 235f
Absorbtometry
  dual energy x-ray. *See* Dual
      energy x-ray
      absorptometry
  photon. *See* Photon
      absorptometry
Accessory (mammillary) process,
      7
Acetaminophen, 143
Achilles (ankle jerk) reflex, 65,
      66f, 67t
Adamkiewicz, artery of, 32
Adductor reflex, nerve root
      innervation, 67t
Adolescent scoliosis, 266–274
Aerobic exercise, 136
Age/aging
  idiopathic scoliosis and, 266
  osteoporosis and, 317
  spinal tumor and, 306
  spondylolisthesis type II and,
      204

at time of spinal cord injury,
      prognosis and, 302
Agenesis
  odontoid, 42
  sacral, 45
AIDS, 229
Alar ligaments, 13, 15f
Alexander technique, 141
Allograft, 160, 161
Alum(a), sacral, 9
Ambulation, level of spinal cord
      injury and, 302
Amphotericin B, 237, 238
Anabolic steroids, in
      osteoporosis, 325
Analgesics, 143
Anal reflex, superficial, 65
Anatomy, 1–34
  anatomic planes, 2, 2f
  articulations, 11–13
    atlantoaxial, 11, 11f
    costovertebral (ribs), 12–13,
        13f
    facet joints, 12, 12f
    intervertebral discs, 11f,
        11–12
    occipitocervical, 10f, 11
    uncovertebral joints, 12, 12f
  bony, 2–10
    cervical spine, 2–7
    coccyx, 9

lumbar spine, 7
sacrum, 7, 9
thoracic spine, 7
intervertebral disc, 11f, 11–12,
      117–118, 119f
key points, 34
ligaments, 13–17
  anterior longitudinal, 14–15,
      16f
  atlantoaxial, 14, 14f
  costal, 17, 18f
  cruciform, 14, 15f
  iliolumbar, 17, 18f
  interspinous, 16, 17f
  intertransverse, 17, 18f
  ligamentum flavum, 16, 16f
  lumbosacral, 17, 18f
  occipitoatlantal, 13, 14f
  occipitoaxial, 13, 15f
  posterior longitudinal,
      15–16, 16f
  supraspinous, 16, 17f
  transverse, 14
muscles, 17–20
  anterior, 20, 21f
  posterior, 17–20, 19f
relation of neural structures to
      bony structures. *See*
      Neuroanatomy
spinal cord, 20, 22–26. *See also*
      Spinal cord

Anatomy (*continued*)
spinal nerves, 23f, 25, 25f
terminology, 2
vascular anatomy, 29–34
cervical spine, 29–30, 30f
intervertebral disc, 33, 34f
lumbosacral spine, 30–32,
31f
spinal cord, 32, 32f
thoracic spine, 30, 31f
Anesthesia, hypotensive, blood
loss and, 166–167
Aneurysmal bone cyst, 306t
Angiography, spinal tumor,
306–307
Ankle clonus, testing, 73, 74f
Ankle jerk. *See* Achilles reflex
Ankylosing spondylitis, 248–252
bamboo spine, 249, 250f
cervical spine, 249, 251, 251f
clinical features, 248–249
lumbar spine, 249, 250f
radiographic features, 249,
249f–250f, 251f
Rome criteria, 248t
thoracolumbar spine, 251–252,
252f
Ankylosis, cervical psoriatic
arthritis and, 253
Annulus fibrosus, 11, 11f, 118
collagen in, 185
in degenerative disease, 173
Anterior cord syndrome, 75–76,
288
Anterior costovertebral ligament
complex, 17, 18f
Anterior (ventral) plane, 2
Antibiotics. *See* Antimicrobial
drugs
Anti-inflammatory drugs
nonsteroidal. *See* NSAIDs
topical application,
phonophoresis,
137–138
Antimicrobial drugs
in disc space infection, 233
in vertebral bacterial
osteomyelitis, 231
Aorta
abdominal, 30, 31f
thoracic, 30, 31f
Apical ligament, 13, 15f
Aplasia, caudal, 45
Arachnoiditis, 255
Arachnoid matter, 22, 23f
Arch, posterior, 7
Arm. *See also* Extremity, upper
cervical herniated disc and, 197

pain
cervical nerve root
compression and, 157
compression-traction test,
52, 53f
Arnold-Chiari malformation, 41,
41f
Arthrodesis, 160
Articular facets
atlas, 4, 5f
axis, 4, 5f
Articular processes
cervical vertebrae, 6f
lumbar vertebrae, 7, 9f
Articulations, 11–13. *See also*
specific articulations
atlantoaxial, 11, 11f
costovertebral (ribs), 12–13,
13f
facet joints, 12, 12f
intervertebral discs, 11f, 11–12
occipitocervical, 10f, 11
uncovertebral joints, 12, 12f
Artificial intervertebral disc, 328,
328f
Aspergillosis, osteomyelitis and,
238, 238f
Aspergillus, 238
Atlantoaxial articulation, 11, 11f
instability, in Down's
syndrome, 42, 43f
Atlantoaxial ligaments, 14, 14f
Atlantoaxial subluxation, in
rheumatoid arthritis,
244f
Atlanto-occipital ligament. *See*
Occipitoatlantal
ligament
Atlas (C1)
arcuate foramen, 42
bony anatomy, 4, 5f
differentiation, 40, 40f
fracture, 119, 120f. *See also*
Jefferson fracture
occipitalization, 42
ossification of posterior arch,
42
surgical exposure, 154, 155f
Autograft, 160, 161
Autonomic dysreflexia, spinal
cord injury and, 301
Autonomic nervous system,
25–26, 26f
parasympathetic, 26, 26f
sympathetic, 26, 26f
Autotraction, 142
Autotransfusion, 167
Axial (transverse) plane, 2

Axilla, examination, 52
Axis (C2)
bony anatomy, 4, 5f
differentiation, 40, 40f
odontoid fracture, 291, 292f
spondylolisthesis, traumatic,
291
trauma, 291

B
Babinski's test, 73, 75f
Back pain
acute, bed rest for, 135
ankylosing spondylitis and, 248
disc space infection and, 232
epidural abscess and, 239
fibromyalgia and, 254
herniated disc disease and
lumbar, 186
thoracic, 196
low
after discectomy, risk factors,
194
lumbosacral orthoses for, 143
traction for, 142
transcutaneous electrical
nerve stimulation for,
139–140, 140f
in scoliosis, 267
spinal tumor and, 306
thoracolumbar stenosis and,
221
vertebral bacterial
osteomyelitis and, 230
Back school, 143
Bamboo spine, 249, 250f
Basilar artery, 30, 30f
Basilar invagination (impression),
41–42
in rheumatoid arthritis,
244–246, 247f
measurement of, 245f, 246f
Batson's plexus, 32
Bed rest, 135–136
in discitis, 234
in herniated disc disease
cervical, 199
lumbar, 191
Biceps muscle, deep tendon
reflexes, 55f, 55t
Biceps reflex, nerve root
innervation, 55t
Biofeedback, 142–143
Biomechanics of spine, 109–134
cervical spine, 116–124
failure mechanisms, 119–122
kinematics, 116–117

kinetics, 117–119
stabilization, 122–124
creep, 114, 115f
force, 109, 110f
key points, 134
kinematics, 116
kinetics, 116
moment, 109, 110f
relaxation time, 114, 116f
stiffness, 109–110, 111f. *See
also* Stiffness
strain, 109, 111f
strength, 112, 114. *See also*
Strength of body
stress, 109, 110f
terminology, 109–116
thoracolumbar spine, 124–134
failure mechanisms, 128–129
kinematics, 124–125
kinetics, 125–128
stabilization, 129, 133
viscoelastic properties, 114
Biopsy, bone mass measurement,
319–320
Bisphosphonates, in osteoporosis,
325
Black disc disease, 176, 176f
Blastocyst, 36
Blastomycosis, osteomyelitis and,
237
Block vertebra, 44, 259
Blood loss, intraoperative,
techniques to
minimize, 166–167
Blood transfusion, autologous,
167
Bone biopsy, 319
Bone graft, 160–161
allograft, 160, 161
autogenous cancellous bone,
160
autograft, 160, 161
harvesting, 160
resorption, infection and, 240,
240f
synthetic, 160
Bone loss, postmenopausal, 317
Bone mass
measurement of, 319–320
biopsy, 319–320
dual energy x-ray
absorptiometry, 319
photon absorptometry, 319
qualitative CT scan, 319
radiographic methods, 319
peak, 318
Bone morphogenic protein
(BMP), 160

Bone scan. *See* Radionuclide
scanning
Bony spur. *See* Osteophyte
Bowstring sign, 66, 69f
Braces/bracing. *See also*
Orthoses/orthotics
chair-back brace, 129, 132f
hyperextension brace, 129,
132f
Milwaukee brace, 273, 274f
Brachioradialis muscle, deep
tendon reflexes, 55t
Brachioradialis reflex, nerve root
innervation, 55t
Breast cancer, spinal metastases,
313f–314f
Brown-Séquard syndrome, 75,
288
Brucella, 236
Brucellosis, osteomyelitis and,
236–237
Bulbocavernosus reflex, in trauma
patient, 76–77
Burst fracture
osteoporotic, 322
thoracolumbar spine, 298, 299f

C
Calcification
intervertebral disc, 179, 179f
intervertebral disc calcification
syndrome, 234
Calcitonin, parenteral
for osteoporosis, 324–325
in osteoporotic vertebral
fracture, 323
Calcium
recommended daily intake, 324
supplementation, 324
Calcium deficiency, osteoporosis
and, 324
Cancellous bone, vertebral body,
126
Carotid tubercle, 6, 6f, 51
Caudad, 2
Cauda equina, 26
anatomy, 22, 22f
compression, 220
Cauda equina syndrome, 195,
195f
surgical management, 195
results, 194
thoracolumbar ankylosing
spondylitis and, 252
Caudal aplasia, 45
Central cord syndrome, 76, 288

Cephalad, 2
Cerebral palsy, scoliosis and, 263
Cerebrospinal fluid, in
meningitis, 239
Cervical rib, 43
Cervical spine
angulation, measurement, 121f
ankylosing spondylitis, 249,
251, 251f
atlantoaxial (A-A) distance,
119, 120f
atlantoaxial articulation, 11,
11f
atlantoaxial ligamentous
complex, 14, 14f
biomechanics, 116–124
failure mechanisms, 119–122
kinematics, 116–117
kinetics, 117–119
bony anatomy, 3f, 4f–6f, 4–7
atlas (C1), 4, 5f
axis (C2), 4, 5f
C3-C6, 4, 6, 6f
lateral aspect, 4f
vertebra prominens (C7),
6–7, 7f
"clunk" test, 52
compression-traction test, 52,
53f
CT myelogram, 104f
CT scan
axial, 91, 92f, 93f
sagittal reformation, 91, 93f
deep tendon reflexes, 54–55,
55f, 55t
degenerative disease, 180–183
clinical presentation,
180–181
CT scan, 182
diagnostic evaluation,
181–182
discography, 182, 183f
facet blocks in, 182
magnetic resonance imaging,
182, 182f
radiographic findings, 181f,
181–182
stenosis and, 216, 217f
treatment, 182–183
nonoperative, 182
operative, 183
degenerative disease and,
121–122
diffuse idiopathic skeletal
hyperostosis, 254
facet joints, 12, 12f
dislocations, 293, 294f, 295f
subluxation, 293–294

Cervical spine (*continued*)
  failure mechanisms, 119–122
    degenerative disease,
        121–122
    trauma, 119
    tumor, 119–121
  fracture
    comminuted, 294, 296f
    hangman's, 291, 293f
    Jefferson fracture, 290, 291f
    odontoid process, 291, 292f
    radiographic findings, 288,
        289f
  herniated disc disease, 197–200
    clinical presentation,
        197–198
    diagnostic evaluation,
        198f–199f, 198–199
    treatment, 199–200
      nonoperative, 199–200
      operative, 200, 200f
  inspection, 50, 50f, 51f
  instability, 119–122
    degenerative disease,
        121–122
    diagnostic checklist, 122t
    measurement, 119, 121f
    trauma and, 119
    tumor and, 119–121
  interspinous (nuchal) ligament,
      16, 17f
  juvenile rheumatoid arthritis,
      247–248
  kinematics, 116–117
    anatomic basis, 116
    kinematic properties,
        116–117
  kinetics, 117–119
    intervertebral disc, 117–119,
        119f
    spinal ligaments, 117, 118f
  L'Hermitte's sign, 52, 52f
  ligaments, 117, 118f
  lower (C3–C7), 116, 117f
    bony anatomy, 4, 6f, 6–7, 7f
    range of motion, 116–117
    rheumatoid arthritis, 245f
    trauma, 292–295
      clay shoveler's injury, 294
      extension injury, 294
      facet dislocations, 293,
          294f, 295f
      facet subluxation, 293–294
      flexion injury, 294, 295f
      fracture of lateral elements,
          294
  magnetic resonance imaging,
      97, 99f

  motor examination, 52–53
  myelography, 102f
  nerve root pathways, 26–27,
      27f
  nerve roots, 25f
    compression, 157, 157f. *See
        also* Nerve roots,
        compression
  occipitoatlantal joint, 10f, 11
    dislocation/fracture, 290
  occipitoatlantal ligamentous
      complex, 13, 14f
  occipitoaxial ligamentous
      complex, 13, 15f
  palpation, 51–52
  physical examination, 50–55
  psoriatic arthritis, 253
  radiography, 80–83
    anteroposterior (AP) view,
        80, 81f
    intervertebral disc space
        height, 80
    lateral view, 80, 81f
    oblique view, 80, 82f
    open-mouth view, 82, 82f
    pillar views, 83, 84f
    soft tissue examination, 80
    swimmer's view, 82–83, 83f
    vertebral body alignment, 80
  range of motion, 50–51, 51f,
      52f, 116–117
  rheumatoid arthritis, 244–246,
      245f
  sensory examination, 53–54
  spinal cord compression
    surgical management, 158,
        159f
    tumor and, 119–121
  spinal cord enlargement, 22,
      22f
  spondylolisthesis, 203–204
  stabilization, 122–124
    anterior plating, 123, 123f,
        165f
    buttressing, 123, 123f
    cervicothoracic orthoses, 122
    collars, 122
    external, 122
    halo devices, 122
    internal, 122f, 123, 123f,
        124f
    lag screw fixation, 123, 123f
    laminar hook fixation, 123,
        125f
    posterior C1-C2 wiring,
        122f, 123
    screw-plate fixation, 123,
        124f

  tension banding, 123
    wiring, 123, 124f
  stenosis, 216–219
    acquired, 216–217, 217t
    clinical presentation, 217
    congenital, 216, 217t
    diagnostic evaluation,
        217–218
    etiology, 216–217, 217t
    nonoperative management,
        219
    surgical options, 218–219
    treatment, 218–219
  subaxial. *See* Cervical spine,
      lower
  surgery, anterior approach,
      149, 153
    incisions, 152f
  tomography, 90, 90f
  trauma, 119
    atlas, 290–291, 291f
    imaging studies, 288, 289f,
        290t
    lower spine, 292–295
    occipitocervical junction, 290
  tumor, 119–121
  uncovertebral joints, 12, 12f
  upper (C0–C2), 116, 117f
    bony anatomy, 4, 5f
    developmental anomalies,
        41–43
    differentiation, 40, 40f
    range of motion, 116
    surgery, anterior approaches,
        154, 155f
    trauma
      atlas (C1), 290–291, 291f
      axis (C2), 291, 292f, 293f
      occipitocervical junction,
          290
  vascular anatomy, 29–30, 30f
  vertebral body, neoplastic
      involvement, 121
  vertebral displacement,
      measurement of, 119,
      121f
  vertebra prominens (C7), 6–7,
      7f
Cervical traction, 142f
Cervicothoracic junction, surgical
    exposure, 157
Chaddock's test, 73, 75f
Chamberlain's line, 41, 80, 244,
    245f
Chance fracture, 298
Check ligaments, 13, 15f
Chemonucleolysis
  contraindications, 192, 192t

indications, 192t
injection technique, 192, 192f
lumbar herniated disc, 192, 192f, 192t
Chemotherapy
    metastatic disease, 315
    in tuberculosis, 235
Chest expansion
    measurement, 56, 58f
    normal minimum, 56
Chest tenderness, thoracic herniated disc and, 196, 196f
Chest wall, pain, thoracic nerve root compression and, 158
Chest x-ray, in spinal tuberculosis, 235
Chiropractic therapy, 141
Chondrification, vertebral development, 39, 39f
Chordoma, 310–311, 312f
Chymopapain. *See* Chemonucleolysis
Claudication, neurogenic, 220
Clay shoveler's injury, 294
Clonus, 73
    testing, 73, 74f
Cluneal nerves, 167
"Clunk" test, 52
Cobb technique, measurement of scoliosis, 272, 272f
Coccidioides sp., 238
Coccidioidomycosis, osteomyelitis and, 238
Coccyx
    bony anatomy, 3f, 9, 10f
    nerve root pathways, 28
Cock-robin deformity, 50f
Collagen
    in annulus fibrosus, 185
    intervertebral disc, 11
Colles' fracture, 320
Commissures, 22, 23f
Compression fractures, 295–298, 320–322
Compression-traction test, 52, 52f
Computed tomography (CT scan), 91–96
    aneurysmal bone cyst, 307f
    breast cancer metastatic to spine, 313f
    burst fracture, thoracolumbar spine, 300f
    in cervical rheumatoid arthritis, 247f
    cervical spine, 91, 92f-93f

cervical stenosis, 218
chordoma, 312f
CT discography
    in degenerative disease
        cervical spine, 183f
        lumbar spine, 177
    in herniated disc disease
        cervical, 198, 199f
        lumbar, 189
        thoracic, 196
CT myelography, 100, 104f
    hemangioma, 308f
    in herniated disc disease
        cervical, 198, 198f
        lumbar, 189
        thoracic, 196, 197f
    in thoracolumbar stenosis, 225, 226f
degenerative disease
    cervical spine, 182
    lumbar spine, 174, 176f
empty nest sign, 301f
giant cell tumor, 310f
hemangioma, 308f
Hounsfield units, 91
lumbar facet joints, in ankylosing spondylitis, 249, 250f
mechanisms of scanning, 91, 92f
myeloma, 311f
osteoblastoma, 309f
osteoid osteoma, 308f
    nidus, 310f
pseudarthrosis, 168f
quantitative, bone mass measurement, 319
spondylolisthesis, 209, 211f
thoracic spine, 91, 94, 94f, 95f
thoracolumbar stenosis, 224–225
vertebral bacterial osteomyelitis, 231, 232f
Conus medullaris, 20, 22f, 26
Cornua, coccygeal, 9, 10f
Coronary artery(ies), 33, 34f
Corsets, 129
Cortical bone, vertebral body, 125
Corticospinal tract, 24t
Costal ligaments, 17, 18f
Costocentral articulation, 13
Costotransverse articulation, 13
Costotransversectomy, 156f, 157
    in herniated disc disease, thoracic, 197

Costotransverse ligament complex, 17, 18f
Costovertebral articulation, 12–13, 13f
Cotrel-Dubousset instrumentation, in scoliosis, 276f
Cotrell traction, 142
Craniosacral therapy, 141–142
Crankshaft phenomenon, 274
Creep, 114, 115f
Cremasteric reflex, superficial, 65, 66f
Crossover test, 67, 71f
Cruciform ligament, 14, 15f
Cryotherapy, 138
Cryptococcosis, osteomyelitis and, 237
Cryptococcus sp., 237
Culture studies
    in disc space infection, 232–233
    in vertebral bacterial osteomyelitis, 231

D
Decompression
    cervical spine, 122
    surgical, 148
Degenerative disease, 173–184. *See also specific spinal segments*
    cervical spine, 121–122, 180–183
    key points, 184
    lumbar spine, 174–178
    thoracic spine, 179–180
    thoracolumbar spine, 129
Dens. *See* Odontoid process
Dermatome, 36
    cervical, 54f
    lumbar, 64f
    sacral, 64f
    thoracic, 59f
Developmental anomalies, 40–47
    arcuate foramen, 42
    Arnold-Chiari malformation, 41, 41f
    basilar invagination (impression), 41–42
    block vertebra, 44–45
    cervical rib, 43
    cervical spine, 41–43
    cutaneous manifestations, 59, 260
    failures of formation, 40–41

Developmental anomalies
(*continued*)
failures of segmentation, 41
key points, 47
Klippel-Feil syndrome, 42–43,
44f
kyphosis, 45
lumbosacral junction, 45
meningocele, 46
myelomeningocele, 46, 47, 47f
neural structures, 46–47
occipitalization of atlas, 42
odontoid agenesis/hypoplasia,
42
os odontoideum, 42, 44f
ossification of posterior arch of
atlas, 42
platybasia, 41
rachischisis, 46–47
sacral agenesis, 45
scoliosis, 44–45
spina bifida, 46
spinal dysraphism, 46–47
thoracolumbar spine, 44–45
torticollis, 42
unilateral unsegmented bar, 45
Diabetes mellitus, diffuse
idiopathic skeletal
hyperostosis and, 254
Diet, calcium deficiency,
osteoporosis and, 324
Disc. *See* Intervertebral disc
Discectomy
cervical, 158f
lumbar, 193–194, 194f
percutaneous
automated, 192–193, 193f
lumbar herniated disc,
192–193, 193f
Discitis, 234
adult. *See* Infections, disc space
infection
Discography
CT scan after. *See* Computed
tomography, CT
discography
in degenerative disease
cervical spine, 182, 183f
thoracic, 180
Disc space infection. *See*
Infections, disc space
infection (adult)
DISH (diffuse idiopathic skeletal
hyperostosis), 254,
254f
Dizziness, in degenerative
disease, cervical, 181
Dorsal root ganglion, 23f, 25, 28

Down's syndrome, atlantoaxial
instability in, 42, 43f
Drug therapy
analgesics, 143
antibiotics. *See* Antimicrobial
drugs
in degenerative disease
cervical spine, 182
lumbar spine, 178
metastatic disease, 315
muscle relaxants, 144
NSAIDs, 143–144, 144t
in spinal tuberculosis, 235
topical
iontophoresis, 140
phonophoresis, 137–138
Dual energy x-ray absorptometry,
319
Duchenne muscular dystrophy,
scoliosis and, 263,
265f
Dural sac compression, 158–160
spinal stenosis, 215, 216f
in spinal tuberculosis, 235,
236f
Dura mater, 22, 23f
Dwyer system, in scoliosis, 274,
277f
Dysphagia
in degenerative disease,
cervical, 181
diffuse idiopathic skeletal
hyperostosis and, 254

E
Ectoderm, 36
Education. *See* Patient education
Elasticity
creep, 114, 115f
elastic range, 114, 114f
modulus of, 110, 111f
viscoelastic properties, 114
Electromyography
in cervical stenosis, 218
in herniated disc disease
cervical, 199
lumbar, 188
in spondylolisthesis, 210
Electrotherapy, 138–140
high-voltage galvanic
stimulation, 138, 139f
in idiopathic scoliosis, 273,
275f
instrumentation, 138, 139f
interferential current,
138–139, 139f
iontophoresis, 140

transcutaneous electrical nerve
stimulation, 139–140,
140f
Embryology, 35–40
differentiation of vertebrae,
35–36, 39f–40f, 39–40
embryonic period, 35, 36, 37f
fetal period, 37
pre-embryonic period, 35, 36,
36f
stages of development, 35
Embryonic disc, 36
EMG. *See* Electromyography
Empty nest sign, 301f
Endoderm, 36
End plate, vertebral, 11–12
Enthesopathy, 248
Epidural space infection (abscess),
238–239
diagnosis, 239
etiology and pathogenesis,
238–239
treatment, 239
Erector spinae muscles, 18–20,
19f
Erythrocyte sedimentation rate,
vertebral bacterial
osteomyelitis and, 230
Escherichia coli, vertebral
osteomyelitis, 230
Estrogen replacement therapy,
osteoporosis and, 324
Ethnicity, osteoporosis and, 318
Evoked potentials
factors affecting, 170
intraoperative spinal cord
monitoring, 169–170,
170f
somatosensory
cortical evoked potentials,
169–170
in herniated disc disease,
lumbar spine, 188
spinal evoked potentials, 170
spinal-spinal evoked potentials,
170
Ewing's sarcoma, 309–310
Exercise, 136–137
aerobic, 136
contraindications, 136
extension, 136, 137f
flexion, 136, 136f
for lumbar herniated disc, 191
osteoporosis and, 324
Extension
ligamentous resistance, 118f
range of motion, cervical spine,
51, 51f

Extension exercises, 136, 137f
Extension injury, cervical spine, 294
Extremity, lower
  autonomous sensory zones, 65f
  deep tendon reflexes, 65–66, 66f, 67f, 67t
  muscles, nerve root innervation, 63, 63t
Extremity, upper
  cervical herniated disc disease and, 197
  deep tendon reflexes, 54–55, 55t
  muscles, nerve root innervation, 53, 54t

F

Fabere test, sacroiliac joints, 72, 72f
Facet block, 177
  in degenerative disease
    cervical, 182
    lumbar, 177
    thoracic, 180
Facet joints, 12, 12f
  degenerative changes, 174
  tropism, 84
Fasciculus(i), 17
Fatigue strength, 114, 115f
Femoral stretch test, 67, 70f
  in herniated disc disease, lumbar, 186
Fenamate, 144t
Fever, vertebral bacterial osteomyelitis and, 230
Fibromyalgia, 254
Fibrositis. *See* Fibromyalgia
Filum terminale, 22, 22f
Finger escape sign, 74, 76f
Fissures, 22, 23f
Flexion
  forward, lumbar spine, thoracolumbar stenosis and, 220, 223f
  ligamentous resistance, 118f
  range of motion, cervical spine, 51, 51f
Flexion exercises, 136, 136f
Flexion injury, cervical spine, 294, 295f
Fluoride. *See* Sodium fluoride
Foot dorsiflexion test, 66, 68f
Foramen transversarium, atlas, 4, 5f
Foraminal stenosis, 220
Foraminotomy, 227

Force, 109, 110f
Fracture(s)
  atlas (C1), 119, 120f, 290, 291f
  burst fracture
    osteoporotic, 322
    thoracolumbar spine, 298, 299f
  cervical spine
    in ankylosing spondylitis, 251, 251f
    radiographic findings, 288, 289f, 291f–296f
  clay shoveler's injury, 294
  flexion-distraction, thoracolumbar spine, 298, 300f
  hangman's, 291, 293f
  Jefferson, 119, 120f, 290, 291f
  lumbar spine
    multiple myeloma and, 322, 322f
    osteoporosis-associated, 320f
  odontoid process, 291, 292f
    lag screw fixation, 123, 123f
  osteoporosis-associated, 318. *See also* Osteoporosis, fractures
    acute kyphosis and, 56, 57f, 323, 323f
    Colles' fracture of distal radius, 320
    hip, 320
    vertebral, 320–324
      classification, 321, 321f
      diagnosis, 321–322
      management, 322–324
  pars interarticularis
    spondylolisthesis and, 204
    thoracolumbar, 297
  sacral spine, 300–301, 302f
  spinous process
    C7, 294
    thoracolumbar, 297
  thoracic spine, 128
  thoracolumbar spine, 128, 295–300
  thoracolumbar stenosis and, 219
  transverse process, thoracolumbar, 297
  wedge compression fracture, thoracic, 297, 297f
Fracture-dislocation
  cervical, 293, 294, 294f
  thoracolumbar, 298
Frontal plane, 2
FSU. *See* Spine, functional spinal unit

Fusion
  lumbar facet joints, in ankylosing spondylitis, 249, 250f
  sacroiliac joints, in ankylosing spondylitis, 249, 249f
  surgical. *See* Spinal surgery, fusion
  in vertebral bacterial osteomyelitis, 231

G

Gadolinium, MRI enhancement, 191, 191f
Gaenslen's test, sacroiliac joints, 72, 73f
Gait
  in spasticity, 73
  in spondylolisthesis, lumbar, 206
Gallium 67. *See* Radionuclide scanning
Gastrocnemius-soleus muscle group
  evaluation, 63, 63f
  in herniated disc disease, lumbar, 186
Gastrointestinal hemorrhage, NSAIDs and, 144
Gender
  ankylosing spondylitis and, 248
  diffuse idiopathic skeletal hyperostosis and, 254
  idiopathic scoliosis and, 266
  osteoporosis and, 317
  Reiter's disease and, 252
  rheumatoid arthritis and, 244
  spondylolisthesis type II and, 204
Genitourinary tract. *See* Urinary tract
Giant cell tumor, 308, 310f
  treatment, 311
Gibbus, in spinal tuberculosis, 234
Gillet's maneuver, 71, 71f
Gluteus maximus muscle, evaluation, 63, 64f
Gout, diffuse idiopathic skeletal hyperostosis and, 254
Graft. *See* Bone graft
Gray ramus communicans, 26
Gray substance, spinal cord, 22, 23f
Grip and release test, 74

H

Halo device, 122
Hamstring reflex, nerve root
        innervation, 67t
Hand, myelopathic, 74
Hangman's fracture, 291, 293f
Harrington, Paul, 162
Harrington rod, 162–164, 163f
    in scoliosis, 274, 276f
Headache, in degenerative
        disease, cervical, 181
Head posture
    cervical spine evaluation, 50,
        50f, 51f
    cock-robin deformity, 50f
Heat therapy, 137, 138f
    contraindications, 137
Hemangioma, 307, 308f
    treatment, 311
Hematoma, central cord
        syndrome and, 76
Hemiepiphysiodesis, 262, 262f
Hemilaminectomy, 193
Hemivertebra, 45
    scoliosis and, 259, 259f
Hiatus, sacral, 9
Hip fracture, osteoporosis-
        associated, 320
History taking, 49–50
    in adult scoliosis, 276–277
    in congenital scoliosis, 260
    in osteoporotic vertebral
        fracture, 322
HLA-B27
    ankylosing spondylitis and, 248
    Reiter's disease and, 252
Hoffmann's sign, 74, 76f
Hooks, for internal fixation, 133,
        133f, 162, 165f, 169f
Hoover's test, 77, 77f
Hormone replacement therapy,
        osteoporosis and, 324
Hounsfield units, 91
Human immunodeficiency virus
        (HIV), tuberculosis
        and, 234
Hydrocephalus, in Arnold-Chiari
        malformation, 41
Hydrosteroids, for metastatic
        disease, 315
Hyperkyphosis, thoracic, 280
Hyperostosis
    diffuse idiopathic skeletal
        hyperostosis, 254
    idiopathic vertebral, lumbar,
        174
Hyperuricemia. *See* Gout
Hypoplasia, odontoid, 42

I

Ibuprofen, 144t
Iliac artery(ies), 31f, 32
Iliacus muscle, 20, 21f
Iliocostalis muscles, 18, 19f, 20
Iliolumbar artery(ies), 31f, 32
Iliolumbar ligament, 17, 18f
Imaging studies, 79–106. *See also*
        specific modalities
    in adult scoliosis, 277
    in basilar invagination, 42
    computed tomography (CT
        scan), 91–96
    key points, 106
    magnetic resonance imaging,
        97–100
    in metastatic disease,
        313f–314f, 313–314
    myelography, 100, 102f–105f
    radiography, 79–90
    radionuclide scanning, 104,
        106
    spinal tumor, 306–307
    tomography, 90
    trauma patient, 288–290, 289f
Immobilization. *See also* Bed rest;
        Orthoses/orthotics
    for pars interarticularis
        fracture, 297
    trauma patient, 287
Immunocompromise, and
        infection, 229, 234,
        238
Immunoglobulin(s), IgM, in
        rheumatoid arthritis,
        244
Implant(s), 162–165
    anterior cervical plating, 123,
        123f, 164f
    artificial intervertebral disc,
        328, 328f
    breakage, 167, 169f
    cervical spine stabilization, 123
    failure, 167, 169f
    Harrington rods, 162, 163f,
        164
    historical perspective, 162, 164
    in idiopathic scoliosis
        Cotrel-Dubousset
            instrumentation, 274,
            276f
        Dwyer system, 274, 277f
        Harrington instrumentation,
            274, 276f
        Zielke system, 274, 277f
    Kostuik-Harrington system,
        anterior, 164f

mechanical disassembly/
        loosening, 167, 169f
    posterior hook and rod system,
        165f
    posterior pedicle screw system,
        166f
    posterior plating system, 165f
    postoperative infections,
        239–240
    thoracolumbar spine
        stabilization, 133, 133f
Indium. *See* Radionuclide
        scanning
Infections, 229–240
    discitis, 234
    disc space infection (adult),
        232–233
        diagnostic findings, 232–233
        etiology, 232
        treatment, 233
    epidural space infection,
        238–239
    intradural, 239
    key points, 240
    meningitis, 239
    myelitis, 239
    nonbacterial, nontuberculous
        osteomyelitis,
        236–238
    postoperative, 239–240
    systemic, Reiter's disease and,
        252
    tuberculosis of spine, 234–236
    vertebral bacterial
        osteomyelitis,
        229–232. *See also*
        Osteomyelitis,
        bacterial
Inflammatory diseases, 243–255
    arachnoiditis, 255
    key points, 255
    rheumatologic. *See also*
        Rheumatic diseases
        diffuse idiopathic skeletal
            hyperostosis, 254
        fibromyalgia, 254
        seronegative diseases,
            248–253
        seropositive diseases,
            244–248
Inspection
    cervical spine, 50, 50f, 51f
    scoliosis, 55
    thoracic spine, 55–56, 56f
    trauma patient, 74
Instability
    cervical spine, 119–122, 122t
    metastatic disease and, 313

thoracolumbar spine, 128–129, 129t
Interbody fusion. *See* Spinal surgery, fusion
Intercostal artery(ies), 30, 31f
Internal fixation. *See* Implant(s)
Interspinous ligaments, 16, 17f
Interstriation angle, 11, 11f
Intertransversarii muscles, 20
Intertransverse ligament, 17, 18f
Intervertebral disc
   anatomy, 11f, 11–12, 117–118, 119f
   artificial, 328, 328f
   biomechanical properties, 117–119
   calcification, 179, 179f
   calcification syndrome, 234
   cervical spine, 117–119
   degenerative disease, 173–174
   embryology, 37, 38f
   excision. *See* Discectomy
   extruded disc rupture, 186, 187f
   herniation, 185–201. *See also specific spinal segments*
      anatomic considerations, 185–186, 187f
      cervical, 197–200
      degrees of, 187f
      herniated nucleus pulposus, 185–186, 187f
      intraspongi nuclear herniation, 186, 187f
      key points, 201
      lumbar, 186–195
      nerve root compression and, 157–158
      thoracic, 196–197
   kinetics, 126–127, 127f, 128
   prolapsed, 186
   protrusion, 186
      sciatica and, 66
   sequestered, 186, 187f
   vascular anatomy, 33, 34f
Intradiscal pressures, 128
Intraoperative monitoring, 167, 168–170
Inverse traction, 142
Iontophoresis, 140

J

Jefferson fracture, 119, 120f, 290, 291f
   odontoid fracture and, 291f

Jendrassik maneuver, 65, 67f
Joint(s)
   atlantoaxial, 11, 11f
   facet, 12, 12f
   of Luschka. *See* Uncovertebral joints
   occipitoatlantal, 10f, 11
   rheumatic diseases. *See* Rheumatic diseases
   sacroiliac, physical examination, 69–72
   uncovertebral, 12, 12f
   zygoapophyseal. *See* Facet joints
Juvenile rheumatoid arthritis, 246–248
   categories, 246–247
   cervical spine, 247–248

K

Kinematics, 116. *See also specific spinal section*
Kinetics, 116. *See also specific spinal section*
Klippel-Feil syndrome, 42–43, 44f
   inspection in, 50, 51f
Knee clonus, 73
Knee jerk. *See* Quadriceps reflex
Kostuik-Harrington system, anterior, 164f
Kyphosis, 2, 280–285
   acute angular, 282, 282f
   adult, 282–283
      classification, 283t
      evaluation, 283, 284f, 285f
      moment arm in, 283f
      treatment, 283
   cervical, in ankylosing spondylitis, 251, 251f
   congenital, 45, 280
   in congenital scoliosis, 260, 261f
   measurement on lateral x-ray, 281f
   multiple levels, 282f
   neuromuscular, 285f
   normal amount, 280
   osteoporotic vertebral fracture and, 56, 57f, 323, 323f
   posture and, 280
   radiographic findings, 283, 284f, 285f
   Scheuermann's, 280f, 280–282
      poor posture vs, 281f
   spinal dysraphism and, 47

spinal tuberculosis and, 235, 237f
   structural excessive, 280
   thoracic, 55–56, 57f, 280–285
   thoracolumbar, 251, 252f, 253f
   tuberculosis of spine and, 284f
   types of deformity, 282f

L

Laboratory tests, in osteoporotic vertebral fracture, 322
Lamellae, intervertebral disc, 11
Laminectomy, 148, 193
   in cauda equina syndrome, 195
   cervical, 158, 159f
Laminoplasty
   cervical, 158, 159f
   in cervical stenosis, 218–219
Laminotomy, lumbar, 193, 193f
Lasègue's sign, 67, 69f
Laser therapy, percutaneous discectomy, 192–193
Lateral bending, range of motion, cervical spine, 51, 51f
Lateral masses
   atlas, 4, 5f
   axis, 4
   cervical vertebrae, 6
Lateral recess
   boundaries, 219, 222f
   stenosis. *See* Spinal stenosis
Lateral rotation, range of motion, cervical spine, 51, 52f
Leg pain, herniated disc disease and, lumbar, 186
Leg raising test
   straight, 66, 68f
      in herniated disc disease, lumbar, 186
      nonorganic pathology, 77
   well-leg raising test, 67, 70f
      in herniated disc disease, lumbar, 186
Leukomyelitides, 239
Levator costae muscles, 19f, 20
L'Hermitte's sign, 52, 52f
Lifting, 127
Ligament(s), 13–17
   alar, 13, 15f
   anterior longitudinal, 14–15, 16f
   apical, 13, 15f
   atlantoaxial, 14, 14f
   biomechanical properties, 117, 118f
   cervical spine, 117, 118f

Ligament(s) (*continued*)
  check, 13, 15f
  costal, 17, 18f
  cruciform, 14, 15f
  iliolumbar, 17, 18f
  interspinous, 16, 17f
  intertransverse, 17, 18f
  ligamentum flavum, 16, 16f
  lumbosacral, 17, 18f
  nuchal, 16, 17f
  occipitoatlantal, 13, 14f
  occipitoaxial, 13, 15f
  ossification
    in ankylosing spondylitis,
      149, 150f
    in thoracolumbar ankylosing
      spondylitis, 252
  posterior longitudinal, 15–16,
    16f
  Sickle. *See* Lumbosacral
    ligament
  stellate. *See* Anterior
    costovertebral
    ligament complex
  supraspinous, 16, 17f
  transverse, 14
    rupture, 290–291
Ligamentum denticulatum, 22,
  23f
Ligamentum flavum, 16, 16f
Load, 112–115
  thoracolumbar spine, 125–127
Longissimus muscles, 19f, 20
Longitudinal fascicles, 14
Longitudinal ligament
  anterior, 14–15, 16f
  posterior, 15–16, 16f
    in central disc herniation,
      195
    ossification, 217, 217f, 218f
Longus capitis muscle, 20, 21f
Longus colli muscle, 20, 21f
Lordosis, 2, 280
Lumbar puncture, in meningitis,
  239
Lumbar spine
  angulation, measurement, 131f
  ankylosing spondylitis, 249,
    250f
  bony anatomy, 3f, 7, 8f, 9f
  compressive loads and lifting,
    127–128
  CT myelogram, 104f
    sagittal reformation, 105f
  degenerative disease, 174–178
    clinical presentation, 174
    CT scan in, 174, 176f

diagnostic evaluation,
    174–177
discography in, 176–177
facet blocks in, 177
magnetic resonance imaging,
    176, 176f, 177f
radiographic findings, 174,
    175f
risk factors, 174, 178
treatment, 177–178
  nonoperative, 177–178
  operative, 178
facet joints, 12, 12f
forward flexion, thoracolumbar
    stenosis and, 220, 223f
fracture
  multiple myeloma and, 322,
    322f
  osteoporosis-associated, 320f
herniated disc disease, 186–195
  central disc herniation, 195,
    195f
  clinical presentation, 186
  CT discography in, 189, 190f
  CT myelography in, 189
  diagnostic evaluation,
    188–191
  electromyography in, 188
  magnetic reaonance imaging
    in, 189–191,
    190f–191f
  pain in, 186
  physical examination, 186
  radiographic findings, 188f,
    189
  risk factors, 186
  somatosensory evoked
    potentials in, 188
  surgical management,
    191–194
    chemonucleolysis, 192,
      192f, 192t
    discectomy, 193–194,
      194f
    indications, 191
    percutaneous discectomy,
      192–193, 193f
  treatment, 191–194
    nonoperative, 191
    operative, 191–194
instability. *See also*
    Thoracolumbar spine
diagnostic checklist, 129t
segmental, 174
kinematics, 124, 126f
kinetics, 128–129. *See also*
    Thoracolumbar spine

magnetic resonance imaging,
    100, 101f, 102f
myelography, 103f
nerve root pathways, 28, 28f
nerve roots, 25f
  compression, 158
physical examination. *See*
    Lumbosacral spine
range of motion, 124–125
retrolisthesis, 205, 207f
spinal cord compression, 158
spinal cord enlargement, 22,
  22f
spondylolisthesis, 204–213
  classification, 204f–206f,
    204t, 204–206
  clinical presentation, 206,
    207f
  diagnostic evaluation,
    206–210
  radiographic findings,
    206–209, 209f–211f
  treatment, 211–213
surgery
  anterior approaches,
    153–154
    anterior retroperitoneal
      approach, 154, 154f
    anterior transperitoneal
      approach, 154, 155f
    anterolateral flank
      approach, 153–154
  posterior approach, 150f
    incisions, 149, 152f
    patient positioning, 149,
      151f
  vascular anatomy, 30–32, 31f
  vertebral displacement,
    measurement, 131f
Lumbosacral junction
  developmental anomalies, 45,
    45f
  cutaneous changes, 59
  segmentation abnormality, 45,
    45f
Lumbosacral ligament, 17, 18f
Lumbosacral spine
  CT scan, 94
    axial, 94, 96f
    sagittal reformation, 94, 97f
  inspection, 59–60, 60f, 61f
  motor examination, 63, 64f
  nerve root tension, tests of,
    66–67, 68f, 69f
  palpation, 63
  pelvic obliquity, 60
  physical examination, 59–69

radiography, 84, 87–88
  anteroposterior (AP) view,
    84, 87f
  Hibbs' views, 88, 89f
  lateral view, 84, 87, 88f
  oblique views, 87–88, 89f
range of motion, 60, 61f, 62f
reflexes, 65–66, 66f, 67f, 67t
Schober test, 60, 61f
sensory examination, 65
spondylolisthesis, 207, 209f
stabilization, 129, 132f, 133
tomography, 91f
Lung. *See also* Pulmonary
    function
  in spinal tuberculosis, 234
Lupus erythematosus, systemic,
    248
Luque technique, in scoliosis, 274
Luschka, joints of. *See*
    Uncovertebral joints
Lymphoma, 310

M
Magnetic resonance imaging
    (MRI), 97–100
  aneurysmal bone cyst, 307f
  aspergillar spinal osteomyelitis,
    238, 238f
  in cervical rheumatoid arthritis,
    246, 247f, 248f
  cervical spine, 97, 99f
  in cervical stenosis, 218
  chordoma, 312f
  in degenerative disease
    cervical spine, 182, 182f
    lumbar spine, 176, 176f, 177f
    thoracic spine, 179, 180f
  gadolinium-enhanced, in
    herniated disc disease,
    lumbar, 191, 191f
  hemangioma, 308f
  in herniated disc disease
    cervical, 198–199, 199f
    lumbar, 189–191, 190f–191f
    thoracic, 196, 197f
  lumbar spine, 100, 101f, 102f
  principles, 97, 98f
  prostate cancer metastatic to
    spine, 314f
  in spondylolisthesis, 209–210
  thoracic spine, 100, 100f
  in thoracolumbar stenosis,
    225–226, 227f
  in trauma patient, 288

T1-weighted image, 97, 100f
T2-weighted image, 97, 99f,
    101f, 102f
  in vertebral bacterial
    osteomyelitis, 231,
    232f
Malignant tumors. *See* Tumor(s),
    malignant
Malingering, reverse sciatic
    tension test in, 77
Manipulation, 140–141
  chiropractic, 141
  osteopathy, 141
Manual therapy, 140f, 140–142
  Alexander technique, 141
  alternate forms, 141–142
  chiropractic, 141
  craniosacral therapy, 141–142
  manipulation, 140–141
  massage, 141
  mobilization, 140
  osteopathy, 141
  physical therapy, 141
  shiatsu, 141
  structural integration (Rolfing),
    142
  Traeger approach, 141
Marie-Strümpell disease. *See*
    Ankylosing spondylitis
Massage, 141
McGregor's line, 244, 245f
McKenzie extension exercises,
    136
Median crest, sacral, 9
Meninges, anatomy, 22, 23f
Meningitis, 239
  cryptococcal, 237
Meningocele, 46, 47, 47f
Mesoderm, 36
Metallic implants. *See* Implant(s)
Metastatic disease, 311, 313–315
  neurologic deficit in, 313
  nonoperative management,
    314–315
  pain in, 314
  patient evaluation, 313–314
  spinal deformity/stability and,
    313
  surgical management, 315
  treatment considerations, 313t
Microdiscectomy, 194
Milwaukee brace, 273, 274f
  in Scheuermann's kyphosis,
    282
Mobilization therapy, 140
Modulus of elasticity, 110, 111f

Moment, 109, 110f
  increasing moment arm in
    kyphosis, 283f
Morula, 36
Motor examination
  cervical nerve roots, 52–53
  lumbosacral nerve roots, 63,
    63f, 64f
Motrin, 144t
Multifidus muscle, 19f, 20
Multiple myeloma. *See* Myeloma
Muscle(s)
  anterior, 20, 21f
  erector spinae, 18
  iliacus, 20, 21f
  iliocostalis group, 18, 19f, 20
  intertransversarii, 20
  levator costae, 19f, 20
  longissimus group, 19f, 20
  longus capitis, 20, 21f
  longus colli, 20, 21f
  lower extremity, nerve root
    innervation, 63, 63t
  multifidus, 19f, 20
  posterior, 17–20, 19f
  psoas, 20, 21f
  quadratus lumborum, 20, 21f
  rotators, 20
  semispinalis group, 19f, 20
  spasticity, 73
  spinalis, 19f, 20
  strength grading, 53t
  thoracolumbar kinetics and,
    127–128
  upper extremity, nerve root
    innervation, 53, 54t
  weakness. *See* Weakness
Muscle relaxants, 144
Muscular dystrophy, scoliosis
    and, 263, 265f
Mycobacterium tuberculosis,
    234. *See also*
    Tuberculosis
Myelitis, 239
  transverse, 248
Myelography, 100, 102f–104f
  CT scan after. *See* Computed
    tomography, CT
    myelography
  hemangioma, 308f
  in spondylolisthesis, 209, 212f
  in thoracic herniated disc
    disease, 196
  in thoracolumbar stenosis, 224,
    225f
  in vertebral bacterial
    osteomyelitis, 231

Myeloma, 308–309, 311f
  lumbar compression fracture
      and, 322, 322f
  osteopenia and, 318f
Myelomeningocele, 46, 47, 47f
  scoliosis and, 263
Myelopathy
  cervical stenosis and, 217
  diffuse idiopathic skeletal
      hyperostosis and, 254
  hand findings, 74
  physical examination, 72–74
  plantar response, 73–74
  spasticity, 73
Myerding technique,
      measurement of
      spondylolisthesis, 206
Myotome, 36

N

Naphthylakanones, 144t
Napoleon's hat, 207, 210f
Narcotic analgesics, 143
Nash technique, determination of
      vertebral rotation, 272,
      273f
Neck. *See* Cervical spine
Nerve conduction studies, in
      herniated disc disease,
      cervical, 199
Nerve root block, in
      spondylolisthesis, 210
Nerve roots
  cervical, 26–27, 27f
  compression
    cervical, 27, 157, 157f, 198,
        198f
    lumbar, 158
      disc herniation and, 186,
          187f
      spinal stenosis and, 215, 216f
      surgical management,
          157–158
      thoracic, 158
  lumbar, 28, 28f
  sacrococcygeal, 28
  spinal, 25, 25f
  tension
    bowstring sign, 66, 69f
    foot dorsiflexion test, 66, 68f
    Lasègue's sign, 67, 69f
    straight leg raising test, 66,
        68f
    tests, 66–67, 68f, 69f
    well-leg raising test, 67, 70f
  thoracic, 27f, 27–28

Neural folds, 36
Neural foramen(ina)
  cervical, 27
  lumbar, 28
  thoracic, 27
Neural tube, 36, 37f
Neuroanatomy, 26–29
  general, 26
  innervation of spine, 28–29,
      29f
  nerve-bone relationships,
      26–28, 27f, 28f
  nerve roots, 26–28
    cervical, 26–27, 27f
    lumbar, 28, 28f
    sacrococcygeal, 28
    thoracic, 27f, 27–28
  posterior primary ramus, 29,
      29f
  sinuvertebral nerve, 28–29,
      29f
Neurocentral synchondrosis, 39
Neuroglia/neuroglial cells, 22
Neurologic examination
  in idiopathic scoliosis, 269
  in osteoporotic vertebral
      fracture, 322
  in trauma patient, 75–77, 288
Neuromuscular kyphosis, 285f
Neuromuscular scoliosis. *See*
      Scoliosis,
      neuromuscular
Night pain, 306
Nociception, cervical nerves,
      53–54
Nonorganic evaluation, 77–78
Nonsteroidal anti-inflammatory
      drugs. *See* NSAIDs
Notochord, 36, 37f
NSAIDs, 143–144, 144t
  side effects, 144
Nuchal ligaments, 16, 17f
Nucleus pulposus, 118
  herniated, 185–186
  intervertebral disc, 11f, 12
Nutrient artery, 33, 34f

O

Observation
  in congenital scoliosis, 261
  in idiopathic scoliosis, 272
  in neuromuscular scoliosis, 263
Occipitoatlantal ligament, 13, 14f
  ossification, 42
Occipitoaxial ligament, 13, 15f

Occipitocervical
      (occipitoatlantal)
      articulation, 10f, 11.
      See also Cervical spine
  malformations, 41–43
Occiput (C0), 116, 117f
Odontoid process
  agenesis, 42
  anatomy, 4, 5f
  fracture, 291, 292f
    displaced, 292f
    Jefferson fracture and, 291f
    lag screw fixation, 123, 123f
    type I, 291, 292f
    type II, 291, 292f
    type III, 291, 292f
  hypoplasia, 42
  os odontoideum, 42, 44f
  ossification, 40
  in rheumatoid arthritis, 244f
Oppenheim's test, 73–74, 76f
Orthoses/orthotics, 143
  cervical, 143
    in degenerative disease, 182
  cervicothoracic, 122
  chair-back brace, 129, 132f
  corsets, 129
  hyperextension braces, 129,
      132f
  in idiopathic scoliosis,
      272–273, 274f
  lumbosacral, 143
    in degenerative disease, 178
  neuromuscular scoliosis and,
      263
  in osteoporotic vertebral
      fracture, 323
  pain relief from, 133
  rigid braces, 129, 132f
  in Scheuermann's kyphosis,
      281–282
  in scoliosis, congenital, 261
  Somi (sternal occipital
      mandibular
      immobilization), 122
  in spondylolisthesis, 211
  thoracolumbar, 129, 132f, 133,
      143
  thoracolumbosacral, 133
Os odontoideum, 42, 44f
Ossification
  atlas, 40, 40f
  axis, 40, 40f
  costal ossification center, 39
  dens, 40
  ligaments
    in ankylosing spondylitis,
        149, 150f

in thoracolumbar ankylosing
spondylitis, 252
occipitoatlantal ligament, 42
posterior arch of atlas, 42
posterior longitudinal ligament
cervical stenosis and, 217,
217f
segmental vs continuous,
218f
primary, vertebral
development, 39, 39f
sacrum, 40
secondary, vertebral
development, 39, 40f
Osteoarthritis, 173
Osteoblastoma, 307–308, 309f
treatment, 311
Osteoconduction, bone graft, 160
Osteogenesis, bone graft, 160
Osteoid osteoma, 307–308, 308f
treatment, 311
Osteoinduction, bone graft, 160
Osteomalacia, 317
Osteomyelitis
aspergillosis and, 238
bacterial, 229–232
clinical presentation, 230
diagnostic findings, 230–231
etiology, 229–230
treatment, 231–232
blastomycosis and, 237
brucellosis and, 236–237
coccidioidomycosis and, 238
cryptococcosis and, 237
nonbacterial, nontuberculous,
236–238
Osteopathy, 141
Osteopenia, 317
differential diagnosis, 309
myeloma and, 318f
Osteophyte
in diffuse idiopathic skeletal
hyperostosis, 254
nerve root compression and,
27, 27f, 157, 157f
Osteoporosis, 317–325
associated medical conditions,
318
calcitonin therapy, 324–325
calcium supplementation in,
324
definition, 317
epidemiology, 317–318
exercise and, 324
fractures, 318, 320–324
hip, 320
rates, 320

vertebral, 320–324
biconcave, 321f
bracing in, 323
classification, 321, 321f
compression, 321, 321f,
322
acute kyphosis and, 56,
57f, 323, 323f
neurologic deficit and,
322
lumbar spine, 320f
management, 322–324
pain and, 321
pain management, 323
wedge (crush), 321, 321f
investigational therapies, 325
key points, 325
prevention, 325
estrogen replacement
therapy, 324
risk factors, 318
safety considerations, 325
treatment, 324–325
vitamin D supplementation in,
324
Oxicam, 144t

P

Paget's disease
cervical stenosis and, 217
thoracolumbar stenosis and,
219, 221f
Pain
in adult scoliosis, 277
arm. *See* Arm, pain
chest wall, thoracic nerve root
compression and, 158
in degenerative disease
cervical, 181
lumbar, 174
thoracic, 179
in fibromyalgia, 254
herniated disc disease and
cervical, 197
lumbar, 186
L'Hermitte's sign, 52, 52f
management, in osteoporotic
vertebral fracture, 323
metastatic disease and, 314
osteoporotic vertebral fracture
and, 321
radicular, 186
relief, orthoses and, 133
in Scheuermann's kyphosis, 281
in spondylolisthesis, lumbar,
206
in thoracolumbar stenosis, 220

Palpation
cervical spine, 51–52
in fibromyalgia, 254, 255f
in herniated disc disease,
lumbar, 186
lumbosacral spine, 63
sacroiliac joints, 69, 71
in spondylolisthesis, lumbar,
206, 207f
in trauma patient, 74
Pannus, 244
Paralysis, epidural abscess and, 239
Parasympathetic nervous system.
See Autonomic
nervous system
Pars interarticularis, 7
fracture
spondylolisthesis and, 204
thoracolumbar spine, 297
spondylolisthesis, 204, 205f
radiographic evaluation, 207,
209, 210f
Pars lateralis, sacral, 9
Patient education
back school, 143
in osteoporotic vertebral
fracture, 322
Patrick's test. *See* Fabere test
Pediatric population
cervical spine radiographs, 80
discitis, 234
Pedicles
lumbar vertebrae, 7, 8f
thoracic vertebrae, 7, 8f
Pedicle screws. *See* Screws,
pedicle
Pelvic obliquity, 60
in neuromuscular scoliosis, 263
Pelvic traction, 142f
Pes cavus, spinal dysraphism and,
260
Philadelphia collar, 122
Photon absorptometry, 319
Physical examination, 49–78
in adult scoliosis, 277
in ankylosing spondylitis,
248–249
bowstring sign, 66, 69f
cervical spine, 50–55
compression-traction test,
52, 53f
deep tendon reflexes, 54–55
inspection, 50, 50f, 51f
L'Hermitte's sign, 52, 52f
motor examination, 52–53
palpation, 51–52
range of motion, 50–51, 51f
sensory examination, 53–54

Physical examination (*continued*)
  chest expansion, 56, 58f
  in congenital scoliosis, 260
  crossover test, 67, 71f
  in degenerative disease
    cervical spine, 181
    lumbar spine, 174
  femoral stretch test, 67, 70f
  foot dorsiflexion test, 66, 68f
  general examination, 50
  in herniated disc disease,
       lumbar, 186
  in idiopathic scoliosis, 268f,
       268–269, 269f–271f
  key points, 78
  Lasègue's sign, 67, 69f
  L'Hermitte's sign, 52, 52f
  lumbosacral spine, 59–69
    inspection, 59–60, 60f, 61f
    motor examination, 63, 63f,
       63t, 64f
    nerve root tension, 66–67,
       68f, 69f
    palpation, 63
    range of motion, 60, 62f
    rectal examination, 67, 69
    reflexes, 65–66, 66f, 67f, 67t
    sensory examination, 64f, 65
  myelopathic hand, 74, 76f
  myelopathy, 72–74
    plantar response, 73–74
    spasticity, 73
  nonorganic evaluation, 77–78
  order of, 50
  in osteoporotic vertebral
       fracture, 322
  in postoperative infections, 240
  rectal examination, 67, 69
  sacroiliac joints, 69–72
    Fabere test, 72, 72f
    Gaenslen's test, 72, 73f
    palpation, 69, 71
    range of motion, 71f, 71–72
    stress test, 72
  in Scheuermann's kyphosis,
       281
  in spondylolisthesis, lumbar,
       206
  straight leg raising test, 66, 68f
  thoracic spine, 55–59
    chest expansion, 56, 58f
    inspection, 55–56, 56f
    range of motion, 56, 58f
    reflexes, 56, 58, 59f
    rib cage asymmetry, 56f
    sensory examination, 58–59,
       59f
  in thoracolumbar stenosis, 221

trauma, 74–77
  inspection, 74
  neurologic examination,
       75–77
  palpation, 74
  trauma patient, 288
  well-leg raising test, 67, 70f
Physical therapy, 141
  in degenerative disease, cervical
       spine, 182
Pia mater, 22, 23f
Plantar response, 73–74
Plasmacytoma, 309
  treatment and prognosis, 311
Plasticity, plastic range, 114, 114f
Plating. *See* Implant(s)
Platybasia, 41
Poliomyelitis, scoliosis and, 263,
    264f
Posterior cord syndrome, 75, 288
Posterior (dorsal) plane, 2
Posterior longitudinal ligament.
    See Longitudinal
    ligament, posterior
Posterior primary ramus, 29, 29f
Posture
  head, cervical spine evaluation,
    50, 50f, 51f
  kyphosis and, 280
  in lumbar herniated disc
    disease, 186
  lumbosacral spine inspection,
    59–60, 60f
  poor, Scheuermann's kyphosis
    vs, 281f
  spondylolisthesis and, 59–60,
    60f
Pott's disease, 234
Propionic acid derivatives, 144t
Prostatic cancer, 311
Proteus sp., vertebral
    osteomyelitis, 230
Pseudarthrosis, 167, 167f, 168f,
    278
Pseudomonas sp., vertebral
    osteomyelitis, 230
Psoas muscle, 20, 21f
  abscess, in spinal tuberculosis,
    234, 235f
Psoriatic arthritis, 252–253
  cervical spine, 253
  thoracolumbar spine, 253
Pulmonary function,
    neuromuscular
    scoliosis and, 263
Pyranocarboxylic acid, 144t
Pyrazalones, 144t

Pyrrole acetic acid derivatives,
  144t

Q
Quadratus lumborum muscle, 20,
  21f
Quadriceps (knee jerk) reflex, 65,
  66f, 67t
Quadriplegia
  C4, 301–302
  C5, 302
  C6, 302

R
Race/racial factors. *See* Ethnicity
Rachischisis, 46–47
rad, 79
Radiation therapy
  metastatic disease, 315
  plasmacytoma, 311
Radicular pain
  epidural abscess and, 239
  herniated disc disease and,
    lumbar, 186
Radiculopathy
  cervical stenosis and, 217
  straight leg raising and, 66
Radiography, 79–90
  in adult kyphosis, 283, 284f,
    285f
  in adult scoliosis, 277
  in ankylosing spondylitis, 249,
    249f, 250f, 251f
  anteroposterior (AP) view
    cervical spine, 80, 81f
    lumbosacral spine, 84, 87f
    thoracic spine, 83–84, 85f
    thoracolumbar stenosis, 221,
       224f
  in arachnoiditis, 255
  aspergillar spinal osteomyelitis,
    238, 238f
  breast cancer metastatic to
    spine, 313f
  burst fracture, thoracolumbar
    spine, 300f
  in cervical rheumatoid arthritis,
    244, 247f
  cervical spine, 80–83, 81f, 82f
    anteroposterior (AP) view,
      80, 81f
    lateral view, 80, 81f
    oblique view, 80, 82f
    open-mouth view, 82, 82f

pillar views, 83, 84f
in trauma patient, 288, 289f, 290t, 291f, 292f–296f
cervical stenosis, 217–218
cervicothoracic junction, swimmer's view, 82f, 82–83
chordoma, 312f
in congenital scoliosis, 259f, 260
degenerative disease
cervical spine, 181f, 181–182
lumbar spine, 174, 175f
thoracic, 179, 179f
discitis, 234
disc space infection, 232, 233f
dynamic, 88, 90
flexion-distraction fracture, thoracolumbar spine, 301f
flexion-extension views, 88, 90
in cervical rheumatoid arthritis, 246
in cervical trauma, 119, 120f
measurement of angulation in lumbar spine, 132f
fracture-dislocation, thoracolumbar spine, 301f
giant cell tumor, 310f
hemivertebra, scoliosis and, 259f
implant failure, 169f
lateral view
cervical spine, 80, 81f
lumbosacral spine, 84, 87, 88f
thoracic spine, 84, 86f
thoracolumbar stenosis, 221, 224, 225f
in trauma patient, 288
lumbar instability, 129
lumbosacral spine, 84, 87–88
anteroposterior (AP) view, 84, 87f
Hibbs' views, 88, 89f
lateral view, 84, 87, 88f
oblique views, 87–88, 89f
in myeloma, 309, 311f
myeloma-induced osteopenia, 318f
Napoleon's hat, 207, 210f
oblique view
cervical spine, 80, 82f
lumbosacral spine, 87–88, 89f
pars interarticularis integrity, 207, 210f

osteoblastoma, 309f
in osteoporotic vertebral fracture, 322
pillar views, cervical spine, 83, 84f
pseudarthrosis, 168f
rads, 79
roentgen-equivalent man (rem), 79
roentgens (R), 79
scotty dog, 210f
skeletal maturity determination, 267
special views, 88, 90
spinal tuberculosis, 235, 236f
spinal tumor, 306
spondylolisthesis, lumbar, 206–209, 209f–211f
stretch films, 90
in trauma patient, 288
thoracic spine, 83–84
anteroposterior (AP) view, 83–84, 85f
lateral view, 84, 86f
thoracolumbar kyphosis, 253f
thoracolumbar spine, in trauma patient, 288, 290t
thoracolumbar stenosis, 221, 224, 224f, 225f
in trauma patient, 288
vertebral bacterial osteomyelitis, 230f, 230–231, 231f
Radionuclide scanning, 104, 106
gallium 67, 104, 106f
indium, 106
technetium 99, 104, 105f
breast cancer metastatic to spine, 314f
discitis, 234
spondylolisthesis, 209
vertebral bacterial osteomyelitis, 231, 231f
Radius, distal, Colles' fracture, 320
Ranawat method, basilar invagination (impression) measurement, 246f
Range of motion
cervical spine, 50–51, 51f, 52f, 116–117
lumbar spine, 124–125
in herniated disc disease, 186
lumbosacral spine, 60, 61f, 62f
sacroiliac joints, 71f, 71–72

thoracic spine, 56, 58f
lower, 124–125
Reactive arthropathy, 252
Rectal examination, 67, 69
trauma patient, 288
Redlund-Johnell method, basilar invagination (impression) measurement, 246f
Reflexes
abdominal superficial skin reflexes, 58, 59f
Achilles (ankle jerk), 65, 66f, 67t
bulbocavernosus, 76–77
deep tendon
grading, 55t
lower extremity, 65–66, 66f, 67f, 67t
upper extremity, 54–55, 55f, 55t
Jendrassik maneuver, 65, 67f
lower abdominal skin reflex, 58
lumbosacral spine, 65–66, 66f, 67f, 67t
midabdominal skin reflex, 58
plantar response, 73
quadriceps (knee jerk), 65, 66f, 67t
superficial anal reflex, 65
superficial cremasteric reflex, 65, 66f
upper abdominal superficial reflex, 58
Rehabilitation, 301–302
Reiter's syndrome, 252
Relaxation time, 114, 116f
rem (roentgen-equivalent man), 79
Research, 327–328
basic science research, 328
clinical research, 328
key points, 328
outcomes research, 327–328
Reticulospinal tract(s), 24t
Retrolisthesis, 205, 207f
Reverse sciatic tension test, 77
Rheumatic diseases, 243–253.
See also specific diseases
ankylosing spondylitis, 248–252
classification, 243
juvenile rheumatoid arthritis, 246–248
psoriatic arthritis, 252–253
Reiter's syndrome, 252
rheumatoid arthritis, 244–246

Rheumatic diseases (*continued*)
  seronegative, 243, 248–253
    ankylosing spondylitis,
        248–252
    psoriatic arthritis, 252–253
    Reiter's syndrome, 252
  seropositive, 243, 244–248
    juvenile rheumatoid arthritis,
        246–248
    rheumatoid arthritis,
        244–246
    systemic lupus
        erythematosus, 148
  systemic lupus erythematosus,
      148
Rheumatoid arthritis, 244–246
  basilar invagination
      (impression) in,
      244–246, 247f
    measurement of, 245f, 246f
  cervical spine, 244–246, 245f
  juvenile, 246–248
    categories, 246–247
    cervical spine, 247–248
Rheumatoid factor, 244
Rib(s)
  articulation with vertebra. *See*
      Costovertebral
      articulation
  cervical, 43
  costal ossification center, 39
Rib cage, asymmetry, 55, 56f
Rib hump, 257
Risser sign, 267, 268f
Roentgenograms. *See*
      Radiography
Roentgen (R), 79
Rolfing, 142
Rome criteria, ankylosing
      spondylitis, 248t
Rotator muscles, 20
Rubrospinal tract, 24t

S

Sacral artery(ies), 31f, 32
Sacral inclination, 208f
Sacral promontory, 9
Sacroiliac joints
  ankylosing spondylitis,
      248–252
  Fabere test, 72, 72f
  Gaenslen's test, 72, 73f
  palpation, 69, 71
  physical examination, 69–72
  psoriatic arthritis, 253
  range of motion, 71f, 71–72

Reiter's disease, 252
  stress test, 72
Sacrum
  agenesis, 45
  bony anatomy, 3f, 7, 9, 9f, 10f
  development, 40
  fractures, 300–301, 302f
  in lumbosacral
        spondylolisthesis, 207,
        209f
  nerve root pathways, 28
  nerve roots, 25f
  vascular anatomy, 31f, 32
Safety issues, in osteoporosis, 325
Sagittal plane, 2
Salicylates, 143, 144t
  substituted, 144t
Salmonella sp., vertebral
      osteomyelitis, 230
San Joaquin fever. *See*
      Coccidioidomycosis
Scheuermann's kyphosis, 280f,
      280–282
Schmorl's node, 127
Schober test, 60, 61f
Sciatica, 66
  herniated disc disease and,
      lumbar, 186
  lumbar nerve root compression
      and, 158
  well-leg raising test in, 67
Scintigraphy. *See* Radionuclide
      scanning
Sclerotome, 36, 37
Scoliosis, 2, 257–280
  in adults, 276–280, 278f, 279f
    evaluation, 276–277
    incidence, 276
    risk factors, 276
    treatment, 277–278
  categories, 258
  congenital, 44–45, 258–262
    associated anomalies, 261
    bracing in, 261
    classification, 258, 258f
    cutaneous lesions in, 260
    evaluation, 260–261
    failure of formation, 258f,
        258–259
    failure of segmentation,
        258f, 259
    kyphotic deformity in, 260,
        261f
    prediction of progression,
        259
    surgical management, 262
    treatment, 261–262

  unilateral unsegmented bar,
      259–260, 260f
  degenerative, in adults, 276,
      278f
  Harrington rod in, 162–164,
      163f
  idiopathic, 258, 266–275
    adolescent, 266
    in adults. *See* Scoliosis, in
        adults
    associated anomalies, 266
    brace treatment, 272–273,
        274f
    Cobb measurement of curve,
        272, 272f
    curve classification, 267t
    curve progression in, 266
      skeletal maturity and, 267
    curve types, 266–267
    double major right thoracic
        and left lumbar curves,
        271f
    electric stimulation, 273
    epidemiology, 266
    etiology, 266
    forward bending test in, 269,
        269f
    infantile, 266
    juvenile, 266
    lumbar curve, 267
      left, 270f
    Nash measurement of
        vertebral rotation, 272,
        273f
    natural history, 266
    neurologic examination, 269
    observation in, 272
    patient evaluation, 267–272
    physical examination, 268f,
        268–269, 269f–271f
    radiographic evaluation, 272
    right thoracic curve in, 269,
        269f, 270f
    structural curve, 267
    surgical management,
        273–274
      anterior spinal
          instrumentation and
          fusion, 274, 277f
      Cotrel-Dubousset
          instrumentation, 274,
          276f
      Dwyer system, 274, 277f
      Harrington
          instrumentation, 274,
          276f
      Luque technique, 274

posterior spinal
 intrumentation and
 fusion, 274, 276f
 segmental fixation, 274,
 276f
 Zielke system, 274, 277f
 thoracic curve, 267
 right, 269, 269f, 270f
 thoracolumbar curve, 267
 right, 271f
 treatment, 272–274
 inspection for, 55
 lumbar herniated disc disease
 and, 186
 metabolic, 258
 myopathic, 258
 neuromuscular, 262–266
 etiology, 262–263
 evaluation, 263
 pelvic obliquity in, 263
 treatment, 263, 266
 neuropathic, 258
 osteogenic, 258
 prevalence, 257
 progression of curve, 257
 rib prominence in, 55
 spinal dysraphism and, 47
"Scotty dog" sign, 207, 209, 211f
Screws
 lag, 123
 pedicle, 133, 133f, 166f
 plate, 124, 124f, 165f
Semispinalis muscles, 19f, 20
Sensation
 cervical, 53, 54f
 lumbosacral, 64f, 65
 thoracic, 58, 59f
Sex. *See* Gender
Shiatsu, 141
Sickle ligament. *See* Lumbosacral
 ligament
Sinuvertebral nerve, 28–29, 29f
Skeletal maturity
 determination of, 267, 268f
 Risser sign, 267, 268f
Skin
 dimples, sacroiliac joints, 71
 manifestations of spinal
 developmental
 anomalies, 59, 260
Slip angle, of spondylolisthesis,
 206–208, 208f
Smoking
 and pseudarthrosis, 167
 and degenerative disease, 178
Sodium etidronate, in
 osteoporosis, 325

Sodium fluoride,
 supplementation, in
 osteoporosis, 325
Soleus muscle. *See*
 Gastrocnemius-soleus
 muscle group
Somatosensory evoked potentials
 cortical, 169–170
 in herniated disc disease,
 lumbar spine, 188
 spinal, 170
Somi (sternal occipital
 mandibular
 immobilization)
 orthosis, 122
Somites, 36, 38f
Spasticity, 73
Spina bifida, 46
Spina bifida occulta, 46, 46f
 cutaneous lesions in, 260, 261f
Spinal artery(ies), 29
 anterior, 32, 32f
 posterior, 32, 32f
Spinal column
 anterior anatomy, 16f
 functional spinal unit, 116,
 116f, 117f
Spinal cord
 anatomy, 20, 22–26
 ascending (afferent) tracts,
 24f, 24t, 25
 autonomic nervous system,
 25–26, 26f
 cross-sectional arrangement,
 22, 23f, 24f, 25
 descending (efferent) tracts,
 24f, 24t, 25
 enlargements, 22, 22f
 general structure, 20, 22, 22f
 gray substance, 22, 23f
 meninges, 22, 23f
 spinal nerves, 23f, 25, 25f
 white matter, 22, 23f
 ascending (afferent) tracts, 24f,
 24t, 25
 cervical damage, hand findings,
 74
 compression. *See also*
 Myelopathy
 anterior, 148f
 cervical, 158, 159f
 tumors and, 119–121
 disc space infection and, 233
 dural sac compression,
 158–160
 lumbar, 158
 thoracic, 159f

 thoracic herniated disc
 disease and, 196
 in tuberculosis, 234
 descending (efferent) tracts,
 24f, 24t, 25
 function, intraoperative
 monitoring, 167,
 168–170
 electrically evoked
 potentials, 169–170,
 170f
 wake-up test, 169
 gray substance, 22, 23f
 inflammation. *See* Myelitis
 spinal nerves, 23f, 25, 25f
 systemic lupus erythematosus,
 248
 tethering, 47
 transverse myelitis, 248
 trauma, 75–77. *See also*
 Trauma
 deep vein thrombosis and,
 301
 defining level of injury,
 301–302
 prognosis, age at injury and,
 302
 rehabilitation, 301–302
 vascular anatomy, 32, 32f, 33f
 venous drainage, 32, 33f
 white matter, 22, 23f
Spinal deformity. *See also specific
 deformity*
 cervical, in ankylosing
 spondylitis, 251, 251f
 key points, 286
 kyphosis, 280–285
 metastatic disease and, 313
 scoliosis, 257–280
 thoracolumbar, in ankylosing
 spondylitis, 251, 252f,
 253f
Spinal disorders
 degenerative diseases, 173–184
 herniated disc disease, 185–201
 infections, 229–240
 inflammatory diseases,
 243–255
 nonoperative management,
 135–145. *See also
 specific disorders;
 specific modalities*
 back school, 143
 bed rest, 135–136
 biofeedback, 142–143
 cryotherapy, 138
 drug therapy, 143–144

Spinal disorders, nonoperative
management
(*continued*)
electrotherapy, 138–140
exercise, 136–137
heat, 137
key points, 145
manual therapy, 140–142
orthoses, 143
phonophoresis, 137–138
traction, 142
osteoporosis, 317–325
research, 327–328
basic science research, 328
clinical research, 328
outcomes research, 327–328
spinal deformity, 257–285. *See
also* Kyphosis;
Scoliosis
spondylolisthesis, 203–213
stenosis, 215–227
surgical management,
147–170. *See also*
Spinal surgery
trauma, 287–302
tumors, 305–315
Spinal dysraphism, 46–47
cutaneous lesions in, 260, 261f
Spinalis muscle, 19f, 20
Spinal nerves, 23f, 25, 25f
anterior root, 25
cervical
innervation of muscles, 53,
54t
sensory distribution, 54f
dorsal root ganglion, 23f, 25
lumbosacral
innervation of muscles, 63,
63t
sensory distribution, 64f
posterior root, 25
thoracic
assessment, 58, 59f
sensory distribution, 59f
Spinal-olivary tract, 24t
Spinal rhythm, 60, 62f
Spinal shock, in trauma patient,
76–77
Spinal stenosis, 215–227. *See also
specific spinal
segments*
central vs lateral, 215, 216f
cervical spine, 216–219
diffuse idiopathic skeletal
hyperostosis and, 254
dural sac/nerve root
compression and, 215,
216f

foraminal, 220
key points, 227
lumbar herniated disc and, 194,
194f
pathophysiology, 215
in thoracolumbar ankylosing
spondylitis, 252
thoracolumbar spine, 219–227
Spinal surgery, 147–170. *See also
specific procedures*
in adult scoliosis, 278
in ankylosing spondylitis,
cervical, 251
approaches, 149–157
anterior, 149, 152f–155f,
153–154
posterior, 149, 150f–152f
incisions, 152f
patient positioning, 151f
biomedical advances, 328
blood loss during, 166–167
in cervical rheumatoid arthritis,
246
in cervical spine facet
dislocation, 293
in cervical stenosis, 218–219
complications, 165–167
correction of deformity, 149
decompressive, 148, 157–160
cervical spine, 157, 158f, 159f
dural sac, 158–160
in metastatic disease, 315
nerve root, 157–158
in thoracolumbar stenosis,
226–227
in degenerative disease
cervical spine, 183
lumbar spine, 178
thoracic spine, 180
discectomy, 193–194, 194f
percutaneous, 192–193, 193f
in epidural abscess, 239
failure, in adult scoliosis, 278
fusion, 149, 160–162
in adult scoliosis, 278
anterior interbody fusion,
161f, 161–162
bone graft, 160–161
cervical, 158f
in cervical rheumatoid
arthritis, 246
circumferential fusion, 162,
163f, 178
complications, 165–167
degenerative disease
cervical spine, 183
lumbar spine, 178
healing, 160

in idiopathic scoliosis, 274
physiology, 160
posterior interbody fusion,
162, 162f
posterolateral, 161, 161f
pseudarthrosis (nonunion),
167, 167f, 168f, 278
rationale, 160
in scoliosis
congenital, 262
neuromuscular, 263, 266
in spondylolisthesis, 212
types, 161–162
goals, 148–149
correction of deformity, 149
decompression, 148
stabilization, 148–149
hemiepiphysiodesis, 262, 262f
in herniated disc disease
cervical, 200, 200f
lumbar, 193–194
thoracic, 196–197
implants, 162–165
breakage, 167, 169f
cervical spine stabilization,
123
failure, 167, 169f
Harrington rods, 162, 163f,
164
historical perspective, 162,
164
mechanical disassembly/
loosening, 167, 169f
postoperative infections,
239–240
thoracolumbar spine
stabilization, 133, 133f
indications for, in spinal
deformity, 149
key points, 170
in metastatic disease, 315
for pars interarticularis
fracture, 297
patient positioning
blood loss and, 166
posterior approaches, 151f
in Scheuermann's kyphosis,
282
in scoliosis
congenital, 262, 262f
idiopathic, 273–274
neuromuscular, 263, 266
spinal cord monitoring, 167,
168–170
electrically evoked
potentials, 169–170,
170f
wake-up test, 169

in spondylolisthesis, 211–212
stabilization, 148–149,
        160–165
    fusion, 160–162
    implants, 162–165
    in metastatic disease, 315
    in tuberculosis, 235–236
    in vertebral bacterial
            osteomyelitis,
            231–232
    wound infections and, 239–240
        diagnosis, 240
        etiology, 239–240
        treatment, 240
Spine
    aneurysmal bone cyst, 307f
    articulations, 11–13
    bony anatomy, 2–10. *See also*
            specific sections of
            spine
    developmental anomalies,
            40–47. *See also*
            Developmental
            anomalies
    embryology, 35–40
    fractures, osteoporosis-
            associated, 320–324
    functional spinal unit (FSU),
            116, 116f, 117f
        kinetics, 126–127, 127f
    innervation, 28–29, 29f
        posterior primary ramus, 29,
            29f
        sinuvertebral nerve, 28–29,
            29f
    instability. *See* Instability
    ligaments, 13–17
    muscles, 17–20
    trauma. *See* Trauma
    tumors. *See* Tumor(s)
    vascular anatomy, 29–34
Spinocerebellar tract(s), 24t
Spinothalamic tract(s), 24t
Spinous process
    axis, 4, 5f
    cervical vertebrae, 6f
    lumbar vertebrae, 7, 8f, 9f
    thoracic vertebrae, 8f
    vertebra prominens (C7), 6, 7f
        fracture, 294
Spondylodiscitis, thoracolumbar
            ankylosing spondylitis
            and, 252
Spondylolisthesis, 203–213. *See*
            also specific spinal
            segments
    cervical spine, 203–204

classification, 204f–206f, 204t,
        204–206
congenital, 204, 204f
degenerative. *See*
        Spondylolisthesis, type
        III
key points, 213
lumbar spine, 204–213
measurement of, 206, 208f
posture and, 59–60, 60f
traumatic, axis, 291
type I (congenital), 204, 204f
type II (isthmic), 204, 205f
type III (degenerative),
        204–205, 206f
    treatment, 212–213
type IV (posttraumatic), 205
type V (pathologic), 205
type VI (postsurgical), 206
Spondylolysis, definition, 203
Spondyloptosis, 206, 209f
Spondylosis, 173. *See also*
        Degenerative disease
Stabilization. *See also specific*
        spinal segment
    cervical spine, 122–124
    surgical, 148–149
    thoracolumbar spine, 129,
            132f, 133
Staphylococcus aureus
    disc space infection, 232
    postoperative infections, 240
    vertebral osteomyelitis, 229,
            230f
Stellate ligament. *See* Anterior
        costovertebral
        ligament complex
Stenosis. *See also* Spinal stenosis
    definition, 215
Sternocleidomastoid muscle, in
            torticollis, 42
Stiffness, 109–110, 111f, 112
    axial, 112, 112f
    bending, 112, 113f
    shear, 112, 112f
    torsional, 112, 113f
Straight leg raising, 66, 68f. *See*
        also Nerve roots,
        tension
Strain, 109, 111f
Strength of body, 112, 114
    elastic range, 114, 114f
    fatigue strength, 114, 115f
    fracture, 114, 115f
    loading to failure, 114, 115f
    plastic range, 114, 114f
    yield strength, 114
Stress, 109, 110f

Stress shielding, in osteoporotic
        vertebral fracture, 323
Stress test, sacroiliac joints, 72
Subarachnoid space, 22, 23f
Subdental synchondrosis, 40
Subdural space, 22, 23f
Substance P, 328
Sulcus, cervical vertebrae, 6, 6f
Supraspinous ligament, 16, 17f
Surgery. *See* Spinal surgery
Swimmer's view, 82, 83f
Sympathetic nervous system. *See*
        Autonomic nervous
        system
Synchondrosis
    neurocentral, 39
    subdental, 40
Syndesmophyte, 174
Synkinesia, in Klippel-Feil
        syndrome, 43
Synovial cyst, thoracolumbar
        stenosis and, 219, 220,
        221f
Systemic lupus erythematosus,
        248

T
Tactile sensation
    abdominal superficial skin
            reflexes, 58, 59t
    cervical nerves, 53–54
Technetium 99. *See* Radionuclide
        scanning
Tectospinal tract, 24t
Tender points, in fibromyalgia,
        255f
TENS. *See* Transcutaneous
        electrical nerve
        stimulation
Tetracycline, prebiopsy labeling
        of bone, 319
Thoracic hyperkyphosis, 280
Thoracic spine
    anatomy, kinematic regions,
            124, 125f
    bony anatomy, 3f, 7, 8f
    costal ligaments, 17, 18f
    costovertebral articulations,
            12–13, 13f
    CT scan, 91, 94
        axial, 94, 94f, 95f
        sagittal reformation, 94, 95f
    degenerative disease, 179–180
        clinical presentation, 179
        diagnostic evaluation,
            179–180

Thoracic spine, degenerative
    disease (*continued*)
  discography in, 180
  facet blocks in, 180
  magnetic resonance imaging,
    179, 180f
  radiographic findings, 179,
    179f
  treatment, 180
  facet joints, 12, 12f
  fracture, 128
  herniated disc disease, 196–197
    clinical presentation, 196
    diagnostic evaluation, 196
    treatment, 196–197
  inspection, 55–56, 56f
  interspinous ligament, 16, 17f
  kyphosis, 55–56, 57f
  lower
    kinematics, 124, 126f
    range of motion, 124–125
  magnetic resonance imaging,
    100, 100f
  nerve root pathways, 27f,
    27–28
  nerve roots, 25f
    compression, 158
  physical examination, 55–59
  radiography
    anteroposterior (AP) view,
      83–84, 85f
    lateral view, 84, 86f
  range of motion, 56, 58f
  reflexes, 56, 58, 59f
  scoliosis, 55
  sensory examination, 58–59,
    59f
  spinal cord compression, 158,
    159f
  surgery
    anterior approach, 153, 153f
    costotransversectomy
      approach, 156f, 157
  vascular anatomy, 30, 31f
Thoracolumbar spine
  abnormal movement patterns,
    129, 130f
  anatomy, kinematic regions,
    124, 125f
  ankylosing spondylitis,
    251–252, 252f
  anterior column, 128, 128f, 295
  biomechanics, 124–134
    failure mechanisms, 128–129
    kinematics, 124–125
    kinetics, 125–128
    stabilization, 129, 133

degenerative disease, 129
developmental anomalies,
    44–45
diffuse idiopathic skeletal
    hyperostosis, 254, 254f
failure mechanisms, 128–129
  degenerative disease, 129
  trauma, 128
  tumor, 129
fracture, 128
  burst fracture, 298, 299f
  flexion-distraction fracture,
    298, 300f
  major fractures, 295,
    297–300
  minor fractures, 295,
    296–297
  pars interarticularis, 297
  spinous process, 297
  transverse process, 297, 297f
  wedge compression fracture,
    297, 297f, 298
fracture-dislocation, 298, 301f
instability, 128–129
  degenerative disease and, 129
  diagnostic checklist, 129t
  trauma and, 128
  tumors and, 129
kinematics, 124–125
  anatomic basis, 124, 125f,
    126f
  kinematic properties,
    124–125
kinetics, 125–128
  contribution of abdomen and
    muscles, 127–128
  intervertebral disc, 128
  vertebral body, 125–127,
    127f
kyphosis, congenital, 45
lateral recess
  boundaries, 219–220, 222f
  stenosis, 220, 222f
middle column, 128, 128f, 295
nerve root foramen
  boundaries, 220, 222f
  stenosis, 220, 223f
posterior column, 128, 128f,
    295
psoriatic arthritis, 253
range of motion, 124–125
Reiter's disease, 252
scoliosis, congenital, 44–45
stabilization, 129, 132f, 133
  anterior fixation devices, 133
  external, 129, 132f, 133
  internal, 133, 133f

pedicle screw vs hook
    systems, 133, 133f
  posterior fixation devices,
    133, 133f
stenosis, 219–227
  central, 219
  classification, 219, 219f
  clinical presentation,
    220–221
  combined, 219, 220f
  congenital, 219
  CT myelography, 225, 226f
  CT scan, 224–225
  degenerative (synovial) cysts
    and, 219, 220, 221f
  diagnostic evaluation, 221,
    224–226
  etiology, 219t, 219–220
  extraforaminal, 220
  foraminal, 220, 223f
  lateral recess, 220, 222f
  MRI, 225–226, 227f
  myelography, 224, 225f
  nonoperative management,
    226
  radiographic findings, 221,
    224, 224f, 225f
  surgical decompression,
    226–227
  treatment, 226–227
trauma, 128, 295–300. *See also*
    Thoracolumbar spine,
    fracture
  classification, 295
  imaging studies, 288, 290t
  major fractures, 295,
    297–300
  minor fractures, 295,
    296–297
tumor, 129
Thoracotomy, 153, 153f
Thrombosis, deep vein, spinal
    cord injury and, 301
Tibialis anterior muscle
  evaluation, 63
  in herniated disc disease,
    lumbar, 186
Tinnitus, in degenerative disease,
    cervical, 181
Tomography, 90, 90f, 91f
  in cervical rheumatoid arthritis,
    247f
  computed. *See* Computed
    tomography
Torticollis, 42
Traction, 142
  cervical, 142f

in cervical spine facet
  dislocation, 293
contraindications, 142
in herniated disc disease
  cervical, 199–200
  lumbar, 191
  pelvic, 142f
Traeger approach, 141
Transcutaneous electrical nerve
  stimulation (TENS),
  139–140, 140f
contraindications, 139
for low back pain, 140f
Transverse ligament. *See*
  Ligament(s), transverse
Transverse myelitis, 248
Transverse processes
  atlas, 4, 5f
  axis, 4, 5f
  lumbar vertebrae, 7, 9f
    fracture, 297, 297f
  thoracic vertebrae, 7, 8f
Trauma, 287–302. *See also*
  specific spinal
  segments
acute management, 287–290
  clinical evaluation, 287–288
  imaging studies, 288–290,
    289f
    algorithm for, 288, 290f
  immobilization, 287
  prehospital care, 287
anterior cord syndrome, 75–76,
  288
Brown-Séquard syndrome, 75,
  288
bulbocavernosus reflex and
  spinal shock in, 76–77
central cord syndrome, 76, 288
cervical spine, 119, 290–295
fractures. *See* Fracture(s)
inspection, 74
key points, 302
neurologic evaluation, 288
neurologic examination, 75–77
palpation, 74
physical examination, 74–77,
  288
posterior cord syndrome, 75,
  288
rectal examination in, 288
rehabilitation, 301–302
sacral spine, 300–301, 302f
sensory examination in, 76
spinal shock in, 76–77

thoracolumbar spine, 128,
  295–300
Trendelenburg test, delayed, 64f
Treponema pallidum myelitis,
  239
Triceps mucle, deep tendon
  reflexes, 55t
Triceps reflex, nerve root
  innervation, 55t
Tropism, facet joints, 84
Tubercles
  atlas, 4, 5f
  cervical vertebrae, 6f
Tuberculin skin test, 235
Tuberculosis, 234–236
  clinical presentation, 234, 235f
  diagnostic findings, 235, 236f
  treatment, 235–236
Tumor(s), 305–315
  aneurysmal bone cyst, 307f
  benign, 307–308
    cell origin, 306t
    giant cell tumor, 308, 310f
    hemangioma, 307, 308f
    osteoblastoma, 307–308,
      309f
    osteoid osteoma, 307–308,
      308f
  cervical spine, 119–121
  malignant, 308–311
    cell origin, 306t
    chordoma, 310–311, 312f
    Ewing's sarcoma, 309–310
    lymphoma, 310
    myeloma, 308–309, 311f
  metastatic, 311, 313–315. *See*
    also Metastatic disease
  primary, 305–311
    age and, 306
    anatomic distribution, 306f
    assessment, 306–307
    benign. *See* Tumor(s), benign
    cell origin, 305, 306t
    clinical presentation, 306
    imaging studies, 306–307
    malignant. *See* Tumor(s),
      malignant
    management goals, 311
    staging, 307
    treatment, 311
  thoracolumbar spine, 129

U

Ultrasonography
  heat therapy, 137

Uncinate processes, cervical
  vertebrae, 4, 6f
Uncovertebral joints, 12, 12f
Undulant fever. *See* Brucellosis
Urinary tract, anomalies, in
  congenital scoliosis,
  40, 43, 45, 261

V

Vascular system
  cervical spine, 29–30, 30f
  intervertebral disc, 33, 34f
  lumbosacral spine, 30–32, 31f
  spinal cord, 32, 32f
  thoracic spine, 30, 31f
Vena cava, inferior, 32, 33f
Vertebrae
  anatomy, 2–10. *See also*
    specific sections of
    spine
  vertebral body, 119f
  bacterial osteomyelitis,
    229–232. *See also*
    Osteomyelitis,
    bacterial
  cervical, 4–7
  compression fracture, in
    osteoporosis, acute
    kyphosis and, 56, 57f
  congenital block vertebra,
    44–45
  differentiation, 35–36, 39–40
    atlas and axis development,
      40, 40f
    chondrification stage, 36, 39,
      39f
    mesenchymal stage, 36, 39,
      39f
    primary ossification stage,
      36, 39, 39f
    sacral development, 40
    secondary ossification stage,
      36, 39, 40f
  embryology, 37, 38f
  end plate, 11–12
  fracture, in osteoporosis. *See*
    Fracture(s),
    osteoporosis-
    associated
  lumbar, 7, 9f
  sacrum, 7
  thoracic, 7, 8f
  unilateral unsegmented bar, 45,
    259–260, 260f

Vertebral artery(ies), 29, 30f
  compression, 181
Vertebral body
  anatomy, 119f, 125–126
  cancellous bone, 126
  cortical bone, 125
  idiopathic hyperostosis,
      lumbar, 174
  kinetics, 125–127, 127f
  spondylolisthesis, 203–213
Vestibulospinal tract, 24t
Viscoelastic properties, 114
Vision, blurred, in degenerative
      disease, cervical, 181
Vitamin D, supplementation,
      324
von Bechterew's disease. *See*
      Ankylosing spondylitis

W
Wake-up test, 169
Weakness
  epidural abscess and, 239
  giving way vs, 77
White matter, spinal cord, 22, 23f
Wiring
  C1-C2 posterior wiring, 122f,
      123
  cervical spine, 123, 124f
Wolff's law, spinal fusion, 160
Wound healing, spinal fusion, 160
  inflammatory phase, 160
  remodeling phase, 160
  reparative phase, 160
Wound infection, surgical. *See*
      Spinal surgery, wound
      infections and

X
X-rays. *See* Radiography

Y
Yellow ligament. *See*
      Ligamentum flavum
Yield strength, 114

Z
Zielke system, in scoliosis, 274,
      277f
Zygoapophyseal joints. *See* Facet
      joints